This book is dedicated to my parents, who taught me the literal and lateral approaches to science, and to my children, who may, one day, pick up the torch. I am indebted also to the many scientific and clinical investigators whose work I have read and cited here. I have tried in this volume to make it accessible to a wider public and incorporate it into a coherent whole.

There are few pieces of incontrovertible evidence in nutrition, few trials which cannot be criticised, refuted or re-interpreted. Much work in the field is underfunded, incomplete or badly designed. Accordingly, and after studying many hundreds of scientific papers, I have tried to step back from the detail of individual studies to build what seems to me to be the most reasonable conclusions, from all the many pieces of evidence, about the links between nutrition and health.

Some of the ideas developed in this book are fast becoming the new consensus. Others are still speculative. My aim is to inform and empower the consumer – and challenge the scientific community to prove or disprove the nutraceutical approach to the prevention and treatment of the chronic diseases outlined in the following chapters.

I would like to thank Professor David Richardson, Dr Steve Hodges and Maurice Hanssen for their valuable comments; Allison Lee for retrieving some of the more esoteric references; Chris Holmes for his work on the illustrations and Lena Young for her marathon work on the manuscript.

C O N T E N T S   Page

PART 3: DIETS WHICH FIGHT DISEASE

PART 4: DIETS WHICH PROMOTE HEALTH

How to read this book

Part One describes the reasons why our bodies run down. This is not so much due to the passage of time, but rather because our natural defences and repair systems are gradually overwhelmed due to chronically inadequate nutritional support.

Part Two describes the solution – the nutrients you need and how to use them.

Part Three looks at the problem from a different angle. It asks why people get the killer diseases, and shows how you can best protect yourself against each of them.

At the end of each chapter in Part Three we have summarised the risk factors that threaten you and which nutritional solutions will counterbalance the threats.

Part Four pulls all the conclusions together and details exactly what should be in your diet and your daily supplement.

Almost 40% of adults now take vitamin and mineral supplements, but the choice in the average health food store or chemist is bewildering, and many products are so poorly formulated that they cannot deliver the benefits you may hope for. You will now have the knowledge to make an informed choice.

Each chapter starts with the highlights and finishes with a summary. You may want to read all these highlights and summaries first to give yourself a 'feel' of the whole story.

I also recommend that you look now at the pages which give a visual summary of some of the key arguments that you need to understand in order to take the action that will, I believe, materially benefit your health.

Paul Clayton

Introduction

THE BIG PICTURE

*A*n overview of the material covered in the book, the issues raised, and the protective nutrient shields that will help to maintain fitness into old age.

THE BIG PICTURE

An overview

The next few pages give you some of the key arguments expanded in the book.

They enable you to grasp the 'big picture' – the core ideas – so that the detail in the rest of the book is easier to understand.

Very few people – perhaps 1 in 10,000 – die of old age. The vast majority of us sicken and die prematurely, picked off by 'natural causes' long before our biological life span has run its course. Average life expectancy in the First World is around 75 years for men and 82 for women; but cell culture studies, and the very few individuals who live on healthily into their second century, indicate that our true life span lies between 110 and 120.

So why is a long and healthy life such a rarity? Why do so few of us live out our biological potential?

We used to die, in the main, of infection or trauma. Twentieth century medicine has scored significant victories against these; and the major causes of ill health and death now are the chronic degenerative diseases such as coronary artery disease and cancer.

What we need is a medicine for the 21st century; a medicine which will prevent these degenerative diseases from making our last years difficult, and extend our healthy middle years.

The foundations for this new medicine have already been published in many thousands of research papers. This book draws the research findings together and translates them into simple guidelines which you can use to improve your chances of living a longer and healthier life.

Reading selected chapters

Each chapter has been designed so that it can be read separately. For this reason, certain topics have been re-visited in different sections and contexts.

In nutrition there are many common themes, elements and connections.

The drugs don't work

Five out of six 60-year-olds have one or more of the chronic degenerative diseases, such as coronary artery disease, arthritis, osteoporosis, Alzheimer's, or cancer. For these unfortunates, the drugs don't work. They may alleviate some of the symptoms, but they do little to alter the underlying disease, which generally continues to deteriorate.

This is because drugs do not address the causes of these diseases. Based on the concept of the 'magic bullet', they are

Health

The usual medical definition:

Absence of clinically defined disease.

My definition:

Noticeable energy, absence of clinically defined disease – **plus** no signs of sub-clinical, ie pending, disease.

designed to block a single step in the generally multifactorial process leading to illness; an inappropriate strategy guaranteeing ineffectuality and a high risk of side effects.

An even more fundamental criticism of modern medicine is that it is practised as crisis management. Wait until the diagnosis, then hammer the patient with drugs. But by the time symptoms of one of these diseases appear, damage has already been done to the body; damage that drugs cannot begin to address.

Drug companies start from the wrong point. They must sell their synthetic, patented molecules – and to a company selling hammers, every problem looks like a nail.

The pre-ill

We now know that the majority of cases of illness in the West are caused by lifestyle factors such as exercise, smoking and nutrition. We also know that these diseases have a long latency period before symptoms appear and a diagnosis can finally be made. Coronary artery disease, cancer, Alzheimer's and osteoporosis do not occur overnight, although the symptoms might do. They are slowly progressing conditions, which develop for years or decades before symptoms finally emerge.

In other words, the majority of apparently healthy people are in fact *pre-ill.* They contain in their bodies the seeds of the illness which will eventually become overt, and perhaps kill them. An artery is beginning to silt up; bone is thinning; brain cells are dying – leading inevitably, eventually, to a heart attack, osteoporotic fracture, or dementia.

But is it inevitable? If we were to focus on the pre-ill, perhaps we could slow or stop these diseases before they became clinical. This is the core of the new medicine; a medicine which concentrates on the pre-ill, analysing the metabolic errors which lead to clinical illness, and correcting them before the first twinge of angina, the first broken bone, or the first shadow on the x-ray.

Prevention or Cure?

A clear equation

The British Health Service is really an 'illness service' – treatment *after* things go wrong. It costs over £750 a year for every man, woman and child in the nation.

The full range of preventative nutritional supplements recommended in this book would cost a fraction of this.

The difference in philosophy is that conventional medicine waits for something to go wrong and then tries to suppress that particular symptom with a chemical with which the body is not familiar.

Preventative nutrition is pro-active and holistic, using compounds which the body is familiar with, and depends on.

It aims to gently boost your body's own repair mechanisms and defences against hostile environmental factors – like pollution, stress, free radicals, toxins, carcinogens, and infectious agents such as bacteria and viruses.

It helps deal with the **causes** of potential problems.

Body maintenance

This approach is based on the fact that the body has significant powers of self-healing and regeneration. If that were not the case, our joints and bones would be worn thin by the age of 20; our arteries solid by the time we reached 30; our brains burned out by 40.

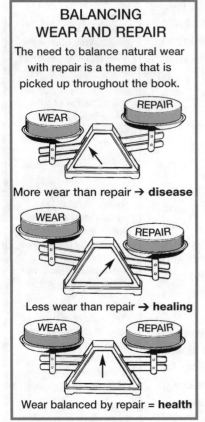

BALANCING WEAR AND REPAIR

The need to balance natural wear with repair is a theme that is picked up throughout the book.

More wear than repair → **disease**

Less wear than repair → **healing**

Wear balanced by repair = **health**

Most of us do better than that. But it is despite our lifestyles, not because of them. Starved of key nutrients, our restorative systems run down, and are eventually overtaken and overwhelmed by the forces of decay.

All biological tissues are dynamic. Their apparent constancy disguises a constant state of flux, with the processes of decay and regeneration going on at the same time. Bones are constantly being built up and worn away, as are joints. Atheroma is constantly accumulating inside the arteries, and just as constantly being removed.

If the processes are in balance the tissue remains intact, and good health is sustained. But if the rate of decay is only a little faster than the rate of repair, there will be a net loss of healthy tissue, a pre-illness growing little by little every day until the clinical illness finally emerges.

This is why we sicken and die prematurely at 75; because in almost all of us, the processes of repair are below par. And the balance of evidence shows that, in the majority of cases, this is due to multiple micro-nutrient depletion.

Surveys, like the one below, show that *most* people are depleted in *most* micro-nutrients.

VITAMIN INTAKES
US DEPARTMENT OF AGRICULTURE (USDA) SURVEY 1994[1]

Vitamin	A	E	C	B1	B2	Niacin	B6	B4	B12
% Population Depleted	55	68	37	32	31	27	54	34	17

It is not the absolute absence of a nutrient that causes a deficiency disease, like Vitamin C and scurvy, but a sub-optimal level of a nutrient or nutrients which slows a restorative process by a mere per cent or two. That is enough to lead, over a period of years, to debilitating or fatal illness.

Drugs cannot remedy this pattern of multiple micro-nutrient depletion leading to illness. Only well-designed nutritional programmes, specifically assembled to support regenerative function and slow the processes of decay, can do this.

The well-balanced, nutritionally <u>deficient</u> diet

Malnutrition is all too common in the developed nations. This is not the calorie and/or micronutrient deficiency associated with developing nations (Type A malnutrition); but mutiple micro-nutrient depletion, often combined with calorific balance or excess (Type B malnutrition).

The incidence and severity of Type B malnutrition is worsened if we include the newer micro-nutrient groups such as the PUFA's, various fibre types, methyl groups, xanthophylls, flavonoids etc. In every case, commonly ingested levels of these micro-nutrients are sub-optimal, to the point where health is compromised.

Increasingly, Type B malnutrition is coming to be considered as the most important cause of the chronic degenerative diseases. Logically, therefore, the prevention and treatment of these conditions must also be couched in micro-nutrient repletion programmes.

Like many doctors, I began my career assuming that you could obtain all the nutrition needed from a well-balanced diet. We evolved without vitamin pills. But the USDA survey, and many other studies[4, 7-10], show that we are not getting the micro-nutrients we need. There are well known reasons for this.

1 We don't eat enough!

We were designed to live active lives, and to consume 3000 to 4000 calories per day. No longer hunter-gatherers, we live sedentary lives, and burn far fewer calories. Our appetites have shrunk, but not quite enough – which explains why so

---

Changing needs

Our nutritional needs are fine-tuned to conditions of life that existed over 10,000 years ago, when we were evolving.

Genetically, our bodies are the same as they were then – but our diet and lifestyle aren't.

Thousands of generations of people were hunter-gatherers, five hundred generations have depended on agriculture, ten generations have lived since the start of the industrial age and only two have grown up with highly processed 'convenience' foods.

This is a nutritional experiment out of control – and is probably the most important reason why so many of us develop degenerative diseases.

Eating badly

Our eating habits are deteriorating. Children in the UK eat less fruit and vegetables than in the 1950s[5]; and only 15 per cent of Americans eat the recommended amounts[6].

Depleted vegetables

The average mineral content of fruits and vegetables has declined dramatically in the last 50 years.

Between 1940 and 1991 magnesium has declined by 25%, calcium by 47%, iron by 36%, and copper by 62%[15].

Importance of chewing

We have even forgotten how to eat. Studies show we obtain fewer calories and nutrients from soft food than from crunchy food we have to chew[14].

Unchewed food is hard or impossible to digest, so its calories and micro-nutrients pass through our systems.

The Victorians recommended chewing every mouthful 20 times; we are in too much of a hurry for that. The less you chew fruits and vegetables, the less their micro-nutrients are released for absorption.

many are overweight. But when we eat less, we're also consuming fewer micro-nutrients.

2 **Too many processed foods**

Many (not all) processed foods are depleted in micro-nutrients – and we're eating more processed foods than ever before.

3 **Depleted soils**

Many soils are low in key minerals, or have become depleted, due to over-intensive farming. Plants or animals raised in these areas are depleted in these minerals. This is why UK intakes of the anti-cancer mineral selenium, for example, are worryingly low.

4 **Bad habits**

Smoking, sunbathing, pollution, excessive drinking or exercise, all deplete the body of anti-oxidants.

5 **Ageing**

We become progressively more depleted in more micro-nutrients as we get older[11, 12].

Reduced finances may mean a restricted diet – as (sadly) does institutionalisation. We become less active – so appetite, food and micro-nutrient intake fall further. We lose teeth and opt for softer foods, with fewer of the fruits and vegetables that supply so many micro-nutrients.

Older digestive systems are also less efficient at absorbing micro-nutrients from whatever food is eaten. Finally, older people take more medications, many of which can make micro-nutrient depletion worse[13].

Only comprehensive nutrition will do

All this explains why, as we get older, we become more likely to get sick and die. It is little to do with ageing, as few of us get even close to our theoretical life span. It is due to a multiple systems failure caused by a cumulative depletion of many micro-nutrients. If you skimp on maintaining your car, it will break down. If you do not give your body the micro-nutrient maintenance it needs, it too will break down.

And as most people are depleted in the majority of micro-nutrients, it doesn't make sense to take a single micro-nutrient.

Think of car maintenance. You need to change the oil every now and then; but you must also replace the spark plugs, tyres, oil and air filters, adjust the fan belt, and so on. And of course a human being is far more complex than a car, and requires much more extensive nutritional maintenance.

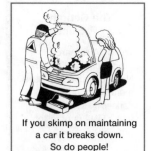

If you skimp on maintaining a car it breaks down. So do people!

Unfortunately, this self-evident truth has been overlooked by many clinical scientists. Wedded as they are to the single agent, 'magic bullet' approach, they find it hard to appreciate the complex relationships between multiple food ingredients and health.

For example, Vitamin E reduces the risk of coronary artery disease; but so do fish oil, Vitamin C, the carotenoid lycopene, betaine, grapeseed flavonoids and many other micro-nutrients. Now we understand that all these compounds work in different but complementary ways, it is logical to combine them; and supremely illogical of scientists and regulatory authorities to refuse to deal with 'nutraceutical' combinations of this sort.

The classical approach says that if you give a compound formula to test subjects and obtain positive results, you cannot know which ingredient is exerting the benefit, so you must test each ingredient individually. In the field of nutrition, this is nonsense. It is like the mechanic who, confronted with a chronically under-maintained car, insists on a test drive after changing the oil filter; another after replacing one of the spark plugs – and so on.

Each intervention on its own will hardly make enough difference to be measured. In any case, this approach to car maintenance would take forever, and be prohibitively expensive. To make the car run noticeably better (and last longer), it requires a comprehensive service. Similarly, to enable humans to live healthier (and longer) lives, **comprehensive** nutritional support is indicated.

So should we analyse each individual's nutritional status and then tailor a formula specifically for him or her? After all, different people have different lifestyles, and eat different foods.

Bottlenecks

Another theme that recurs in this book is the problem of bottlenecks.

As we get older, we become less efficient at absorbing or forming the nutrients we need.

So it's sometimes necessary to bypass a metabolic bottleneck and consume the nutrient 'ready made'.

Supplementing with Omega 3 rich fish oil is a well-known example, but glucosamine and Co-Enzyme Q10 are equally valid candidates.

Accordingly, one person may be depleted in Vitamin E, methyl groups and Omega 3 oils. Another may be depleted in Vitamins C and B12, copper and selenium. A third may be consuming sub-optimal amounts of isoflavones and lycopene.

We do not have the resources to analyse millions of individual cases, but in any case there is no need to do so. The vast majority of people are consuming sub-optimal amounts of most micro-nutrients; and most of the micro-nutrients concerned are very safe. So if we wish to improve the general health of the nation, a comprehensive and universal baseline programme of micro-nutrient support should be the most cost-effective and safest way of achieving this.

In most cases, therefore, wide-spectrum nutritional programmes are recommended. But equally, it is apparent that as we age, bottlenecks form in key metabolic pathways, and lead directly to the metabolic run-down to illness.

By-passing the bottleneck may be enough to increase the rate of regeneration to the point where it outstrips the forces of decay, and the disease can be slowed, stopped or forced into reverse. This may be true, for example, in the treatment of osteoarthritis with glucosamine. So to a 'baseline' of wide-spectrum nutrients you may need to add one or two specialist nutrients for specific conditions – as well as a physician's support, of course.

The twin themes of restoring metabolic balance, and overcoming metabolic bottlenecks, recur throughout the book. The nutritional strategies outlined here represent the next wave of health care; no magic bullets, and no friendly fire either, but a health care based on the gentle correction of multiple metabolic imbalance with comprehensive nutritional support, and a health care which, I believe, will make the degenerative diseases a rarity.

Complex data – simple solutions

The sheer complexity of nutrition explains why there have been so many conflicting trial results. For example, although several high profile studies show that Vitamin E protects against heart attacks, a recent trial found no such effect. A logical explanation is that different populations have different nutritional baselines.

Where anti-oxidant intake is low (eg much of America), Vitamin E supplements are protective; whereas in areas such as the Mediterranean countries, where anti-oxidant intakes are already high, they can have little additional effect. Similarly, supplements of 200mcg selenium appear to be highly cancer-protective in the American Mid-West, where dietary selenium is very low (See Chapter 13, Cancer); but the same supplement will have no effect in Greenland, where the diet already contains 2000mcg selenium a day!

Scientists are used to the idea that most drugs are equally effective (or ineffective) wherever they are used. But as you can see, nutritional intervention with a single micro-nutrient has different effects in different populations. Nonetheless, because of their superior safety, almost all micro-nutrients can be given to almost all people. And if a nutritional programme is sufficiently comprehensive, it will remedy whatever dietary defects the individual or population may have.

Completing the nutritional jigsaw

The nutrients you need provide a series of overlapping lines of defence. Each defence affords some protection, but unless you have *all* the defences in place you remain vulnerable. The nutrients can also be visualised as pieces in a jigsaw. To complete the big picture all the pieces need to be in place. Broadly, there are nine pieces in the nutritional jigsaw.

 The first piece is composed of anti-oxidants to protect your cells against free radical damage (see Chapter 4).

Vitamin C and Vitamin E are two of the best known, but what are the optimum levels of these and other anti-oxidant nutrients? Research is now providing some clear answers.

A daily intake of 267mg (400IU) of Vitamin E has been shown to reduce the risk of heart disease by 50%. Yet the Recommended Daily Allowance (RDA) for E is only 10mg; and the typical Western intake of Vitamin E is just 9.3mg!

Another study indicates that a daily intake of 500mg of Vitamin C can also cut death rates by 50%. The RDA for Vitamin C is 60mg; the average person's intake of Vitamin C is 58mg.

> **Overlapping functions**
>
> The concept of a nutritional jigsaw simplifies a quite complex subject and makes it easier to understand.
>
> It also underlines the fact that there is an inter-relationship between the pieces – they don't act independently, but each contribute to the whole.

INTRODUCTION: **The big picture**

Never too late!!

The focus of these nine lines of defence, or nine pieces in the jigsaw – and indeed the whole book – is on **preventing** degenerative disease in the first place.

However, the same basic nine-step nutritional plan is valid even for people who have already started to exhibit some symptoms of incipient disease. In addition to a physician's care, you will find advice on additional nutritional strategies for specific diseases in later chapters.

There is evidence that smokers should **not** supplement with beta carotene, or with other carotenoids unless combined with Vitamin C, see page 182.

The average dietary intake of these nutrients, therefore, is lower than the RDAs, even though the RDAs are much lower than optimum – because RDAs are designed to prevent deficiency symptoms from appearing, not to optimise health.

Since most vitamin and mineral supplements on the market use the RDAs as their baseline, it follows that most supplements are inadequate. It makes no sense to take less than the therapeutic dose.

Although Vitamins C and E are important, many other anti-oxidants are every bit as powerful and, when combined, have additive and complementary protective effects. The flavonoids, Q10 and the anti-oxidant mineral selenium are good examples.

The average intake of selenium is 35mcg and, although there is no official UK RDA, the optimum intake is likely to be 120-200mcg. This depletion is serious because selenium has a vital role in protecting against heart disease, stroke, and cancer. Flavonoids have a similar function; yet the average intake of these nutrients is 140mg, there is as yet no RDA and optimal daily intake is probably around 500-1000mg.

You not only need the right nutrients, you also need them in the right amounts – and in a form that the body can most easily absorb and use. So as the book progresses, we will use the conclusions from thousands of studies to try and define the ideal nutrients and their optimum levels.

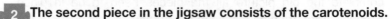

The second piece in the jigsaw consists of the carotenoids.

Carotenoids, such as beta carotene, lutein and lycopene, are derived from vegetables and fruits, and have anti-oxidant and anti-cancer properties. The RDA has not yet been determined.

A less well known carotenoid, lycopene, is a powerful cardio-protectant and anti-cancer agent. A third, cryptoxanthin, appears to reduce the risk of cervical cancer. A fourth, lutein, appears to confer very significant protection against age-related blindness; a fifth, astaxanthin, may improve gastric function and fertility.

The available data indicates that intakes of all these carotenoids are much lower in the average diet than the probable optimum intakes. (The typical diet provides just 2mg of beta carotene a day against an optimum of 10 to 15mg.)

3 **The third piece in the puzzle is composed of the flavonoids.**

Flavonoids (such as grapeseed extract, green tea extract or pycnogenol) are powerful anti-inflammatory agents and are defensive against heart disease, cancer, and inflammatory conditions such as asthma and arthritis. They are also anti-ageing compounds for skin. At present there is no RDA.

4 **The essential Omega 3 oils found in oily fish and certain plant oils provide a fifth piece.**

These oils protect against heart disease, and have a role to play in defending against inflammatory conditions like asthma and arthritis. The average person's intake of Omega 3 is about 150mg a day; far below the level that the UK Government is currently considering recommending, which is 350mg a day.

5 **Recently we have discovered a related, puzzle piece – isoflavones.**

Isoflavones (like genistein), are found in soy, and have remarkable defensive powers against cancer. They can not only force cancerous cells to revert to normal, but can also help choke off the blood supply to emerging tumours. In addition, they have an important role to play in minimising problems linked to the menopause.

While there isn't as yet an RDA, the average daily intake of isoflavones in the West is as low as 5mg. The level that I recommend (40mg) will provide you with an intake similar to the diet eaten in countries like Korea, where the rates of some of the major cancers are very much lower than in the (non soy-eating) West.

6 **The sixth piece is a comparatively new one – methyl groups, best supplied by the 'quasi-vitamin' betaine.**

Betaine lowers levels of a toxic amino acid (homocysteine) that can build up in the body, and which is a direct cause of heart disease and is implicated in Alzheimer's.

Betaine, at the correct levels, also increases the body's resistance to stress, toxins, carcinogens and infection; and enhances liver and kidney function by supplying essential

> **ORAC Units**
>
> The US Government, working with the world-famous Tuft's University in Boston, measure the anti-oxidant protection provided by foodstuffs in ORACs (Oxygen Radical Absorbance Capacity)[2,3].
>
> Typical diets provide 1400-1500 ORACs a day: optimal intakes are reckoned to be between 3-5,000 ORACs. To achieve that, you would need to eat 10-15 servings of fruits and vegetables a day – or add a high ORAC scoring supplement to your diet (see page 335).

methyl groups (see Chapter 11). While as yet there is no RDA, an estimated 95% of people are depleted in methyl groups.

 The seventh piece in the jigsaw is formed by another new class of nutrients called pre-biotics.

Pre-biotics include FOS (Fructo-Oligo-Saccharide), and inulin, members of a family of non-digestible fibres found in chicory, leeks, onions and some other vegetables and grains.

These pre-biotics are considered to protect against bowel and colon cancers, and probably liver and breast cancers also. They also help to normalise bowel function.

The estimated average intake of this type of non-digestible fibre is about 3g a day. You need 8g or more, but the RDA has not yet been agreed.

 The eighth piece consists of a broad spectrum A-Z type multi-vitamin and mineral supplement.

Sadly, most A-Z supplements are based on Recommended Daily Amounts (RDAs) which, I believe, need updating. Optimal levels for some of the vitamins and minerals are much higher.

 The ninth piece consists of Co-enzyme Q10 and glucosamine.

These are nutrients which maintain the inner and outer health of the trillions of cells that make up the body.

Q10 supports the mitochondria (the vital 'energy factories' inside every body cell) and has an important role in maintaining a healthy heart.

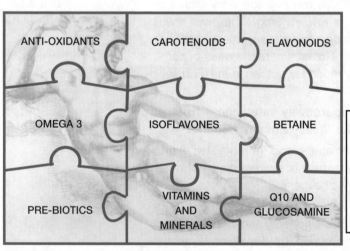

ANTI-OXIDANTS | CAROTENOIDS | FLAVONOIDS
OMEGA 3 | ISOFLAVONES | BETAINE
PRE-BIOTICS | VITAMINS AND MINERALS | Q10 AND GLUCOSAMINE

You can visualise the ideal nutritional defence plan as interlocking pieces in a jigsaw. Any one on its own has a value, but comprehensive protection comes only when all the pieces are securely in place.

Glucosamine strengthens the connective tissues in the body and helps protect joints and skin.

Both nutrients are important in delaying the process of ageing by protecting the cellular structures of the body.

Wellness

The basic source of the nine pieces in the nutritional jigsaw must be a healthy diet. So start with a diet rich in fruits, vegetables, soy, and oily fish, plus herbs like thyme, rosemary and oregano, and spices like turmeric, garlic and ginger.

But even a healthy diet needs a core of supplements in order to reach the **optimum** nutritional levels that research shows can provide a real defence against degenerative disease. So add a well-designed supplement programme that ensures that all nine pieces of the nutritional jigsaw are in place – in the optimum amounts.

Top off with some moderate exercise, stop smoking (if you haven't already done so), and now your repair mechanisms should be working as they were designed to do, to keep you well.

The result is a programme that should help protect against almost all of the major diseases, including cancer, stroke, heart disease, Alzheimer's, osteoporosis and diabetes.

The focus is on maintaining 'wellness' rather than treating illness.

The aim of this book is to close hospitals, and put doctors out of work – by helping you live a healthier and longer life!

Website update

I have tried to incorporate the very latest research on nutrition and health available at the date of publication.

Inevitably, however, important new data is appearing all the time. Consequently, I am making free updates available on the following website:

www.healthdefence.com

Part 1

*L*ife expectancy has nearly doubled since 1900, largely thanks to better public health and the control of the major infectious illnesses. You might think that more people would be dying of old age: but the truth is that virtually nobody dies of old age. What kills us are the diseases associated with old age.

Various pieces of evidence suggest that our maximal life span is over 120 years, but few of us ever reach that point. Systems and organs falter, break down and finish most of us off before we reach 80.

However, with a combination of new developments in medicine, and a more thorough approach to looking after ourselves, more and more of the illnesses of old age could be postponed – and our healthy middle age extended for many decades.

Chapter 1

Extending your lifeline

They say that life begins at 40, but new research into ageing has shown that for many, the fourth decade is a period of accelerated ageing. This is a time when many of us stop taking regular exercise, and the stresses of work or family push us into smoking and drinking more, sleeping less, eating junk foods.

According to Canadian gerontologist Dr Richard Earle, women on the threshold of 40 can expect to age a staggering 18.8 biological years by the time they make 50, while their menfolk put on 15.2 years.

That's the bad news. The good news is that not everybody ages this fast. Even better news is that if you combine diet, exercise and lifestyle changes, together with a little medical help, you too can beat the clock.

Sex, stress and sustenance

Even within groups of similar people, there are huge differences in the rates of ageing. Some look old before their time, others retain youthful looks and good health into their 50s and beyond. What's the secret? How can you get into the slow lane?

Edinburgh-based clinical psychologist Dr David Weeks has been studying a group of people he terms the 'Super Young' – people who look and act at least 10 years younger than their age. One thing his 3,500 volunteers had in common was an active and varied sex life. "Slow agers make love more than other people. They are very carnal – they come across as very happy people who enjoy sex both in terms of quality and quantity," says Dr Weeks.

It's highly complex!

You have about 60 trillion cells in your body.

In **each** cell thousands of different chemical reactions are taking place every single minute of every day!

Each of these reactions depends upon an individual specialist enzyme. And most enzymes depend upon your intake of adequate vitamins and minerals.

The British Geriatric Society take a similar line, pointing out that sexual activity boosts the heart (it is, after all, a form of exercise), and the immune system. The biological effects of happiness and pleasure are increasingly coming under study. We know, for example, that sex stimulates the brain to release Growth Hormone, which has reparative and anti-ageing effects on the body.

Attitude is also important. "The Super Young tend to be optimists," says Weeks, "and the recipe for slow ageing would include staying active, curious, involved and stimulated. A younger partner helps!"

Stress, on the other hand, is one of the most important causes of over-rapid ageing. "Worriers age more quickly," says Dr Stephen Webster of the British Geriatric Society, "Someone with worry lines etched in their face almost certainly has prematurely old arteries."

Then there's nutrition. Three meals a day is being replaced, in anti-ageing circles, by grazing – providing this is not on snack foods. Snacking on nuts, cereals and pulses, plus plenty of fruit and vegetables, with the odd fish thrown in, puts less stress on the body, is easier to digest and may be better for bone and muscle development.

Next add anti-oxidant supplements – but with a twist. Nutritionists have abandoned the idea that it's enough to take just one anti-oxidant such as Vitamin C. The secret is synergistic anti-oxidant combinations. It's no coincidence that when the traditional (ayurvedic) Indian 'Pot of Immortality' (Amrit Kalash), was analysed recently, it was found to contain a host of plant-based anti-oxidants and adaptogens.

If you're interested in slowing the clock, this book will show you how in detail. To get you started, check how healthy your lifeline is currently looking using the guide below. It's designed to show you how your life literally lies in your hands. And how a simple regime of moderate exercise, de-stressing, a sensible diet with supplementation and an active sex life can make all the difference.

Slower ageing

Simply increasing lifespan isn't the objective. Almost all families have an example of elderly relatives clinging to a poor quality of life that distresses themselves and their carers.

My objective in writing this book is to show how to slow the ageing process **and** maximise a healthy life span.

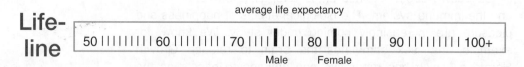

ELIMINATE THE NEGATIVE

Smoking — 6 years
It ages the heart, circulation, skin and lungs, and can contribute to an early menopause, osteoporosis, heart disease and cancer.

Junk food diet — up to 4 years
Too much fat and salt and not enough vitamins, minerals, flavonoids and fibre leads to heart disease, hypertension and cancer.

Alcohol — 1 to 10 years
Over 2 units a day (with the exception of red wine) is bad news. Really heavy drinking loses up to 10 years. Ages the liver, kidneys, heart and brain.

Overweight — 3 years
More than 10% overweight increases the risk of diabetes and hypertension.

Unfit — 1 to 2 years
Heart rate: if not normal within 10 minutes of vigorous exercise, you're so unfit it's going to cost you 1– 2 years. If it's over 80 beats per minute at rest, lose another year.

High cholesterol — 2 years
If over 6.7 mmol/l it will increase your risk of a heart attack.

Stressed out — 4 years
You're over-stressed if you are always tired, sleep badly, and are often worried or irritable. Stress drives up blood sugar and lipids, contributing to heart disease; and depresses the immune system, leaving you vulnerable to infection and cancer.,

High blood pressure — 3 years
If over 135/95, strokes, heart attacks and kidney failure are on the cards.

Sun-worship — 2 years
Lose up to 10 years in appearance. Too much sun ages the skin and can cause skin cancer.

Excessive exercise — 3 years
While exercise is very beneficial, over-exercising increases free radical damage and speeds ageing.

ACCENTUATE THE POSITIVE

Alcohol
+ 1 to 5 years

While more than 2 units of alcohol a day speeds up ageing, less than 2 units a day helps to make blood platelets less sticky, cutting the risk of heart attacks and adding a year to life expectancy. Red wine is the exception – it contains flavonoids and if your daily intake is between 2 and 3 glasses a day, add up to 5 years.

Nutrition
+ 7 to 10 years

Low calorie diets increase the life span of lab animals, and are associated with long life in human communities too – so no more than 1800 calories a day unless you're physically very active. The diet should consist mostly of carbohydrate (pasta, bread, potatoes), plenty of green, red and blue fruits and vegetables, plus nuts, pulses, olive and peanut oil, and relatively little animal protein – preferably fish or game.

Anti-oxidant and micro-nutrient supplements
+ up to 20 years

Vitamins A, C and E, plus a mix of carotenoids, flavonoids and the minerals copper, manganese, zinc and selenium slow down the ageing process in a number of organs including the heart and blood vessels.

Vegetarian diet
+ 2 to 5 years

Since vegetarians eat more fruit and vegetables containing anti-oxidants, fibre and no animal fats, they live longer.

Regular exercise
+ 1 year

Moderate exercise is not only de-stressing and slimming, but life-extending too. It tones up the cardiovascular system, and a 60-year-old who exercises regularly can retain up to 80 per cent of the strength and stamina he or she had at 25.

Sex
+ 2 years

An active (safe) sex life can be an excellent form of exercise, and good for morale too, boosting the cardiovascular and immune systems. A good sex life is one of the common factors found in slow agers.

Stress-reducing techniques
+ 3 years

Whether it's yoga, an hour in the garden or an evening's worth of your favourite soap, relaxation is the key. There are many other de-stressing techniques.

Social interactions
+ 2 years

A good social life with plenty of opportunities to see your friends is associated with slower ageing and a longer life.

(Data from actuarial tables and published scientific papers)

- Millions in the West are malnourished. You're probably one of them

- The modern diet is so low in nutrients that even a balanced diet can't provide all the micro-nutrients we need

- Malnutrition impairs the body's natural defences which guard against common degenerative diseases like cancer, arthritis and heart disease

- Modern medicine attacks disease 'from the outside' – often causing side effects. Nutritional therapy enhances the body's inner natural defences and is the strongest and safest form of preventative medicine

Chapter 2

Malnutrition – the biggest killer in the West?

Breast cancer risk

The risk of breast cancer is increased as much as tenfold by a diet deficient in Vitamin E and the mineral selenium. Isoflavones and the carotenoid lycopene are also important; see Chapter 13, Fighting cancer with food.

For most people, malnutrition means TV images of emaciated figures from the Third World. But malnutrition also occurs closer to home: not the acute lack of calories that can kill within weeks but a chronic depletion of micro-nutrients such as vitamins and minerals, essential fatty acids and certain other substances such as dietary fibre. These chronic deficiencies may not cause obvious short-term effects, but they nonetheless leave a legacy of lasting ill-health and premature death.

The victims aren't necessarily underweight. They could be (and often are) overweight. They may look the picture of health, but meanwhile, some section of their metabolism is going subtly awry, or one of the body's defence systems is beginning to fail. There may be no warning signs until one day a chest pain, a positive cervical smear, a broken bone or loss of vision reveals that something has gone terribly wrong.

There are genetic factors involved, and also environmental elements, such as exposure to pollutants like tobacco smoke – but malnutrition is the key. For example, cataracts are far less likely if you take the right anti-oxidant vitamins and flavonoids; whereas the incidence of heart disease is much higher in people who eat a good deal of meat and dairy products, but don't eat much oily fish, and whose diet is low in anti-oxidant rich fruit and vegetables.

A few diehards maintain we get everything we need in a balanced diet. An eminent UK professor made a notorious speech only a few years ago, saying that the only effect of vitamin pills was expensive urine.

Ironically, it was a research team from his own hospital which subsequently proved that folic acid supplements given to pregnant women reduced the risk of spina bifida babies.

Babies, in fact, are particularly well catered for. Read the list of ingredients on any box of baby food, and you'll see that manufacturers pack their products with as complete a range of vitamins and minerals as they can. But for older consumers, who need just as many micro-nutrients (and, in many cases, more), it appears that the food industry couldn't care less.

Over-processed foods, convenience foods, depleted soils, prolonged food storage and inappropriate cooking techniques mean that the vast majority of us do not get enough of a whole range of micro-nutrients. British and American Government surveys have borne this out. Study after study has shown the need for the beneficial effects of supplements – and conversely, the damaging effects of the average diet.

As a result, there has been a dramatic turnaround in the opinions of medical experts. Dr Tom Sanders, Professor of Nutrition at King's College, London, believes it is almost impossible to select a diet which supplies every nutrient needed for health.

Anthony Diplock, former Professor of Biochemistry at Guy's Hospital, advises everybody who wants to reduce their risk of heart disease to take up to 250IU (International Units) of Vitamin E daily (or 167mg) – but nobody on an average diet would get anything like that dose. You would have to eat over half a pound of wheatgerm every day, which is not a realistic option. In fact, the average intake of Vitamin E is 5-15IU per day. Supplements are practically the only way of guaranteeing that you're getting enough of the right stuff.

A TYPICAL BABY FOOD PACK

NUTRITION INFORMATION TYPICAL VALUES		Per 100g Powder	(% LRV)	Per 100g as fed*	(% LRV)
Energy	kJ	1806		452	
	kcal	429		107	
Protein	g	12.3		3.1	
Carbohydrate	g	66.7		16.7	
of which: sugars	g	29.8		7.5	
Fat	g	12.5		3.1	
of which: saturates	g	5.6		1.4	
Fibre	g	1.8		0.5	
Sodium	g	0.1		0.03	
Vitamin A	µg	450	113	110	28
Vitamin D	µg	10	100	2.5	25
Vitamin E	mg	6.0		1.5	
Vitamin C	mg	30	120	7.5	30
Thiamin	mg	0.5	100	0.13	25
Riboflavin	mg	0.9	113	0.23	28
Niacin	mg	9.0	100	2.3	25
Vitamin B6	mg	0.8	114	0.2	29
Folic Acid	µg	100	100	25	25
Vitamin B12	µg	0.7	100	0.18	25
Calcium	mg	470	118	120	30
Iron	mg	7.0	117	1.8	29
Zinc	mg	4.0	100	1.0	25

*when reconstituted as directed.
LRV Labelling Reference Value for infants and young children.

Irresponsible?

The food industries produce many foods which are nutritionally shoddy and responsible for much ill health.

What if the petro-chemical industry sold fuel so poor it wore out car engines long before their life span? Wouldn't there be an outcry?

For example, trans-fats (hydrogenated fats) and salt are responsible for many cases of heart disease and stroke – yet the food industry continues to produce foods containing excessive levels of these.

It's irresponsible; and consumers pay the price.

A consensus statement, issued in 1997 by the Department of Human Nutrition at Utah State University, declared that it is now impossible for women to obtain their Recommended Daily Allowances (RDAs) for all vitamins and minerals from the average American diet.

And as we'll see in the next chapter, many of the RDAs are too low to maintain optimum health.

Supplementary benefits

Many scientists who still state in public – as a result of peer pressure – that we don't need supplements acknowledge, in private, that they take them themselves. Their decision to take supplements is based on a substantial body of trials which have demonstrated the benefits of taking additional vitamins and minerals. The American Physicians Trial, the Zutphen Trial, the University of California Trial, the Basle Study, the Beijing Trial, and many more have shifted the balance of evidence to the extent that the pro-supplement team no longer have to prove that supplements can help your health.

In fact, I would say that you're gambling with your health if you **don't** supplement. Because … whether we like it or not, we're all guinea pigs.

We are all taking part in a vast, unplanned dietary experiment with unknowable long-term consequences. Our diet has changed beyond recognition from the hunter-gatherer type food that we evolved with, and on which our metabolism was designed to run. And the process of dietary change has speeded up considerably since the end of World War II. That's mainly due to the multinational food processors and distributors who have a financial interest in selling processed, and value-added (but often micro-nutrient-depleted) products.

Another 'experimental' factor is the creation of new environmental pollutants in the water, the air and the food chain (the American Chemical Society recently announced the synthesis of the 10 millionth new chemical).

It's not an experiment in any scientific sense. It's not controlled. No-one is in charge. But the limited amount of information that we

---

Degenerative diseases are the First World killers

Because the degenerative diseases are mostly diseases of affluence, they are relatively uncommon in the developing countries.

In the Third World, most people still die of infectious diseases or trauma, although tobacco-related cancers and heart problems are increasing.

All over the world, however, death is generally hastened by diseases with predominantly social causes.

Just as Third World death rates could be slashed by improved sanitation, vaccination programmes, better food storage, fairer land allocation, and restrictions on cigarette advertising, so Western health could be radically improved by a little social tinkering, more sophisticated agricultural policies, improved nutrition, and better health education.

do have suggests we may be laying the seeds of health problems to come which can only be made worse by the general greying of the populations of the Western countries. In short, we may be looking towards a huge increase in degenerative diseases. Some of the most recent surveys of public health suggest that this trend may already have begun.

Who is at risk?

Various activities or conditions can either increase our requirements for micro-nutrients, or reduce the body's ability to absorb them from food.

Dieters
When food intake is reduced, the intake of micro-nutrients is also reduced; and yet the body's requirements for certain vitamins and minerals may actually increase during periods of weight loss. Anorexics and bulimics are also at increased risk of multiple micro-nutrient deficiency.

Smokers
Each cigarette uses up large amounts of Vitamin C and other anti-oxidants, which is one reason why smokers are more vulnerable to heart disease and cancer.

Drinkers
Too much alcohol depletes the body of B vitamins, and the minerals zinc, magnesium and calcium.

Athletes
Heavy exercise burns more oxygen and therefore increases the requirements for anti-oxidants. Large quantities of zinc and other minerals can be lost through perspiration and need to be replaced.

Sun-worshippers
Too much sun uses up anti-oxidants. If you take Vitamins A, C and E and increase your carotenoid and flavonoid intake, your skin will be better protected against the ageing effects of ultra-violet radiation.

Vegans and vegetarians
Need to plan their diets carefully. Vitamins at risk include D and B12.

The Pill
Oral contraceptives are thought to increase the need for folic acid, Vitamins B and C, and zinc.

Accidents, illness and surgery
All increase the need for vitamins and minerals, including calcium, zinc and magnesium and Vitamins A, B, C and E.

Pregnancy and breast-feeding
The metabolic demands of providing for a growing child increase the need for B complex vitamins, folic acid, Vitamins A D and probably E, and minerals such as iron, calcium and magnesium.

Post-menopausal women
Need more calcium, magnesium and other minerals to save their bones, and Vitamins A, D, B, C, E and K. Other vegetable-derived compounds are important too.

The elderly
Digestion is less efficient in the elderly, who generally have multiple micro-nutrient depletion. A properly designed multi-vitamin and mineral programme is strongly recommended in the over-60s.

Micro-Nutrient Depletion Symptom Checker

Depletion of some micro-nutrients such as Vitamins E and K and the minerals selenium and magnesium are difficult to spot until, eventually, some serious illness develops. Lack of other nutrients can be detected early, because there are often obvious depletion symptoms.

SYMPTOM	POSSIBLE LACK OF
Cracking at corners of mouth	iron, folic acid, Vitamins B2 & B6
Recurrent mouth ulcers	iron, folic acid, Vitamin B12
Dry, cracked lips	Vitamin B2
Cracked tongue	Vitamin B3
Red/sore taste buds at tip of tongue	Vitamins B2 or B6
Bruising/enlargement of veins under tongue	Vitamin C
Red, greasy skin on face, esp. side of nose	Vitamins B2, B6, zinc, EFAs (essential fatty acids)
Rough, red or pimply skin on thighs and arms	Vitamin B complex, Vitamin E, EFAs
Scrotal and vulval dermatitis	Vitamin B2, zinc
Eczema, dry rough cracked skin	zinc, EFAs
Poor hair growth	iron or zinc
Bloodshot or gritty eyes	Vitamins A, B2
Night blindness	Vitamin A or zinc
Dry eyes	Vitamin A, EFAs
Brittle or split nails	iron, zinc or EFAs
White spots on nails	zinc
Pale, anaemic	iron, Vitamin B12, folic acid
Restless legs at night	iron, folic acid
PMS (pre-menstrual syndrome)	zinc, magnesium, Vitamin B6
Gingivitis/gum disease	co-enzyme Q10 and other anti-oxidants
Low energy	many nutrients, including Co-enzyme Q10

Many of the above problems can be caused by other medical conditions or by certain medications. If symptoms are severe or persistent, consult your doctor.

From S Davies & S Stewart *Nutritional Medicine*, Pan Books 1987

Victims of affluence

The human body is incredibly resilient, and can take a good deal of punishment. We can survive injury, infections and periods of starvation; we can even go without water for a few days. With luck cuts heal, broken bones mend, and the stomach upset brought on by unwise eating fades away after a few days.

It's hardly surprising that our immune defences and self-repair systems are so good – after all, we evolved in a tough and unforgiving environment. Our Stone Age ancestors had to get by without the social security, intensive medicine and post-traumatic counselling we take for granted.

What we have to fear is not so much the hard times, but the good times. We have become the victims of our own affluence, and the comforts that we depend on are the very things that make us ill.

The horsemen of our apocalypse are no longer war, famine and plague, but cigarettes, hamburgers and the motor car.

The universal diet

The consensus is that the anti-heart disease diet, the anti-cancer diet, the anti-diabetes diet and the anti-obesity diet are all the same – ie: we should be eating more fruit and vegetables, more carbohydrates and fibre, less fats and sugars, and less animal proteins.

To that I would add well-designed supplements.

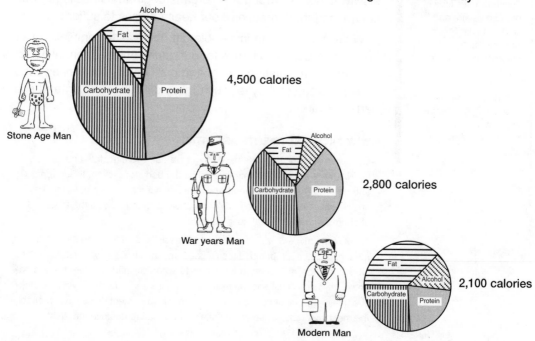

Estimated % of calories by source – from Stone Age to Present Day

Stone Age Man — 4,500 calories

War years Man — 2,800 calories

Modern Man — 2,100 calories

WHY DISEASE STRIKES : **Malnutrition**

We are, of course, more than just what we eat, but conversely the foods we eat and the supplements we take have a profound influence on whether we live out our allotted life spans, and in what sort of health.

The heart of the problem is that we have moved too far away from our evolutionary origins. I'm not recommending a return to a hunter-gatherer diet of roots and grubs. I'm partial to many of the luxuries our society affords – I like Chinese restaurants, the cinema, good design and better ice cream. When I get a headache I take paracetamol or ibuprofen.

But we didn't evolve with central heating, or junk food. Our ancestors had no knowledge of tobacco, and they ate proportionately less fat, and little sugar or salt. If they wanted to eat at all, they had to do a certain amount of physical work to get the food. These are the conditions that formed us.

In marked contrast we take too little exercise, we smoke too much, we eat too many calories in the form of rich, processed foods, and we don't get enough of the vital micro-nutrients that many of these same processed foods are so deficient in. And so, slowly, things go wrong. Our organs begin to fail, cells run out of control and then, gradually, our health begins to suffer.

We're born with an incredible gift, this vastly complex physical body which acts as a house for our genes and our central nervous system. We maintain our cars and our homes, but we neglect our bodies – and yet they're much more difficult to repair, and spare parts are rare!

Vitamin C leads to a longer life?

Recent studies indicate that people who take Vitamin C supplements live longer[3, 56].

Like all research, interpretation and other factors are important. Such people are likely to be more health conscious generally, eg. take other supplements and exercise.

Nevertheless it seems that people with high levels of Vitamin C generally have lower blood pressure and, since Vitamin C helps prevent the oxidation of cholesterol, they are, therefore, less vulnerable to strokes and heart attacks. Vitamin C also seems important in reducing the risk of many forms of cancer.

WHY MICRO-NUTRIENTS ARE VITAL

Good nutrition encompasses everything we eat. Proteins, fats and carbohydrates are the main elements used by the body for growth, tissue repair and energy. The vitamins and trace minerals act mainly as catalysts. They are essential in helping the body's metabolism to regulate all the thousands of chemical reactions that keep us alive.

Think of the micro-nutrients as a kind of specialised oil, keeping the machinery turning. A lathe or pump doesn't need much oil but if you skimp on the lubrication, the machinery soon starts to wear out and will eventually break down. If you don't get enough essential vitamins and minerals in your diet, then eventually your health will break down too. Micro-nutrient depletion is probably the most important cause of ill-health and premature death in the West.

The global diet

According to a recent World Health Organisation (WHO) report, Irishmen and Scotsmen are three times more likely to die of coronary artery disease than their French counterparts.

Their partners are even worse off: women in Belfast or Glasgow are nine times more likely to die of a heart attack than their French sisters. In fact, British women are at the top of the International Ladies' League Table of Heart Attacks, and British men are in the number one position in the male league.

The fact that Aberdonians are so much more at risk than the citizens of Toulouse is known as the French Paradox. French cuisine, after all, is at least as rich as Scottish food. A diet replete with full fat cheese, cream and pâté de foie gras is not at all what the doctor ordered – and yet the French seem to be able to get away with it.

The relative immunity of the French is due to various components in their diet, including the mono-unsaturated fatty acids (and flavonoids) in olive oil, the flavonoids in red wine, and other anti-oxidant compounds such as lutein in kale and other green leaf vegetables[21, 22] and lycopene in tomatoes [25, 26].

In terms of other diseases, however, such as breast and prostate cancer, the French don't do nearly as well as the Koreans, who seem to be protected from these illnesses due to their high consumption of soy products (see Chapters 6, Plant magic, and 13, Fighting cancer with food). And in African cultures where a high fibre diet is still consumed, the incidence of colon cancer is far lower than it is in the USA – or, for that matter, in France and Britain (see Chapter 7, Gut reactions).

Every country and every culture has its own strengths and weaknesses. If we could take the good from each one, we could assemble a diet that would enable far more people to live long and healthy lives, and to reach their biological potential.

The charts that follow show some major national and regional differences. What is it about the lifestyle and diet of Morocco (for example) that results in an 80% lower rate of heart attack than, for example, the UK and Finland?

The best of the best

The common demoninators of the food intake in countries with low cancer, heart attack and stroke rates are high levels of:

- fruit and vegetables
- oily fish
- soy products
- fibre
- pulses, beans and chick peas
- nuts
- olive oil
- red wine

And low in:

- processed food

Pick of the planet

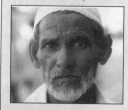

Moroccans have a heart disease rate that is one fifth of the UK. Their diet is high in dried fruits, pulses, vegetables and olive oil – ie high in flavonoids and mono-unsaturates.

WHY DISEASE STRIKES : **Malnutrition**

These are the data and the issues on which I base my belief that you can minimise your risk of heart attack, stroke, cancer and many other diseases with the right lifestyle and nutritional supplements.

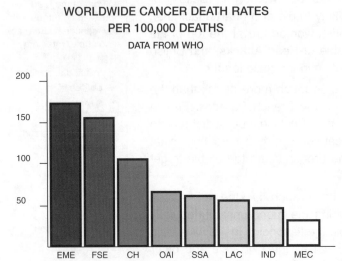

WORLDWIDE CANCER DEATH RATES
PER 100,000 DEATHS
DATA FROM WHO

EME = Established Market Economies

FSE = Formerly Socialist Economies

CH = China

OAI = Other Asian countries and islands

SSA = Sub-Saharan Africa

LAC = Latin America & Caribbean

IND = India

MEC = Middle Eastern Crescent

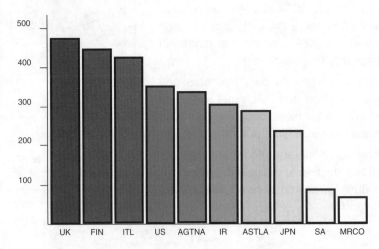

COMPARATIVE DEATH RATES FROM HEART DISEASE
BY SELECTED COUNTRIES PER 100,000 DEATHS
DATA FROM BRITANIA YEAR BOOK 1997

UK = United Kingdom

FIN = Finland

ITL = Italy

US = United States of America

AGTNA = Argentina

IR = Iran

ASTLA = Australia

JPN = Japan

SA = South Africa

MRCO = Morocco

COMPARATIVE DEATH RATES FROM STROKES BY SELECTED COUNTRIES PER 100,000 DEATHS
DATA FROM CANADIAN HEART/STROKE ASSOCIATION

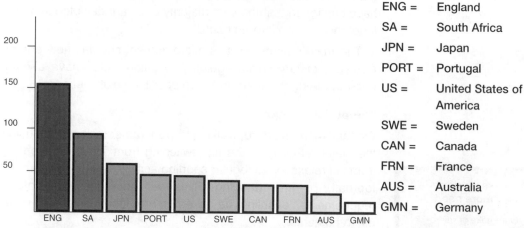

ENG =	England
SA =	South Africa
JPN =	Japan
PORT =	Portugal
US =	United States of America
SWE =	Sweden
CAN =	Canada
FRN =	France
AUS =	Australia
GMN =	Germany

VITAMIN C INTAKE

The term 'deficient' is traditionally used by nutritionists to describe the situation where a micro-nutrient in the diet is so low that a characteristic 'deficiency' disease appears, such as scurvy in those lacking Vitamin C.

We now know that long before a *deficiency disease* like scurvy appears, our cells and organs are already being damaged, increasing the risk of long-term health problems, such as coronary artery disease [5,16,17]. This condition is known as *depletion*, and is far more common than deficiency.

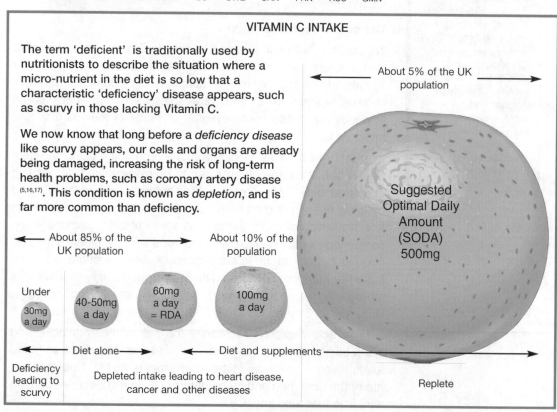

About 5% of the UK population

Suggested Optimal Daily Amount (SODA) 500mg

About 85% of the UK population

About 10% of the population

Under 30mg a day

40-50mg a day

60mg a day = RDA

100mg a day

◄── Diet alone ──►   ◄── Diet and supplements ──────────────►

Deficiency leading to scurvy

Depleted intake leading to heart disease, cancer and other diseases

Replete

The food failure

We don't get enough of all the things we need in our food, no matter how carefully balanced our diets. Many major surveys have confirmed that the vast majority of us are depleted in many, if not most, key micro-nutrients[43].

The main reasons for this micro-nutrient shortfall (low energy lifestyles, dietary shifts, ageing populations, etc.) have already been outlined. There are only two possible solutions.

The purist solution

We take more exercise; walking to work rather than driving, using the stairs rather than the lift, switching from TV and sedentary forms of relaxation to regular sporting activity, whether swimming, football, or line dancing. This will increase our calorie requirements, enabling us to eat more food containing more micro-nutrients.

The convenience solution

We continue with our current low-energy lifestyle, but eat a more micronutrient-rich diet. This can be achieved by opting for 'functional foods', or taking supplements. Some consumers choose organic fruits and vegetables, although there is no evidence that these contain higher amounts of the vitamins and minerals (although see Chapter 5, Anti-oxidants).

In fact the old idea of eating more vegetables being the best way to obtain micro-nutrients has to be re-examined: absorption of carotenoids from green leaf vegetables is not good, and certainly not as good as from supplements[5]. A second trial came to a similar conclusion: the bioavailability of beta carotene when consumed as carrots, the traditional food source, is only a third as good as beta carotene in supplements[6]. Beta carotene in certain fruits like mangoes is stored differently from the way in which it is stored in vegetables, and is more easily absorbed[7] . Unfortunately, mangoes are not as widely eaten as carrots!

Folic acid depletion increases the risk of heart attacks and spina bifida babies. Eating a 'better' diet has little effect on blood folate levels – whereas folate supplements do[4, 33]. Supplements are better absorbed and more stable[28, 37]; stale vegetables contain very little folic acid anyway.

Less nutrients – more need

Our intake of micro-nutrients is dwindling. At the same time our requirements for micro-nutrients are growing. Elements in our lifestyle (exposure to sunlight, cigarettes, pollution, and, for some, excessive exercise) increase the need for vitamins and minerals, including the anti-oxidants.

Fortified foods

Many breakfast cereals contain six to eight added micro-nutrients, and there's good evidence that eating breakfast cereal does improve nutritional status. Professor Malcolm Crawford at the Institute of Human Nutrition at the Hackney Hospital in London showed that the risk of a mother having a baby with cerebral palsy (which is increased by foetal malnutrition, caused by maternal malnutrition during pregnancy) is reduced if she regularly eats breakfast cereal[45, 46].

But six to eight essential micro-nutrients out of a total which may be more than 50 is far from perfect; and the doses the manufacturers include, usually expressed as fractions of the Recommended Daily Allowances (RDAs), are stingy and out of date.

Why don't doctors tell you these things?

The Magic Bullet trap

Nutrition is not taught at medical school, other than a paltry six hours of lectures in a five- or six-year course. This is one reason why many doctors have not until recently been interested in nutrition – they simply don't know much about it. Indeed, many of them find it difficult to cope with patients who may know more about vitamins and minerals than they do.

However, the situation is improving. Even if doctors don't read the women's magazines laid out on their own waiting-room tables (a mine of information regarding the latest health findings), most of them do read specialist medical journals. And in the last few years these journals have begun to publish articles on the health benefits of anti-oxidants and other micro-nutrients. This explains why an increasing number of doctors are becoming interested in nutrition and beginning to change their attitudes.

But don't underestimate medical conservatism. For every doctor who takes vitamins, there are many more who think the whole thing a waste of time and money. There are even some medical scientists who still maintain, against all the evidence, that supplements are a 'con'. This is not due to medical ignorance, but to medical and pharmaceutical bias.

> **Depletion is widespread**
>
> B Vitamin depletion is extremely common, and is a significant cause of coronary artery disease[8-10, 18-21].
>
> Other vitamin and mineral depletions appear to be common, even in well-to-do communities[11-17, 23, 24, 27, 28, 38-40, 42], where vitamin and mineral supplements routinely produce improvements in immune function and health.
>
> The picture is clear: many of us are not getting enough of the micro-nutrients we need to live an optimally healthy life.
>
> Supplements are an easy way of rectifying that problem.

One cause of bias is the fact that most medical research depends on finance from pharmaceutical companies. These companies make their money from designing new drugs, based on novel compounds which they can patent and sell at good margins. They cannot afford to support unprofitable research into nutrients which cannot easily be patented. And because most medical research is restricted to testing new drugs, this moulds the way many doctors and medical scientists think. They don't think in terms of nutrients – they think in terms of developing newer and ever more sophisticated and expensive drugs.

I trained as a medical scientist, and I'm not against modern medicine. This century has seen many medical triumphs, and the pharmaceutical industry's development of new drugs continues to make an important contribution.

For example, Salvarsan, an arsenic compound known as the first 'magic bullet', killed off syphilis in the sense that it was no longer a fatal punishment for 'sexual sin'. After Salvarsan, and the anti-biotics which followed, syphilis became just another illness which could be easily treated.

However, the very success of the first antibiotics, and some of the early hormone replacement therapies such as insulin, became a trap, setting limits to medical thinking. Doctors became obsessed with magic bullets – obliterating or killing the disease was the order of the day. Look through the medical literature and you'll see that metaphors of war and struggle are still prevalent.

But when doctors wage war on disease, patients can be in as much danger from 'friendly fire' as they were from the original disease. In countries such as the USA, as many as 15 per cent of hospital beds are occupied by patients suffering from iatrogenic illness – illness caused by the side effects of their medications.

Bullets, even magic ones, are based on a fundamentally destructive idea. This may be wholly appropriate when dealing with an invading micro-organism, but in other illnesses an easier alternative for the patient may well be to encourage his or her own powers of recuperation.

Degenerative diseases are the end stages of a slow deterioration caused by some mechanism being tipped off balance.

Friendly fire and vicious circles

Painkillers, ironically, can cause gastro-intestinal pain and ulceration. Anti-ulcer drugs can cause impotence. One widely used treatment for impotence (pre Viagra) can cause structural damage to the penis, leaving its owner permanently incapacitated.

The therapies used in the so-called war against cancer, which is where the front-line action is hottest, are the most debilitating, painful and disfiguring treatments of all.

Does it have to be this way? Probably not. In the view of many who study degenerative disease and the ageing process, nutrition could provide kinder answers.

An ounce of prevention is better than tons of cure, particularly in medicine. Protection against degenerative diseases is increasingly being seen as a matter of getting the nutritional balance right.

For example, coronary artery disease develops when the rate that fats are oxidised and deposited in the artery walls is consistently greater than the rate at which the body can remove them.

Osteoporosis develops when the rate of calcium loss from bone is consistently greater than the rate at which the body can replace it.

A cancer grows when its ability to multiply overruns the normal limits to cell growth, and the checks of the immune system.

Problems arise when we overload or undernourish the body's natural defence mechanisms – even by a small margin.

A slight negative imbalance, if continued for many years, will eventually lead to trouble 20 or 30 years down the line. And our self-destructive lifestyles do just that: they tip the balance away from self-repair, and towards gradual self-destruction.

The good news is that minor dietary and lifestyle changes can redress those potentially lethal yet marginal imbalances, tipping them away from illness and towards prolonged good health. Accentuate the positive, eliminate the negative, and you too can look after Mr (and Ms) In-between.

Accentuating the positive means increasing your intake of a range of vital micro-nutrients and taking a bit of exercise.

Eliminating the negative means kicking the cigarette habit, cutting down on fats and sugars, trimming the amount of salt you eat, and drinking no more than moderate amounts of alcohol (although up to half a bottle of red wine a day appears beneficial, see Chapter 6, Plant magic).

It's a small price to pay for a long and healthy life.

My general approach, and the main theme of this book, is that nutritional therapy is usually the best (preventative) form of medicine. It gives the body a gentle and precise helping hand by boosting its own internal repair mechanisms, rather than attacking disease from the outside as drugs generally do.

Research shows that the nutritional approach can work wonders. It can dramatically reduce the risk of heart disease; it can open blocked arteries, improve a failing immune system, speed up the body's ability to heal wounds. It can increase energy, raise intelligence, boost the sex drive. And it can do more. Life extension is no longer over the horizon. It's here.

Our in-built repair kit

The processes of bodily repair are constantly active. They have to be – if we didn't grow new cartilage, our joints would seize up before we reached middle age.

If we didn't have a self-clearing mechanism in our arteries, they would fur up and block before we left our teens.

If we didn't have guard cells to spot and kill off tumour cells before they could become a threat, we'd all die of cancer at a very early age.

The fact that this doesn't often happen is a testimony to the body's ability to police, repair and regenerate itself.

Mr Micawber

"Annual income twenty pounds, annual expenditure nineteen pounds, nineteen and six, result happiness. Annual income twenty pounds, annual expenditure twenty pounds nought and six, result misery."

from 'David Copperfield' by Charles Dickens

EMERGENCY NUTRITION

The nutritional approach is generally slow-acting, because self-repair is slow. It's not often suited to emergency medicine; although even here it has its uses.

The death rate from acute pancreatitis has been cut from 90 per cent to 5 per cent with Antox, which contains anti-oxidant vitamins and the mineral selenium[29-32]. These results are so dramatic that in future all GPs will probably be required to carry a supply of Antox in their black bags.

Co-enzyme Q10 is a micro-nutrient widely used to treat gingivitis and raise energy levels. But in the USA, Japan and Italy, it is a licensed medicine used to improve cardiac function in patients with heart failure – see Chapter 9, The Q Factor.

Why prevention is better than cure!

Some of the most common treatments can have undesirable side effects:

Anti-depressants can cause nausea, headaches and insomnia.

Antibiotics also kill the healthy gut bacteria and, worryingly, are leading to drug-resistant super-bugs.

Decongestants may increase the risk of strokes.

Nutritional therapy

Nutritional therapy is about the safe, gentle and specific mending of tissues by encouraging the body's own repair processes.

The results are being verified by an initially sceptical, but increasingly enthusiastic scientific establishment.

Good health and long life – the simple answer

The literature on nutrition has grown into a forest of information, and one which is becoming increasingly difficult to hack through. But if you're interested in the idea of living a long and healthy life, the way ahead is actually quite simple. It starts with four recent key research findings: together, they provide most of the information we need to increase our life expectancy and decrease the risk of illness.

1 Healthy at 100 years old

A recent investigation set out to find out just what makes a healthy centenarian. There aren't too many healthy hundred-year-olds about, but a dedicated team of scientists combed Italy in search of these paragons of health and long life, and eventually found 37 people who fitted the description. After clinical investigations, they concluded that one thing that all these healthy pensioners had in common was an effective immune system[1].

That makes sense, because it's the immune system which protects us against infections, cancer, and other diseases. To find a healthy immune system in people so old was surprising, because it is well known that the immune system declines with age and becomes less effective.

This is why the elderly are more prone to infections, and why they take longer to recover. It is also one reason why the risk of cancer increases in old age. But why does the immune system run down?

2 Good nutrition

Professor Ranjit Chandra at the John Hopkins University in Baltimore believed that the cause of the weakened immune system so common in the elderly was not old age, but the depletion of the minerals and vitamins that the immune system needs to work effectively.

His elderly subjects were indeed found to be deficient in many key nutrients, and their immune responses were correspondingly below par. He gave them a daily nutritional supplement. Within 12 months their immune systems had recovered. Moreover, their days off sick were reduced by an amazing 50 per cent[2], a finding since replicated by other researchers[12].

3 Anti-oxidants

A second study of the healthy Italian centenarians found that in addition to their strong immune systems, they all had good anti-oxidant defences, with both of these advantages due to their excellent diet[36].

4 Good health at any age

As we have seen, by the time we get into our sixties, a staggering five out of six of us have one or more of the chronic diseases: heart disease, diabetes, arthritis, cancer or osteoporosis. This is a damning indictment of our unhealthy lifestyles, and much of the blame can be laid at the door of poor nutrition.

How can we support such a claim? Because extensive work by Professors Emanuel Cheraskin and Warren Ringdorff, at the University of Alabama Medical College, found that the one thing that was different about the one in six who stayed healthy at age 65 and beyond, was that they consumed more vitamins and minerals.

Healthy old age

Studies show:

1) The common denominators in healthy 100-year-olds are a healthy immune system and good anti-oxidant defences.

2) When elderly people were given vitamin and mineral supplements their weakened immune systems recovered and their anti-oxidant defences improved.

3) The 20% of people aged 60 and over who **don't** have heart disease, arthritis, cancer, diabetes or osteoporosis consume more vitamins and minerals.

What is our diet depleted in?

A few examples ...

- Vitamin C; the main sources are citrus fruits and berries. Intake has fallen by 90% since the Neolithic period[4].
- Carotenoids; main sources are fruits and vegetables. Intake has fallen by about 50% in the last century[47-49].
- Flavonoids; the main sources are fruits and vegetables, especially skins. Intake has fallen by about 75% since Neolithic times[47-49].
- Omega 3 PUFAs; the main source is sea foods. Intake has fallen by 75% since Neolithic times[50].
- Phospholipids; intake has fallen by 50% in the last century[51].
- Prebiotics; the main sources are artichokes, oats, leeks and onions. Intake has fallen by 50% in the last century[derived from MAFF data].
- Selenium; grains are the main source. Intake has fallen by 50% in the last fifty years[52].
- Silicon; oats and hops are the main sources. Intake has fallen by 50% in the last century[53 and MAFF data].

The evidence

The four research findings cited on the previous pages are a distillate of hundreds of trials, millions of pounds-worth of scientific studies, and hundreds and thousands of hours of lab work and analysis.

For the benefit of more technically minded readers, and for anyone who wants to know more about what the scientific community has been getting up to, many of the most important research papers are listed in the reference section.

But for a shorthand introduction to health enhancement and life extension, the preceding four studies show the way ahead.

Conclusion

The research findings assembled here all tell the same story. Most of us are inadequately nourished, and our nutritional profile has worsened in the last 50-100 years. The result is that we pay a high price in terms of chronic, debilitating illness.

A few of us live long, healthy lives; and it seems clear that two of the essential requirements for life extension are an effective immune system and good anti-oxidant defences, both of which are directly related to improved nutrition.

Vegetarianism is a step in the right direction. A 12-year study reported in the 1995 issue of the British Medical Journal showed that vegetarians, whose diet is likely to contain higher amounts of many micro-nutrients, as well as more fibre and less saturated fats, are 30 and 40 per cent less likely to die of heart disease and cancer respectively than meat eaters[55].

This is progress. But to ensure optimal immune and anti-oxidant defences, you need to add a programme of nutritional supplements.

Why RDAs are not enough

When it drew up the Recommended Daily Allowances (RDAs), the National Academy of Sciences never claimed these represented nutrient intakes designed to achieve optimal health. They were never more than a safety net, with the specific purpose of preventing deficiency diseases.

The real mystery is why so many doctors still mistakenly believe that the RDAs have any bearing on the health of their patients, few of whom, in the developed countries at least, are at risk of the classically described deficiency diseases.

The first RDAs were set in May 1941, by a committee of the USA National Academy of Sciences, to prevent scurvy (Vitamin C), pellagra (niacin) and beriberi (Vitamin B1). They were very effective – in that taking 30mg of Vitamin C a day will stop you getting scurvy – but we now know that this dose is not enough to prevent many reactions in the body from going subtly wrong[20, 21, 34].

Even early on it was clear that the RDA concept suffered from two major weaknesses:

1 They are average values and do not take into account the needs of the individual, which may be much higher in many circumstances.

2 The dose sufficient to prevent depletion states is not high enough to guarantee sustained optimal health.

The latest RDAs, issued by the USA National Academy of Sciences in 1989, begin to take individual differences into account. They acknowledged, for the first time, that smokers need more Vitamin C. (Smoking uses up anti-oxidants and many smokers have such low levels of Vitamin C in their blood that they could be regarded as having borderline scurvy.)

Vitamin E

The **minimum** dose of Vitamin E which protects against heart disease (over 100IU of Vitamin E in men and probably over 200IU in women) is far larger than the British and American RDAs, which is a measly 15IU (10mg)!

Vitamin C

Various studies have shown that Vitamin C becomes cardio-protective at doses of between 200 and 600mg a day[1-3].

Our Stone Age diet probably supplied about 400mg a day[4].

The Americans are now considering increasing the RDA to 200-300mg a day.

The EU RDA for Vitamin C is still a mere 60mg a day.

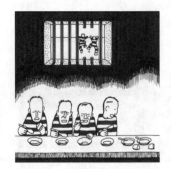

The initial study on requirements for Vitamin C was done on six convicts for a period of nine months – and two convicts escaped before the study was complete!!

RDAs don't always prevent B vitamin depletion

Even people who are consuming the RDAs of the B vitamins are suffering, from a biochemical viewpoint, from a type of depletion, where the resulting changes in their metabolism dramatically increase their risk of coronary artery disease and other problems[34-39].

But smokers suffer from more than low Vitamin C: they also have low levels of Vitamin E, beta carotene, zinc, and Vitamin B6. It seems obvious that the RDAs for these nutrients should also be increased in smokers – but we'll have to wait for years before the RDAs are next re-examined.

What about drinkers? Heavy drinkers tend to have a poor diet and don't absorb nutrients as well as they should. They often have low levels of folate (folic acid), Vitamins B1 and B6, beta carotene, zinc and Vitamin C. The RDAs for these nutrients should be higher for drinkers, as well as smokers.

And what about athletes, pregnant and nursing women, and the elderly who eat less food and don't absorb nutrients so well? What about people exposed to common environmental risks such as increased lead, mercury, traffic fumes, solvents and pesticides? What about the millions of people on fad diets, who are depleted in many nutrients either because they are not eating enough food, or because they are eating crazy combinations of food?

We need a new measure to answer the question, "What are the optimum levels to maintain health, rather than the minimum levels to prevent disease?" One version of this measure is called the SODA – **S**uggested **O**ptimum **D**aily **A**mount.

On the next page I have given SODAs for many of the nutrients which research shows are capable of cutting the risk of heart disease, strokes, certain cancers and Alzheimer's.

POOR EVIDENCE

Since 1951, critics have attacked the way in which the RDAs were drawn up. The American RDA for Vitamin C, for example, is based on a study of just four prisoners (there were six, but two escaped!). They were eating a diet low not just in Vitamin C but in other nutrients too.

Even more seriously, the studies involved in setting the RDAs only lasted six to nine months – about one per cent of the human life span.

Many scientists feel that these short tests could not possibly give any accurate idea about lifetime nutrient requirements.

Animal experiments have shown that although small doses of nutrients may be just enough to maintain health for short periods of time, they are often far too small to maintain health over the life span of the animal.

Suggested <u>Optimum</u> Daily Amounts (SODAs) versus average intakes and RDAs of some key nutrients

Vitamins

	A	B1	B2	Niacin	B6	B12	Folic Acid	C	D	E
SODA	1800mcg	12mg	12mg	60mg	12mg	16mcg	400mcg	550mg	15mcg	275mg
Av. Intake	1012mcg	1.7mg	2.0mg	39mg	2.4mg	7.2mcg	252mcg	58mg	2.9mcg	9.3mg
Sup'mt level	800mcg	7.5mg	7.5mg	15mg	7.5mg	6.7mcg	200mcg	500mg	15mcg	265mg
RDA	800mcg	1.4mg	1.6mg	18mg	2.0mg	1mcg	200mcg	60mg	5.0mcg	10mg

Minerals

	Selenium	Zinc	Calcium	Iron	Magnesium	Chromium	Copper	Manganese
SODA	185mcg	20mg	980mg	10mg	300mg	150mcg	3.5mg	10mg
Av. Intake	35mcg	11mg	917mg	13.2mg	308mg	30mcg	1.5mg	4.6mg
Sup'mt level	150mcg	10mg	100mg	Nil*	50mg	120mcg	2mg	4mg
RDA	75mcg	15mg	800mg	14mg	300mg	125mcg	2.5mg	5mg

Other Nutrients

	Carotenoids			Essential Oils	Vitamin K	Phyto-chemicals	
	Beta Carotene	Lycopene	Lutein	Omega 3		Flavonoids	Isoflavones
SODA	15mg	7.5mg	7.5mg	750mg	75mcg	400mg	45mg+
Av. Intake	1.9mg	2.5mg	1.5mg	150mg	25mcg	140mg	5mg
Sup'mt level	10mg**	5mg	6mg	600mg	50mcg***	250mg	40mg
RDA	N.A.	N.A.	N.A.	N.A.	N.A.	N.A.	N.A.

mg = milligram   mcg = microgram

Source for average intake . . . . Council for Responsible Nutrition and industry sources
Source for RDA . . . . (Recommended Daily Amounts) EU
Source for optimum intake (SODA). . . . . . . Author's estimates based on survey of over 4,000 studies.
The SODA allows for the average intake from food.

* Except in women of child-bearing age.
** Smokers should **not** supplement with beta carotene
*** Except for patients taking warfarin or similar drugs

Note: As we progress through this book you will see that some of the nutrients in which the average person is most depleted are some of the key elements in maintaining the balance between wear and repair, and therefore health. In particular, most people consume inadequate Vitamins C, E and folic acid, too little of the carotenoids, Omega 3 and the flavonoids.

Sources of nutritional research

One way of determining the optimal doses of the various nutrients is to look at trials where high doses of vitamins have been given to large numbers of people to try to reduce the risk of illness.

One of the most significant is the American Physicians Trial[44]. This indicated that the risk of coronary artery disease could be cut almost in half by a daily dose of over 400IU Vitamin E. At this dose, Vitamin E is ten times more effective (not to mention safer and cheaper) than cholesterol-lowering agents.

Studies like these have helped to discredit the idea that RDAs define adequate nutrition and give us valuable pointers as to how much Vitamins C and E we should take. They *don't* tell us about the dozens of other nutrients necessary for long-term health, such as zinc, manganese, the B vitamins, copper. The list goes on and on.

Furthermore, nutritionists are looking at whole new classes of nutrients, which in many ways resemble the vitamins and are probably as important for our overall health. The hydroxycarotenoids, for example, are closely related to beta carotene and Vitamin A. There are hundreds of compounds in this family and several of them have profoundly positive effects on our health.

Two of them, lutein and lycopene, are probably at least as effective as Vitamin E in protecting against heart disease. Others have pronounced immune-enhancing and anti-cancer effects.

Then there are the flavonoids, found in many fruits and vegetables. Some help to maintain the normal function of the blood vessels; others protect against inflammation; others are used to treat Reynaud's Syndrome and cerebral insufficiency (insufficient blood/oxygen supply to the brain) Several flavonoids have been linked to a decreased risk of coronary artery disease.

The carotenoids and flavonoids are called phytochemicals (meaning chemicals from plants). There are over 4000 compounds in these two classes of phytochemicals alone, and we know of at least five other classes of nutrients which also act to protect our health. (See Chapter 13, Cancer, and Chapter 14, Heart disease.)

A new approach

So how can the scientists keep track? How can doctors identify the optimal diet, with the optimal levels of all these nutrients? Basically, they can't. The problem is too complex to solve completely. But one major study, carried out by Professors Emanuel Cheraskin and Warren Ringdorff, at the University of Alabama Medical College, has provided the first concrete step towards optimal nutrition.

They started with one appalling fact. In America, despite the best medical care that money can buy, five out of six people in their 60s have one or more of the major degenerative diseases.

As an indication of the probable accuracy of Cheraskin and Ringdorff's work, their SODA for Vitamin C is around 400mg/day.

This is almost exactly the same as the figure which has recently been calculated for the daily intake of primitive man, who ate a diet with a much higher content of fruits and vegetables than we do[4].

The SODA, for Vitamin C at least, seems to be very much in line with the nutritional content of the diet we evolved with, and were 'designed' to live on.

However, just 1 in 6 remain healthy through their 60s – and many of these people continue to be healthy into their 70s and beyond. The authors were concerned to discover just what was different about this 1 in 6 and spent 15 years examining the lifestyles and health of over 13,500 subjects in six different areas of the USA.

The $2 million study produced an amazing amount of information: 49,000 pages of data, bound into 153 volumes, which have been presented in over 100 scientific papers during the last 20 years or so. This enormous database is still generating papers, and there is undoubtedly more to come; but the interim message is blindingly clear.

The one thing that was different about the healthy folk was that they ate a diet which consistently contained higher levels of nutrients.

Cheraskin and Ringdorff analysed the nutrient content of the diet of the healthy group, and used this as the basis for their new recommended dietary allowances – SODAs: **Suggested Optimal Daily Amounts.**

These SODAs do not take into account some of the more recently discovered phytochemicals described above, but they do give us clear guidelines for a first step towards optimal nutrition and optimal health.

How nutrient levels are determined

There is no one way to determine the optimum levels of any one nutrient. Nutritional information is drawn from a number of sources.

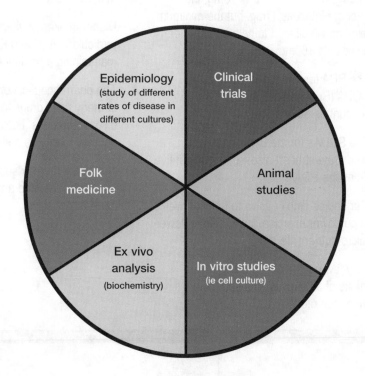

Epidemiology
(study of different rates of disease in different cultures)

Clinical trials

Folk medicine

Animal studies

Ex vivo analysis
(biochemistry)

In vitro studies
(ie cell culture)

SUMMARY

- The RDAs (Recommended Daily Allowances) were established as the level to prevent disease, NOT to achieve optimum health. Moreover, they assume you are in good health, lead a stress-free life, are under 60 and have a perfect digestion.

- Some RDAs were based on small, unscientific samples.

- The RDA for Vitamin E is 10mg, the average intake is 11mg, but the minimum level now indicated to help prevent heart disease is 160mg.

- The RDA for Vitamin C is 60mg, the SODA (Suggested Optimum Daily Amount) is 500mg.

- The SODAs for the B vitamins, which help prevent heart disease, are about five times the RDAs.

- Our bodies didn't evolve to function well in our lower exercise, lower calorie, lower micro-nutrient life style.

- Very few people obtain an adequate intake of all the vitamins and minerals from their diet.

- The effects of vitamin and mineral depletion are not immediate.

- Our defence systems gradually deteriorate until, by the age of sixty, 80% of us find ourselves victims of one of the degenerative killers – cancer, heart disease, diabetes, strokes, osteoporosis.

- A common denominator in the 20% who stay disease-free is a higher vitamin and mineral intake.

- Higher intakes of vitamin and minerals – particularly A, C and E – are essential in maintaining a healthy immune system.

- The pharmaceutical or 'magic bullet' strategy uses drugs to block a step in the disease process. Lack of specificity often causes toxicity as a side effect.

- Nutritional therapy supports the body's own defences, and any side effects are generally positive.

Chapter 3

Inner defences – the immune system

Some people never seem to fall ill, while others come down with coughs and colds every time there's a bug in the neighbourhood. Some individuals live long and healthy lives, but others wither and die in middle age.

Luck? Not entirely. Luck or genetics may play a part, but the important difference is that the lucky ones have better defences against the two most important threats to health: invasion by foreign organisms and attack by dangerous free radicals.

These are two quite different kinds of threat and to counter them we need two quite different forms of defence. To protect against invading micro-organisms we depend on an efficient immune system. And to neutralise destructive free radicals, we need a well-designed anti-oxidant shield.

This chapter looks at the immune system, a highly complex, many-layered defence mechanism. It is designed to protect us, both against the teeming hordes of micro-organisms (bacteria, viruses, parasites and fungi) that see us as food and shelter; and against our own cells that have become cancerous.

The immune system's outer defences consist of millions of free-ranging cells which circulate the whole body, constantly on the lookout for invaders. These cells are pumped round the body in the bloodstream and are drawn back to the heart via the lymphatics – a network of small vessels, rather like veins, that drain through lymph glands in the neck, groin and under the armpits before emptying back into the bloodstream.

If the cells spot an invading bug on their rounds, they bring it back to the lymph glands where other immune cells swing into action.

The immune cells multiply (which is why swollen lymph glands are a sure sign of infection) and release special molecules called antibodies. These search out the bugs and stick to them like glue. This is enough to stop some invaders altogether, but the immune system can also send in the back-up troops – killer cells which zoom in on the combination of 'bug plus antibody' and gobble them up.

Most of the time, very little gets past these defences. Most of the time, despite living in an environment full of potentially disease-causing organisms and carcinogens, we remain healthy.

Problems occur, however, if our immune system is overwhelmed – and that may be an increasing danger. There has been an increase in external threats to our health, including environmental pollution, smoking, viruses which attack the immune system (such as HIV) and the growing use of immuno-suppressant medications. At the same time, there has been a decline in our intake of vital micro-nutrients. The daily intake of selenium, for example, has fallen by half in Britain since the '40s.

New cases of cancer have increased significantly and, unless we change our ways, the figures may continue to worsen. So what should we do to reduce our risk of premature illness? And how can we strengthen our immune systems?

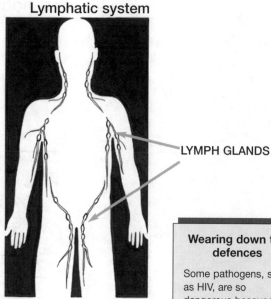
Lymphatic system

LYMPH GLANDS

KURT

Wearing down the defences

Some pathogens, such as HIV, are so dangerous because they can break down our defences. Similarly, if the body is consistently exposed to high levels of carcinogens, as in smoking or excessive sunbathing, and if the immune system is impaired by stress and/or poor nutrition,then eventually a cancer will break through.

Increased cases of cancer

New cases of cancer rose by 10% in Britain between 1979 and 1989 alone.

YOUR BODY'S DEFENCE SYSTEM

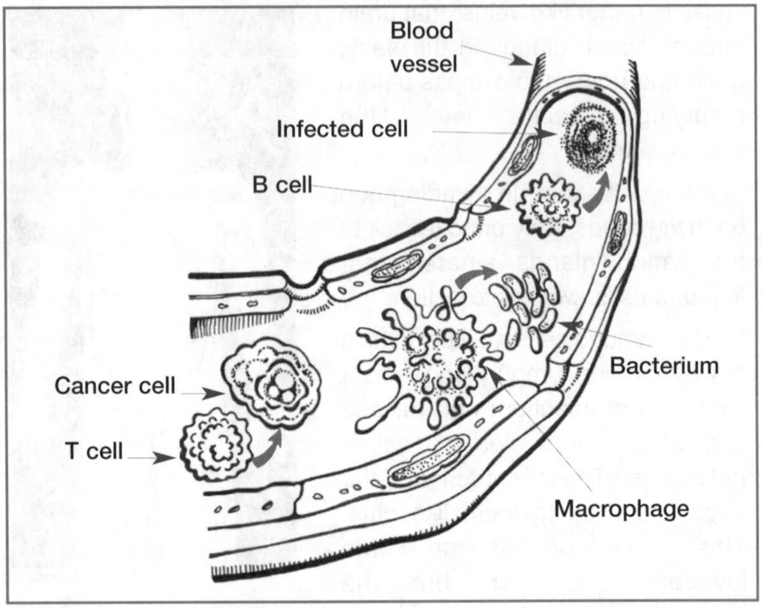

Blood vessel

Infected cell

B cell

Cancer cell

T cell

Bacterium

Macrophage

Boosting the defences

There are three major elements that can affect our immune system: nutrition, our psychological and emotional well-being, and, unexpectedly, the kind of society we live in. Each of these elements can be manipulated to enable us to live healthier, longer lives.

The diagram above shows B cells, T cells, and macrophages dealing with bacterium, cancer and infected cells.

B cells produce antibodies which destroy infected cells. T cells and natural killer cells destroy cancer cells. Macrophages surround and 'gobble up' bacteria. All these defence cells need vitamins and minerals in order to function well.

Supplementing the immune system

The immune system needs well over 20 different micro-nutrients to function properly. Dieting is an all-too-common cause of increased vulnerability to infection, not only because calorie restriction results in a general slowing down of the metabolism, but also because many diets lead to micro-nutritional depletion.

Under attack

It is thought that cancers start to grow relatively frequently in our bodies.

They don't, for the most part, become a problem. This is probably because the immune system spots that the cells are different, reacts to them as if they were foreign, and dispatches killer cells to nip the cancer in the bud.

Even a well-balanced full-calorie diet is unlikely to provide optimal amounts of all of the essential micro-nutrients. As we saw in Chapter 2, this is even more important in middle and old age, when malnutrition is probably the main cause of a faltering immune system.

A number of studies have now shown that supplements of vitamins and minerals can improve immune function, particularly in the elderly where micro-nutrient depletion is more common[19-26]. Vitamin E and the carotenoids are important, but a well-balanced, broad spectrum vitamin and mineral formula is likely to be more effective. However, there's more to supplementation than vitamins and minerals.

There's a wealth of research into natural products which have the ability to support and strengthen the immune system, including such well-known herbs as Siberian ginseng (Eleutherococcus senticosus), and Echinacea. These herbs contain a complex range of ingredients, and researchers are not yet clear as to *how* they work, but there is a general agreement that they *do work*.

> **Extra ingredients for a healthy immune system**
>
> - Micro-nutrients: vitamin/mineral supplement – for general support
>
> - Adaptogen: ie Siberian ginseng – if suffering from stress
>
> - Stimulants: Echinacea OR Shiitake mushrooms OR Pears
>
> - Glutamine – especially for athletes or after trauma

HERBAL IMMUNE SYSTEM BOOSTERS

Eleutherococcus (Siberian ginseng) has a variety of beneficial effects, which have been frequently described in the scientific journals[80-93].

It is an adaptogen, which means it helps people cope with stress. The Russian cosmonauts took the herb to help them with their gruelling training and the rigours of working in space.

This herb also has positive effects on the immune system. It is widely used to counteract infections such as flu and the common cold, and to speed recovery from infection. (Eleutherococcus and Echinacea, another powerful herb, can squash the beginnings of flu overnight.)

In healthy people, Eleutherococcus raises the levels of T-Helper cells and Natural Killer cells in the blood stream; and boosts levels of the immune substance gamma interferon. It also blocks the immuno-suppressant action of the stress steroid hormones. All these changes are important in warding off infection[95-119].

Eleutherococcus also contains anti-oxidants, which is why it is used in Eastern Europe to reduce the side effects of cancer treatment (see Chapter 5, Anti-oxidants). Then there are shiitake mushrooms, which contain polysaccharides that can boost elements in the immune system. The same polysaccharides are found in the skin of pears, so these are also worth considering[1].

Mind and Body

Everybody knows that when times are really tough, and you're stressed beyond endurance, you're more likely to fall sick. But why does the body suffer just because the mind is under pressure? What's the connection?

Chronic worries, repressed anger and depression have all been shown to impair the workings of the body's immune defences by reducing the ability of immune cells to form antibodies, by slowing down the killer cells and by interfering with coordination between the various immune cell types.

The end results can include insufficient immune responses and possibly even auto-immune problems where the immune system attacks the body itself.

Wound healing is also slowed by stress. A recent study in the prestigious *Lancet* journal demonstrated that in people suffering from psychological stress, wound healing is slowed by up to nine days or longer, compared to non-stressed individuals[2].

Many of the Eastern religions have emphasised stress-reduction (via techniques such as meditation) as a key to health for centuries. Modern science is in full agreement with this.

Society

If you want to develop your immune strength to the full, you have to step outside your own door and take a critical look at the society you are a part of. Social status, job security, and even 'social inequality' have an important and direct influence on your life and health.

To begin with, you're better off if you're better off. In class-conscious Britain, socio-economic gradients exist for nearly every chronic illness and disability[4]. The lower down the social scale, the higher the rate of infant mortality[7], childhood death[6], and serious illnesses in adult life[5].

Blue-collar workers are twice as likely to get angina as white-collar types[3] and two to three times more likely to die of heart disease or cancer than their non-manual contemporaries[8]. In fact, nearly all the main causes of death are more prevalent, which is why the least privileged have shorter lives than their

---

Are you stressed?

It's not always easy to tell, because one of the first things to go is your sense of judgement. But the odds are you're suffering from stress if you:

- Get irritable and short-tempered

- Lose your sense of humour

- Burst into tears at inappropriate moments

- Start sleeping badly

- Start smoking (again!)

- Are drinking more than usual

- Are eating far more (or less) than normal.

social betters: they lose out by a startling eight years, roughly 15 per cent of their lifespan.

In the USA, the latest research from the National Centre for Health Statistics shows a depressingly similar pattern – and it's getting worse. Although there was an overall decline in death rates between 1960 and 1986, the health gap between rich and poor grew steadily wider.

Other countries show a similar pattern of poorer health among the poor, but the health difference between the classes is often far less than it is in Britain or in the USA.

Wealth alone does not confer health. Within the developed world, life expectancy in the richer countries is no greater than in poorer countries. Higher living standards do not result in longer life. The one factor that does relate to increased life expectancy is greater social and economic equality.

Could something as abstract as social inequality really damage your health? The evidence strongly suggests that this is indeed the case. If you take one country and make things more unequal, the health of that nation suffers as a result.

This is what happened in Britain after the election of the Thatcher Government. Its policies caused an abrupt increase in social inequality: the rich got richer, and the poor got poorer. Even though the average British income increased by more than a third in the years between 1979 and 1990, death rates for men and women under 45 showed no decline – against the general trend. Indeed there was a marginal increase. This increase in death rates could not be caused by any simple dietary factor, because practically all the main causes of death showed an increase.

And so did many other signs of people in distress: crime, depression, suicide, addiction, falling scholastic standards and family break-up.

This is not an isolated finding. These signs of social problems and weaknesses usually rise and fall in parallel with the health figures. That's the second clue; and it was at Sussex University's Trafford Centre for Medical Research that Dr Richard Wilkinson, who had been studying this conundrum for 20 years, made the breakthrough.

Does wealth buy health?

If you look through 17th- and 18th-century British navy recruiting records, a disturbing pattern emerges. The men aged, or wore out, more quickly than the officers – so much so, that each generation of officers typically outlived two generations of seamen.

The combination of stress, adverse working conditions, drink, disease and malnutrition accelerated the ageing process – a seaman was old at 40 and few reached 45. The officer on the other hand, unless killed in action, might celebrate his 60th or even 70th birthday still in service.

Family doctors who work in deprived areas confirm that by the time their patients reach their mid-40s the signs of degenerative illness are all too often present: damaged and diseased hearts, lungs, livers and kidneys, high blood pressure, raised cholesterol, poor dentition and so on.

His studies confirmed that the countries with the longest life expectancy are not the richest countries; people live longest in countries such as Sweden, Iceland and Japan, where there is the greatest social equality, and the least spread of incomes. This has relatively little to do with better social services in more egalitarian countries; instead, it is closely linked to income distribution[18].

Mixed results in the UK war on cancer

The total number of new cases of cancer rose by 10 per cent between 1979 and 1989.

The largest increases were in cancers of the skin (which doubled), bladder and kidney (which rose by a third), and certain cancers of the blood and lymphatic system.

Lung cancer in women rose by nearly half, and cases of early-stage cervical cancer doubled.

The only bright spot was that the incidence of stomach cancer fell, probably due to an increased intake of fruit juices, rich in Vitamin C.

Lung cancer in men fell also, due to anti-smoking campaigns.

(UK Government figures)

HOW THE MIND AFFECTS THE BODY

Exploration of the mind-body link is a science known as psychoneuro-endocrinology. (Psycho = mind; neuro = nerves in the brain and elsewhere; endocrinology = the hormones controlled by those nerves.)

As this new science advances, it's becoming clear that the reason why long-term stress kills is that it damages the cardiovascular system, the digestive system, the hormonal system and the immune system amongst others.

One example of the mind-body link is seen in depression. The mental state of depression is linked to changed activity in the nerves in a part of the brain called the hypophysis.

During depression, the nerves stimulate the hypophysis to release more of a hormone called ACTH. This hormone increases the activity of the adrenal glands, which release more glucocorticoids into the blood. These steroids have various effects, including a weakening of the immune system, and are linked to an increased risk of osteoporosis and Alzheimer's disease.

Stress is also linked to heart disease. The effects of stress include an increase in blood sugars and lipids and an increase in blood pressure: all of which, if sustained, are considered to increase the risk of coronary artery disease.

Your immune system and general health will benefit if you practise a few tried and tested stress-busting routines.

The Health-Utopia equation

How can living in an unequal society affect your health? You would expect the national health average to be brought down by the poorest of the poor, the underclass, people living meagre and shortened lives in the inner cities. However, the shortened life expectancy in unequal societies affects over half the population.

According to the best evidence we have, this is due to widespread immuno-suppression (depressed immune systems) which in turn lead to increased infectious illnesses, and contribute to an increase in cancer.

So what is the most important cause of immuno-suppression? The answer is almost certainly stress. Stress isn't related to wealth or poverty so much as relative, or perceived status. For example, in a recent study of many thousands of civil servants, most of whom were middle class and reasonably well-off, there was a pronounced difference in health between the ranks.

The 'monkeys' at the top of the tree were healthier than those on the branch below them, and so on down the career structure to the unfortunate occupants of the lowliest positions, who suffered the worst health.

You might think that the senior executives, the high achievers with heavy responsibilities, would experience the most stress. However, the key factor isn't simply the stress itself, but how you experience that stress.

If you're in a position to do something positive about the situation, there's a sense of achievement – and a reduction of stress. But when you don't feel in control, and can't do anything to resolve the stressful situation, the immune system goes into a nose dive.

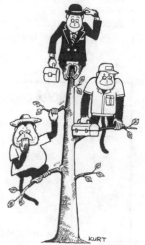

The 'monkeys' at the top of the Civil Service tree are healthier.

In an unequal society, the combination of increased stress and widespread feelings of powerlessness may be the most potent cause of ill health of all. More job insecurity, more unemployment, more house repossessions – the resulting sense of insecurity and loss of control may be more common in the poorer classes, but it spreads to affect the population as a whole.

If job security fades, pension plans evaporate, the health care and educational systems fray; and as the incidence of crime rises, more and more people become affected by insecurity and social unease. As the welfare state shrinks, there is further to fall if something does go wrong. With jobs changing at an increasing rate these pressures are unlikely to diminish.

Nutrition plays a part too, and in urban societies, poorer people undoubtedly eat less well. Scientists used to think the increased risk of heart attacks in the lower socio-economic groups was because of increased consumption of saturated fats and cholesterol; but this has been disproved[11, 12, 15, 16].

WHY DISEASE STRIKES : **Immune system**

People living higher up the social scale eat more fats, and more saturated fats, and have higher serum cholesterol levels than manual workers – yet are **less** at risk from coronary artery disease[15]. A relative lack of fresh fruits and vegetables in the lower groups' diet is probably far more important[9, 10]; and higher rates of smoking also make a significant contribution.

However, poorer people have additional risk factors unrelated to diet and smoking, such as certain blood-clotting factors[12], which are thought to be stress-related. This is one way in which stress (especially stress related to lack of control) could lead to an increased risk of heart disease[13]; and how social improvements could lead to a major reduction in coronary artery disease[14, 17].

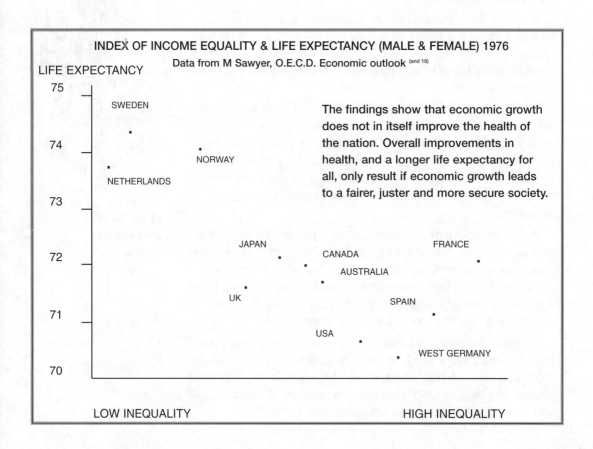

INDEX OF INCOME EQUALITY & LIFE EXPECTANCY (MALE & FEMALE) 1976
Data from M Sawyer, O.E.C.D. Economic outlook [and 18]

LIFE EXPECTANCY

75

SWEDEN

74

NORWAY

NETHERLANDS

73

The findings show that economic growth does not in itself improve the health of the nation. Overall improvements in health, and a longer life expectancy for all, only result if economic growth leads to a fairer, juster and more secure society.

JAPAN   CANADA   FRANCE

72

AUSTRALIA

UK   SPAIN

71

USA

WEST GERMANY

70

LOW INEQUALITY   HIGH INEQUALITY

SUMMARY

The immune system

▶ Your immune system is a key defence against external threats such as bacteria and viruses, and internal threats such as cancers.

▶ Disease breaks out only when your immune system is finally overwhelmed by the attacking organisms.

▶ The health of your immune system depends upon nutrition, psychological well-being and, it seems, the 'fairness' of the society in which you live.

▶ You can strengthen your immune system by ensuring you have an adequate range of nutrients; combined, during periods of stress, with an adaptogen such as Eleutherococcus or Withania (Siberian and Indian ginseng respectively); or, during strenuous exercise, with the anti-oxidants and amino acid glutamine.

> Free radicals are particles which attack the body's cells, damaging or killing them

> Your own metabolism, smoking, sunbathing and strenuous exercise all produce free radicals

> Free radical damage is a major cause of ageing. It leads to the gradual deterioration of organs and to illness such as cancer, arthritis, cataracts and heart disease

> The better your defences against free radicals, the longer you tend to live

> Anti-oxidants reduce free radical damage

> New anti-oxidant drugs are being used to treat stroke, ulcerative colitis, pancreatis and other diseases

Chapter 4

Under attack – the battle against free radicals

Ten years ago, hardly anyone outside specialised research areas knew very much about free radicals. Now you'll find them all over the popular press, from health magazines to the covers of *Time* and *Newsweek*.

From all the publicity, you'd think they were the cause of all illness, ageing and disease. That's taking things too far, but it's true that free radicals are involved in many of the diseases which ultimately kill most of us. It's also becoming clear that they are deeply involved in the ageing process.

As a result, many scientists now believe that anti-oxidants will make as big an impact on public and individual health as did antibiotics half a century ago.

Chain reactions of destruction

Our bodies are built up from many hundreds of thousands of different types of molecules. These molecules are built, in turn, out of rather less than a hundred different kinds of atom.

All atoms consist of a nucleus at the centre surrounded by a shell of electrons spinning round the nucleus, like planets round a sun. Generally the electrons in the outer shell are paired, which is a stable arrangement; but certain processes such as radiation or oxidation may knock an electron out of the shell, leaving an unpaired electron. Atoms with unpaired electrons, and the molecules of which they form a part, are free radicals. Stable radicals are safe; but unstable free radicals behave very aggressively towards biological tissues, ransacking them for replacement electrons.

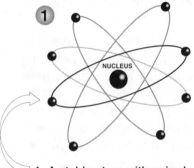

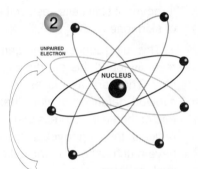

1 A stable atom with paired electrons round it.

2 An unstable atom with an unpaired electron (arrowed). This becomes a free radical and will try to 'grab' an electron from another atom – setting off a damaging 'chain reaction'. Anti-oxidants work by neutralising these free radicals, thus stopping the chain reaction.

Burning wood in a fire produces useful heat, but also potentially dangerous sparks and smoke. Burning petrol in an engine produces useful energy also, but dangerous exhaust fumes are given off. When you 'burn' glucose in your body cells, free radicals are the potentially dangerous by-products of the energy producing process.

Cells are attacked by unstable free radicals many thousands of times every day. Unstable radicals will grab an electron from wherever they can; thus creating more free radicals. Chain reactions occur where thousands of free radicals can be generated in seconds, unless the body's defences catch them in time.

If a chain reaction takes off it can kill the cell. At lower levels, it may damage the cell membrane, making the cell less able to

---

Free Radical poisoning

In the face of sustained attack by free radicals, unprotected biological tissues turn rancid and die.

Free radicals can be thought of as a subtle poison which is constantly weakening us, and contributing to our eventual demise in a slow death of a thousand million cuts.

Free radical damage:

- **Exacerbates inflammation in the joints (rheumatoid and osteo arthritis)**

- **Oxidises the cholesterol in our blood (leading to heart disease)**

- **Damages our eyes (leading to cataracts and blindness)**

- **Degrades the DNA in our body cells, which can either kill them or turn them cancerous**

- **Is deeply involved in most major non-infectious diseases and inflammation**

- **Plays a major role in gingivitis, arthritis, Alzheimer's, pancreatitis and ulcerative colitis**

handle nutrients, less reponsive and less efficient. If free radicals attack the cell's genetic material (DNA) this can, if not repaired in time, lead to cancer. If free radicals attack the mitochondria (the cell's power generators), they can impair the cell's energy balance to such an extent that the cell eventually commits 'suicide'.

If that cell is in the kidney, kidney function will gradually be impaired. If the affected cell is in the skin, it will mean a slower turnover of skin cells, less collagen deposition, and a gradual loss of skin tone and texture.

This all sounds pretty grim – but just because we've only recently found this out doesn't mean free radicals are something new. They are as old as life itself, and all living species have evolved defences against these destructive agents. In fact, the rule of thumb in nature is that the better your defences against free radicals, the longer you live: humans and elephants, for instance, have much better anti-radical defences than shorter-lived species such as mice.

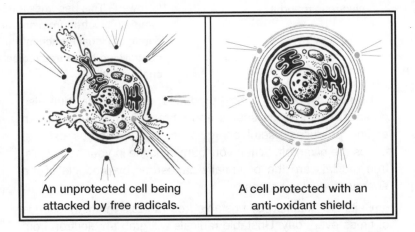

| An unprotected cell being attacked by free radicals. | A cell protected with an anti-oxidant shield. |

There are some rare human genetic conditions where the anti-radical defences are damaged, and in these cases, accelerated ageing, early illness and death is the outcome. Certain nutritional deficiencies, where one or more of the micro-nutrients used in the body's anti-radical defence shield are missing from the diet, have similar results; the victims are far more prone to age-related diseases, such as heart disease, cancer and blindness.

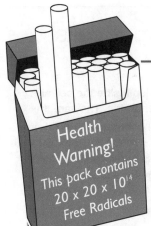

Health
Warning!
This pack contains
20 x 20 x 10^{14}
Free Radicals

Smoking – a free radical production line

Smoking loads the body with trillions of free radicals.

Each puff of cigarette smoke produces 10^{14} free radicals – that's 100,000,000,000,000 – which is why half of all smokers die before their time.

It's been calculated that each cigarette reduces the life expectancy of a smoker by 10 minutes, because of the damage caused by all those free radicals.

The link between smoking and premature death was first discovered by statisticians, but it is the free radical theory which explains why cigarettes are linked with heart disease and cancer.

The increased free radical load uses up the body's anti-oxidants, such as Vitamin C. Smokers (even passive smokers) typically have subnormal Vitamin C levels in their blood[1] – many of them could be said to be suffering from borderline scurvy. Low levels of anti-oxidants cause damage to the lining of the arteries.

At the same time, the free radicals cause lipids (fats) in the blood to oxidise and turn rancid. These rancid lipids attack the damaged artery walls and start building atheromatous plaque (furring of the arteries). This helps to explain why smokers are so prone to heart attacks.

Free radicals also damage the DNA in a smoker's body cells, leading to mutations which may eventually give rise to cancer.

So what about the few smokers who defy the odds and live out a reasonably normal life span? It is almost certainly because they have better anti-oxidant defences.

There may be a genetic factor: some individuals may be better at making anti-oxidant enzymes. Long-life smokers may eat a better diet, containing higher levels of anti-oxidant nutrients.

This suggests that if you cannot (yet) give up smoking, you should at least try to minimise the damage by supplementing with a well-designed mix of the key anti-oxidants.

A threshold of 100mg of Vitamin C reduces the amount of DNA damage[11] and should reduce the risk of cancer. Vitamin E, Co-enzyme Q10, anti-oxidant minerals and the flavonoids are equally important.

EVERYDAY FREE RADICAL DAMAGE

Take the milk out of your fridge in the morning, put it somewhere warm, and by the evening it's sour. Cut an apple in half, and watch it turn brown. Leave butter exposed to air (oxygen) and the fat turns rancid. Leave a scratch on your car untreated, and you'll soon see the exposed metal corroding.

These are all very similar chemical processes. In each case free radicals do the damage – it's called 'oxidative stress' and it's basically rusting.

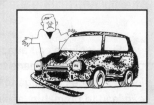

How anti-oxidants protect your cells

1 This is a cross section of the inside of a body cell magnified approx. 10,000 times.

2 Inside the cell is the nucleus which contains most of the cell's DNA. DNA itself contains the genetic codes that make you a unique human being – determining your hair colour, size, shape, features etc.

3 Also inside the cell are mitochondria. They are the energy factories of the body – where the energy in food is converted into energy for you to use.

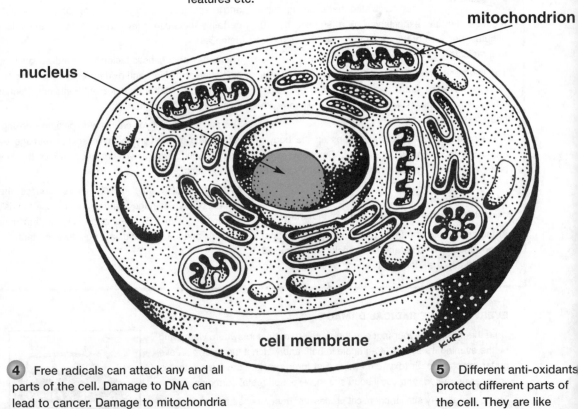

mitochondrion

nucleus

cell membrane

KURT

4 Free radicals can attack any and all parts of the cell. Damage to DNA can lead to cancer. Damage to mitochondria can lead to premature ageing.

5 Different anti-oxidants protect different parts of the cell. They are like specialist defence troops.

6 Vitamin C is water-soluble, and protects against free radicals in the blood and the watery fluids that bathe our cells.

7 Vitamin E and other fat-soluble anti-oxidants such as the carotenoids and Co-enzyme Q10, protect fatty structures such as cholesterol particles in the blood and cell membranes.

Glutathione is an important anti-oxidant inside the cell.

8 Large amounts of free radicals are produced in the mitochondria. Q10 acts inside the mitochondria, and beta carotene protects the mitochondrial walls.

9 Anti-oxidant enzymes neutralise free radicals in almost all areas. They depend on trace elements (see opposite column).

10 When free radicals damage DNA in the cell nucleus that cell may start to grow out of control, and become a cancer.

11 Some flavonoids may bind to DNA, and could provide a local anti-oxidant line of defence.

Other flavonoids can protect other parts of the cell.

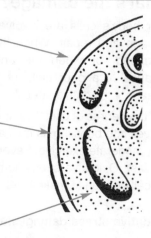

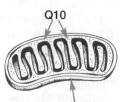

Q10

Beta carotene

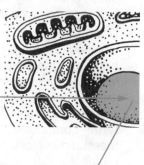

Flavonoid shield

Free radical attack

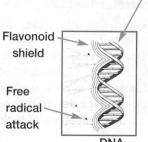

DNA

THE SECRET IS A COMBINATION OF ANTI-OXIDANTS

These diagrams show why it's so important to use a supplement that contains a broad range of anti-oxidants in the right amounts and in the right form.

No single anti-oxidant can provide comprehensive protection, as different vitamins and minerals provide different defences in different places.

For example, anti-oxidants that locate in the mitochondria help protect against mitochondrial ageing. And anti-oxidants that protect lipids (fats) slow the process that leads to strokes and heart attacks.

In addition, certain anti-oxidants only function properly in combination with other anti-oxidants. Vitamin E and carotenoids protect fats in your body from oxidation – but only if sufficient Vitamin C is present.

The body can't make vitamins or minerals, but it does make its own anti-oxidant enzymes. Production of these enzymes depends upon there being enough trace elements like selenium, copper, zinc, manganese and iron present in your diet.

What's the damage?

Your body's cells are involved in a running battle of oxidative damage and repair. When the rate of free radical formation is increased, or when the anti-oxidant defences are impaired because of a poor diet, the result is uncontrolled free radical damage – 'oxidative stress'.

If the degree of oxidative stress is relatively mild, it can stimulate the cell into boosting its own anti-oxidant defences. This happens after moderate exercise. Severe oxidative stress, however, kills the cell fast. Oxidative stress somewhere in the middle can damage the cell enough to make it self-destruct – a slightly slower process.

Oxidative stress damages a cell in a number of ways:

- If a free radical attacks a DNA base, the cell's DNA repair enzymes try to cut out the damaged part and replace it with a new one. The damaged, oxidised DNA base is excreted in the urine, so the rate of DNA damage can be estimated by measuring oxidised DNA base levels in the urine. Non-smokers experience roughly 1,000 DNA base 'hits' a day; smokers between three and ten times as many

- When a protein is oxidised it becomes less efficient, or completely dysfunctional. The body is constantly breaking down and replacing its proteins, so damaged proteins are eventually replaced by newly made protein molecules. The oxidised proteins form compounds which can also be measured in blood or urine.

- When the fatty acids (lipids) in a cell are oxidised by free radicals, they form toxic Lipid Oxidation Products (LOPs), and lipofucsin. Lipofucsin accumulates in the tissues at such a constant rate that it has been suggested that lipofucsin levels are an accurate measure of biological ageing[12,13,70].

Thymol

The anti-oxidant drug Centrophenoxine concentrates in lipids, slows lipid oxidation, and allows the body to clear away deposits of the lipid oxidation end-product lipofucsin (otherwise known as the 'ageing pigment')[12, 13].

Age spots in elderly skin disappear and the mental function of elderly rats and humans improves[14, 15].

The highly potent lipid-soluble anti-oxidants such as thymol, extracted from the herb thyme, are reported to have similar effects[16, 17].

The effects of the build-up of lipofucsin depend on which tissues are affected. In skin, lipofucsin forms so-called liver spots, which are merely unsightly. Inside nerve cells, however, the accumulation of lipofucsin contributes to a steady decline in nerve function, and eventually to cell death. In fact, lipofucsin accumulation is one of the factors which causes the steady loss of brain cells which occur as we age.

In certain conditions the rate of lipofucsin build-up is accelerated. Severe deficiency of the anti-oxidant Vitamin E, for example, leads to a rapid build-up of lipofucsin and symptoms of nerve damage such as unsteadiness and slurred speech[18-20]. Vitamin E therapy improves these symptoms, suggesting that lipofucsin can be removed by the body's normal clearance mechanisms[18].

LOPs (lipid oxidation products), the other main products of lipid oxidation, are also bad for your health. LOPs in the bloodstream are a potent cause of coronary artery disease[21] (See Chapter 14, Heart disease). In other tissues LOPs are thought to trigger inflammation, contributing to conditions such as asthma and arthritis.

Anti-oxidants such as Vitamin E which can get into the lipids in the cells, protect them from oxidation and reduce the rate of LOPs formation.

Of all the different lipids in the body, poly-unsaturated fatty acids (known as PUFAs) are the most vulnerable to oxidation, and can only be replaced from the diet.

In nature, foods rich in PUFAs like nuts and grains always contain high levels of fat-soluble anti-oxidants. With modern processed foods, however, these anti-oxidants are often stripped away.

If we eat too many foods containing refined PUFAs (ie vegetable oils and the poly-unsaturate-rich margarines), without protecting ourselves with anti-oxidant supplements, we put ourselves at risk of producing more lipofucsin and more LOPs[22] (see Chapter 8, Essential oils).

Balance your fish oil supplement

Because PUFAs are so prone to oxidation, PUFA supplements such as fish oil or evening primrose oil should always be combined with lipid-soluble (ie fat-soluble) anti-oxidants.

These include Vitamins A and E, Co-enzyme Q10, Vitamin K, beta carotene, lutein, lycopene, garlic, rosemary, thyme and others.

These, in turn, must be supported by Vitamin C.

REJUVENATED RODENTS

Bruce Ames, the distinguished biochemist at the University of California, has shown that the DNA in each cell of a rat is hit by about 100,000 free radicals a day.

Damaged DNA can either kill a cell, or turn it cancerous, which is why all life forms have DNA repair kits. The rat's DNA repair enzymes work constantly to remove the damage, but they can't keep up.

A young rat has about one million sites of damaged DNA in each cell; old rats have about two million. The DNA repair processes slow down with age because they too accumulate oxidative damage. As a result, older rats have a high cancer rate.

The cancer rate is much lower in humans because, as Richard Cutler at the USA National Institute of Ageing has shown, we have better anti-radical defences – one reason we live so much longer than rats.

In 1993 John Carney at the University of Kentucky Medical Center found that, as expected, levels of oxidised proteins in the brain and other tissues of gerbils increased with age. He gave his elderly, oxidised gerbils an anti-oxidant called phenlybutylnitrone (PBN). This had two important effects – it reduced the oxidative damage in the brain to youthful levels, and it improved the gerbils' short-term memory.

Elderly gerbils lose their memory just like many elderly folk do. On PBN their ability to navigate through a maze shot up until they were doing as well as gerbils half their age – indicating considerable restoration of brain cell function.

Mice and men

Anti-oxidant supplements are good for elderly humans too. Two research groups showed that long-term anti-oxidant supplements given to old folk improved their mental and physical well-being[72, 73].

Not all bad

We can't avoid free radicals altogether, nor would we want to. Some free radicals are good for our health.

Significant numbers of radicals are generated by immune cells as an essential part of the body's defences against invading micro-organisms.

It is when free radicals are produced *in excess* that they spill over from these physiological functions, and cause tissue damage, illness and accelerated ageing.

Free radicals and ageing

The theory that ageing is caused by free radical damage is backed up by a great deal of evidence. For example, Drs Sohal and Rose at the University of California recently succeeded in breeding a mutant super-fly, known as the Methuselah fly, which lives twice as long as its normal brothers and sisters.

When they examined the super-fly, it was different from normal flies in one respect: it was producing extra SOD (super-oxide dismutase) and catalase[3-7] – two key anti-oxidant enzymes whose function is to mop up free radicals.

At more or less the same time, Thomas Johnson at the University of Colorado discovered a super-worm, with a life span 70 per cent longer than normal. This long-lived mutant, like the super-fly, was producing larger than normal amounts of the same two anti-oxidant enzymes: SOD and catalase. So here was a common link – two mutants, two very different species, both with a significantly extended life span and both with better than normal free radical defences.

Higher up the evolutionary tree, one experimenter claimed that mice fed on the anti-oxidant Co-enzyme Q10 increased their life span by up to 50 per cent (see Chapter 9, The Q Factor). The various anti-oxidants work in tandem, and the addition of other anti-oxidants to the mice's diet might have extended their life span still further.

From mice to men is a relatively small step, evolutionarily speaking. Mice are mammals and their metabolism is in many ways similar to our own. It's not identical, but there are more similarities than differences. It follows that much of what is known about free radical damage and ageing in rodents, the most commonly used lab animals, probably has a direct bearing on the human condition.

Check your supplement

The anti-oxidant protection offered by foods is now measured in ORACs (Oxygen Radical Absorbance Capacity).

A diet of five servings of fruit and vegetables a day typically provides 1500 ORACs a day: the evidence suggests we need 3-5000 to stay really healthy[69].

But don't rely on the A-Z type supplements to boost your anti-oxidant status much. A typical 'one-a-day' A-Z supplement provides under 100 ORAC units a day. My recommendation for a supplement provides you with a much higher ORAC score – and hence protection (see Chapter 21, Selecting the right supplements).

EXTREME EXERCISE: DON'T OVERDOSE

When you exercise, you breathe faster, and use more oxygen. The more oxidation going on in the body, the more free radicals are formed as a metabolic by-product.

Moderate exercise stimulates the production of the body's anti-oxidant enzymes, which slow the ageing process. This explains why moderate exercisers live longer than 'couch potatoes'[23].

Top athletes, however, have shorter lives and, probably due to their depressed immune systems[66, 74, 75], are frequently ill[24, 25]. Their very high level of exercise creates more free radicals than their defences can cope with so, like smokers, they tend to die prematurely with heart disease, cancer, etc. This is why many athletes today supplement with high dose anti-oxidants (called 'tanking'.) This is not just an insurance policy: a welcome side effect is reduced muscle damage pain and stiffness after an event, and a faster recovery time [24-38, 40].

N.B. Excessive Vitamin E or carotenoids, if taken without Vitamin C, may be counterproductive[39].

Excessive exercise depresses the immune system.

The powerhouses run down

A significant part of the ageing process is due to damage caused by free radicals to nuclear DNA and to the lipids in cell membranes. However, some experts believe that the key to free radical ageing occurs elsewhere – in the mitochondria, the power generators which are found in each cell of the body.

DNA in the cell nucleus is protected by DNA repair enzymes and anti-oxidant substances such as the histones. DNA inside the mitochondria, however, is unprotected. This is where the cell's oxidative fires burn most fiercely, and where DNA is most vulnerable. The only safety factor is that each mitochondrion has multiple copies of DNA, so that when one strand of DNA is burned out, another takes over. But there are only a limited number of copies, so eventually the mitochondrion starts to break down.

This is why mitochondria become less efficient with age. This was proven by Gino Cortopassi and Norman Anaheim at the University of South California, and Douglas Wallace at the Emory University School of Medicine, who showed that the loss of efficiency in ageing mitochondria is directly related to the steadily increasing number of DNA defects. As the mitochondria run down they produce less energy for the cells, which leads directly to cell and organ decline, systems failure, illness and death.

Co-enzyme Q10 is an anti-oxidant which enters the mitochondria, where it mops up free radicals and slows the rate of oxidative damage. But it has another, equally important role. It is a link in the process whereby energy from the food we eat is transferred to ATP, the energy molecule. By adding Q10, a faltering mitochondrion can produce more energy, thereby giving elderly cells a strong anti-ageing boost. (See Chapter 9, The Q Factor).

That mice fed on Q10 lived half as long again as other mice, suggests that something very profound is going on. Q10 is one of the first nutritional interventions that seems capable of slowing down the hands of the biological clock to such an extent. It is unlikely to be the last.

The superoxide radical

The free radical most commonly formed in the body is the superoxide radical, H_2O_2.

It's not particularly destructive but, in the presence of free iron or copper, it produces hydroxyl radicals, which are much more active and dangerous.

Anti-oxidant defences

Anti-oxidant defences can be increased by taking anti-oxidant vitamins; together with the vital mineral co-factors – zinc, copper, selenium and manganese.

Because micro-nutrient depletion is so prevalent [2, 41-68] anti-oxidant supplements improve the body's defences in most cases.

Rancid people!

Some nutritionists and geriatricians have remarked that old people smell differently from younger folk.

This is nothing to do with hygiene. What the experts are talking about is a sour smell, which, it has been claimed, is the smell of rancid oil. They say this is especially common in elderly folk who, either for preference or because they have dental problems, eat a diet low in fruit and vegetables. This means they aren't getting enough anti-oxidants, leaving themselves vulnerable to free radical attack[71].

The smell of rancid oil is simply a symptom of an unhealthy rate of oxidation taking place in the body, which will, sooner or later, culminate in serious illness.

It is fairly widely accepted that these people are at increased risk of many from the major diseases, and some companies are, even now, developing diagnostic tests which will give an instant 'rancidity' reading, and tell exactly who needs rapid anti-oxidant help.

These test kits should be commercially available in the next few years. In the meantime, a well-designed anti-oxidant supplement should be an essential part of anyone's health and longevity programme. Similar supplements have been shown to reduce 'rancidity' in the elderly[8, 9].

Why older people need supplements

When you reach 50, many micro-nutrients are less well absorbed – especially Vitamins D and B. Also many older people are on prescription drugs which can significantly affect vitamin and mineral levels. Appetite and food intake often fall – reducing micro-nutrient intake further.

Fighting off free radicals

Our defences are reasonably good at keeping free radicals at bay. The body can adapt to a moderately increased free radical load by making more anti-oxidant enzymes[3,4,8]. But when the free radical load gets too heavy, as in smokers or those who live in intensely polluted areas, it overrides the body's defences and leads to illness and premature death, **unless the defences are built up with supplements.**

The next section shows you just what that means.

Iron alert

Be careful with iron supplements!

High iron intake is linked to an increased risk of colo-rectal cancer – and iron supplements increase free radicals in the colon[10, 67].

Make sure your supplement does not contain iron unless you really need it.

BREATH OF LIFE/DEATH OF LIFE

A fire can't thrive without oxygen and neither can we. We need oxygen in order to be able to 'burn' the food we eat, releasing its energy and converting it to ATP, the 'energy molecule' which fuels the activities of cells, such as growth, movement and repair.

Around 95 per cent of the oxygen we breathe forms ATP. The remaining five per cent forms free radicals.

By measuring how much oxygen we take in we can calculate that about two kilograms of free radicals are formed in the body every year.

Oxygen, the colourless, odourless gas essential for life, is eventually responsible, via the formation of free radicals, for many of the ills which plague and eventually kill us.

SUMMARY

Free radicals

▶ Free radicals are atoms or molecules with unpaired electrons that attack other atoms in your body. They can be highly damaging to DNA, which can lead to cancer.

▶ They damage mitochondria (the power plants in each cell), which can cause premature ageing.

▶ They oxidise lipids in cell membranes, leading to cellular dysfunction and death.

▶ They oxidise the cholesterol in the blood which can cause furring up of the arteries and heart disease.

▶ Anti-oxidants protect against the oxidative damage that free radicals cause.

▶ Evidence from animal experiments shows that better anti-oxidant defences are associated with a longer life span.

▶ A comprehensive anti-oxidant strategy needs to involve a combination of anti-oxidant nutrients as each nutrient has its own specialist function, and may protect a different part of the body and its cells.

▶ We can now measure the anti-oxidant power of foods and supplements. Many A-Z type supplements that contain nutrients at just their RDA levels provide a disappointingly low level of anti-oxidant protection.

Part 2

*T*wentieth-century diets are low in many essential nutrients. The solution is simple – put the nutrients back into our bodies. But which ones?

This section looks at four vital groups of nutrients which strengthen our body's own defence systems. They form a series of shields that should constitute the basis of your positive health care strategy:

1) *Antioxidants, which fight free radical damage;*

2) *Flavonoids and isoflavones, plant compounds, which protect the heart and circulatory system and defend against cancer;*

3) *Fibre, which is essential for a healthy digestive system and resistance to infection;*

4) *Fats, which form part of every cell in the body.*

We then look at three other nutrients – and a couple of lifestyle factors – that can add significantly to the effectiveness of your health care strategy.

- Anti-oxidants are the first line of defence against free radical damage and could add many years to your life span

- Studies show that the doses of anti-oxidants needed for good health are far larger than current Recommended Daily Allowances

- Anti-oxidants come in vitamin, enzyme and compound forms. These can all help slow the ageing process

- Trace metals are vital for anti-oxidant enzymes to work

- No single vitamin or mineral is sufficient – our bodies need combinations of anti-oxidants which work in harmony

- The risk of heart disease, blindness, cancer, asthma, dementia and arthritis can all be reduced with anti-oxidants

Chapter 5

Anti-oxidants to the rescue

If free radicals cause illness and premature death, boosting anti-radical defences should improve health and life span.

In animal studies, high doses of anti-oxidants have prolonged life significantly.

We don't yet have enough human data, but a well-designed anti-oxidant programme will probably extend our healthy lives too. Even a modest increase in anti-oxidants and other phytochemicals (compounds found in fruit and vegetables) makes a difference: vegetarians live longer than their meat-eating fellow citizens. Taking larger amounts of the right compounds would almost certainly give us even longer and healthier lives.

Animal experiments suggest that it might be possible to live to the age of 120 or so. Humans tend to have somewhat better anti-oxidant defences, so there might not be quite as much room for improvement in humans as there is in mice. On balance, an additional 20 years or so of good health seems achievable – although many nutritionists and life scientists would say that was too conservative.

The slow burn

Seen as an energy equation, the only difference between an explosion, a fire and a human being is the rate of burning.

An explosion is an extremely fast fire – but humans are on fire too, albeit in a very slow and controlled manner, consuming oxygen and carbon compounds, and burning them to produce water, carbon dioxide, ATP (the energy molecule),and free radicals. The low heat produced in this slow fire keeps us warm and alive.

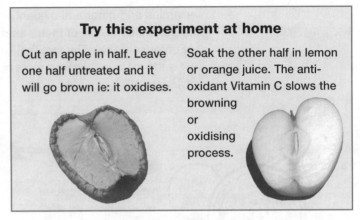

Try this experiment at home

Cut an apple in half. Leave one half untreated and it will go brown ie: it oxidises.

Soak the other half in lemon or orange juice. The anti-oxidant Vitamin C slows the browning or oxidising process.

To stop it from burning out of control and damaging us, we tend the fire very carefully: we parcel it up into tiny, enzyme-regulated steps, surround it with firebreaks, and place fire extinguishers in every corner to douse the excess free radicals. The 'fire extinguishers' are anti-oxidants.

There are basically three lines of anti-oxidant defences:

1st line **Anti-oxidant enzymes** are made in the body and contain an atom of selenium, zinc, manganese, copper or iron. Small amounts of these metals are vital to our health.

2nd line **Anti-oxidant micro-nutrients** are obtained from our diet. These include Vitamins A, C and E, and the B vitamins. Co-enzyme Q10, flavonoids and carotenoids are important vitamin-like compounds which have anti-oxidant properties.

3rd line **Anti-oxidant compounds** are formed in the body, and are made up from elements in the diet. These include melatonin, glutathione, oestrogen, lipoic acid, Q10 and others.

Hardly anyone eats a diet containing enough of all the anti-oxidant minerals,

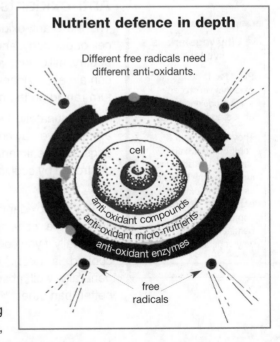

Nutrient defence in depth

Different free radicals need different anti-oxidants.

cell

anti-oxidant compounds

anti-oxidant micro-nutrients

anti-oxidant enzymes

free radicals

vitamins and other anti-oxidant compounds[169-173, 199]. It's important to get enough of all of them, as they work best together in a kind of defence shield. The fact that we don't get enough of them[169, 265-272] is the main reason why most of us die of free radical-related disease.

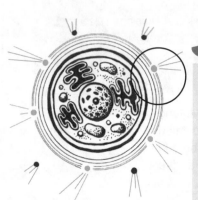

When a cell is protected by an anti-oxidant shield – the right combination of anti-oxidant enzymes, vitamins, minerals and other components – the 'shield' absorbs most of the free radicals.

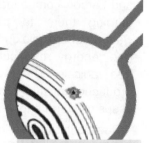

Having been absorbed (or 'quenched') by the anti-oxidant shield, the free radical loses its destructive energy and is neutralised.

Anti-oxidants in the diet

There are anti-oxidants in every living tissue, in every organ and cell of our body, and in almost every food that we eat. Meat, fish, poultry, milk, egg, vegetables and fruit, nuts, grains and pulses all contain anti-oxidants: if they didn't they would rapidly oxidise and turn rancid on the hoof, or on the vine.

Unfortunately, the major anti-oxidants in meat[1], milk and eggs[2] are destroyed by cooking. Nor is there much point in ordering raw eggs and steak tartare, because even if the anti-oxidants weren't destroyed by cooking, they would be broken down in the digestive tract.

The anti-oxidants in fruits and vegetables are more likely to survive the cooking process (although you will destroy them eventually if you cook your fruit and vegetables to a pulp, so lightly cooked is best). Anti-oxidants in fruits and vegetables are generally well absorbed – though some people absorb them better than others[123].

Why vegetarians live longer

Plant foods contain anti-oxidants which can survive cooking to be absorbed by the body.

They also contain compounds which stimulate the body into increasing the levels of its own anti-oxidant enzymes[240], and other compounds which benefit our health. This is why vegetarians live longer.

Anti-oxidants in the body

Dietary factors exert an enormous influence on the levels of free radicals in our bodies. But there are many non-dietary lifestyle factors, such as smoking, sunbathing and aerobic exercise, which increase the amount of free radicals in our bodies.

Chronic infection, whether bacterial, viral or fungal, is another cause of increased free radical formation. This too is linked to increased DNA damage and an increased risk of cancer. Some bacteria appear to be more dangerous than others in this respect: helicobacter pylori as a cause of stomach cancer and papilloma virus as a cause of cervical cancer are among the best documented.

The body's first response to increased amounts of free radicals, whatever their origin, is to defend itself by increasing the levels of its anti-oxidant enzymes[3, 4]. This same defence response is found throughout the animal kingdom, and in plants also[11].

Most dietary advice concentrates on the health benefits of an increased intake of the anti-oxidant vitamins – but the major anti-oxidant enzymes are diet-dependent too. Each enzyme requires an atom of either zinc, iron, selenium, copper or manganese; and all of these must be obtained from our food. This can be a real problem, because there is good evidence of widespread depletion in one or more of these vital trace elements[169-173, 199, 265-272].

Shoring up the defences

Because micro-nutrient depletion is so prevalent[169-173, 265-272], many of us have sub-optimal anti-radical defences.

There's good evidence that our impaired anti-oxidant defences are a significant cause of ill health[164] – and a good case for saying that our governments should spend less money on treating illness and more on preventing it with better nutritional education.

Together with improved food labelling, properly thought-out food fortification programmes and a health-orientated agricultural policy which would shift subsidies from meat and dairy production to fruit and vegetable growers, this would improve the health of the entire nation.

Anti-oxidants are even more vital if you:

- **Smoke**[226] **– even passive smokers**[166]

- **Sunbathe**

- **Exercise excessively**

- **Suffer chronic infections**

- **Suffer chronic inflammatory disease**

- **Have had a heart attack**[179]

Free radicals and national disease prevention

Free radicals are involved in many diseases, including coronary artery disease, Alzheimer's, arthritis, cataracts and some cancers[120].

A minor part of the National Health Service budget spent on nutritional education could make a big impact on health statistics.

THE DEFENCE BOOSTERS: **Anti-oxidants**

Surgery

Tissue damage during surgery is exacerbated by free radicals[20, 93]. Anti-oxidants reduce oedema, speed healing and improve recovery [18, 19].

Full range = Full protection

In the light of recent clinical trials, our improving knowledge of anti-oxidant mechanisms in the body, and the imperfect state of late 20th-century nutrition, the optimal anti-oxidant programme should include Vitamins C, D, E and the B group, Co-enzyme Q10, and a range of carotenoids (including alpha and beta carotene, cryptoxanthin, lutein and lycopene); **plus** flavonoids; **plus** the full range of anti-oxidant trace metals.

Alpha-lipoic acid and melatonin are also important anti-oxidants.

But don't hold your breath. Waiting for governments to make sensible decisions can take a long time, and in this area of policy-making there is strong opposition to change from groups with a vested interest in the status quo.

In the meantime, there's one simple nutritional step we can all take to improve our anti-oxidant defences, which would greatly increase our chances of living a long and healthy life: eat more fruit and vegetables. But even this is no guarantee of achieving optimal nutrition.

OFFAL MEATS CONTAIN THE MOST ANTI-OXIDANTS

With the exception of Co-enzyme Q10, most micro-nutrients are predominantly derived from plant foods, which is why it's a good idea to eat more fruit, vegetables, nuts, grains and pulses.

This is not to say that meat is intrinsically unhealthy. The trace anti-oxidant metals, and some anti-oxidant compounds, including the carotenoids, are not exclusive to plants, and can be found in meat too. Unfortunately, they tend to concentrate in parts of the animal that we do not often eat.

Liver and kidney (and testes and brain) are among the best sources of trace metals, and of some vitamins like A, K, E and Co-enzyme Q10.

However, offal meats are becoming more unpopular for human consumption, and in many affluent cultures are predominantly used for pet food. The meat we eat is mostly skeletal muscle, which is not as good a source of many micro-nutrients.

Trace metals

Depleted soils produce crops low in specific minerals. This is particularly important in the case of selenium, and is the main cause of the selenium depletion which occurs throughout much of Northern Europe, mainland China, parts of Africa and elsewhere.

If you live in an area where the soil is depleted, or you eat foods imported from regions with depleted soils, or you eat a lot of processed foods, your anti-oxidant enzyme defences are probably sub-optimal. The combination of impaired anti-oxidant defences and increased exposure to free radicals is a recipe for premature ageing and illness[84].

Stone Age clues to 20th-century living

Humans evolved eating an omnivorous diet, and a quick glance at eating habits on different continents, in different countries, even in members of the same family, shows that we are capable of getting by on a bewildering variety of foodstuffs. A poor diet, however, will pick us off sooner rather than later.

Although this is something of a generalisation, people who live in the developed countries eat too much meat and dairy produce, too much sugar and white flour, too many empty calories and not enough micro-nutrients. From this starting point, what we need in order to thrive is more refined plant foods.

When you consider how life evolved, it's not so surprising. The first living cells which needed to be able to absorb energy from sunlight, also had to mop up excess free radicals which would have otherwise killed the cells. The green pigment chlorophyll does both of these things; but it is more efficient to have separate compounds, some to absorb energy (photosynthetic) and some to neutralise radicals (anti-oxidants). This is why most plants produce chlorophyll **and** a range of other, more effective anti-oxidants.

Many of these anti-oxidant compounds are coloured, ranging from purples, blues and greens to yellows, oranges and reds. These anti-oxidant compounds are responsible for most of the colours in the plant kingdom, from the bright coloration of flowers and fruit to the rust of autumn leaves.

Some time later in evolutionary history, the first animals appeared. Animals don't photosynthesise. They don't need to produce anti-oxidants in quite the same way as plants; they don't need sunlight for energy, and can afford to block it out with physical barriers such as pigmented skin or shell.

They still need anti-oxidants, however, to neutralise the free radicals produced by the oxygen they breathe; and the easiest way to get anti-oxidants is to eat plants – taking in both their calorie energy and their anti-oxidants. (Carnivores solve the problem in a different way, gaining their anti-oxidant metals and vitamins from offal meats.)

Glasgow gloom

There's a particularly high incidence of heart attacks in young Scottish smokers in their 30s and early 40s[84].

This is due to the huge free radical load imposed by their tobacco habits and a diet singularly lacking in fresh fruits and vegetables. Hence they are low in anti-oxidant compounds and in the trace anti-oxidant metals.

Super mice

Mice fed on lycopene, a carotenoid found in tomatoes, are protected against radiation injury[13].

Vitamins C and E are similarly protective at large doses (ie 1,000IU of Vitamin E a day and 2,000mg of Vitamin C a day[14, 241, 242]), as are other carotenoids[118,119].

THE DEFENCE BOOSTERS : Anti-oxidants

When we eat plant foods we take in their anti-oxidant defences. The carotenoids and flavonoids are a good example of this borrowed (or stolen) defence system. These compounds protect plant cells from free radicals caused by exposure to solar radiation and save them from free radical damage.

When we eat these compounds they protect our skin (and other tissues) from free radical damage in exactly the same way as they protected the original plant[12, 118, 119]. Similarly, the anti-oxidant Vitamins E, C and beta carotene protect against free radical damage caused by ionising radiation in patients receiving radio-therapy[92].

Other animals gain exactly the same benefits. Pigs are very like humans in their metabolism; free-range pigs, which forage for their own food, have better anti-oxidant defences, and are less rancid than their factory-farmed cousins who eat depleted diets[15].

Finding the right combination

Anti-oxidants work best to prevent disease when given together, rather than as monotherapies[60-62, 77, 230, 273]. Our foods contain complex mixtures of anti-oxidants, and, before the arrival of the supplement industry, we obtained all our anti-oxidants from food.

For example, many supplements contain beta carotene, but there are over 600 carotenoids in fruits and vegetables, so why supplement with just one?

Although beta carotene is the main carotenoid in most diets, our bodies also contain, and probably need, alpha carotene (from carrots or pumpkins), lutein (green leaf vegetables, especially kale and broccoli), lycopene (tomatoes), cryptoxanthin (oranges), zeaxanthin (red pepper and spinach) and others[78, 243-245].

The many studies which have looked at the effects of single anti-oxidants are, in part, an unfortunate hangover from the pharmaceutical mind-set. Despite the headlines, it is not very helpful to single out any one micro-nutrient (such as lycopene or selenium) as being 'anti-cancer': it is the general nutritional status that is important. For example, low selenium has been linked to arthritis and myocardial disease in China, coronary artery disease in Finland, breast cancer in New Zealand, and goitre in Zaire.

Each country has a typical nutritional profile through which the low selenium filters, causing a characteristic pattern of illness in each different territory.

The section at the end of this chapter is an attempt to design anti-oxidant and nutritional programmes for specific illnesses; but what about the healthy person who just wants to stay healthy? Which anti-oxidants should they take?

Scientists use a number of different tests to measure the anti-oxidant effectiveness of different compounds, but have not yet reached any general agreement as to which test is the most meaningful. This is not an ideal state of affairs, but nevertheless a few general patterns have emerged.

Many tests show that Vitamin C tends to be used up first. When the C is gone, the carotenoids go next, then Vitamin E; and when the E has all been used up, lipid oxidation begins[248]. Adding either C or E will prevent the lipid oxidation but does not protect proteins from oxidative damage. To protect proteins you must add other anti-oxidants such as flavonoids or glutathione (of which more later). So when it comes to anti-oxidants, monotherapy (ie: attempting to prevent free radical damage with a single anti-oxidant) is both theoretically and demonstrably wrong.

The anti-oxidant cycle

Free radical formed in body

Lipid — Lipid

Vitamin E — Vitamin E

Carotenoid — Carotenoid

Vitamin C — Vitamin C

Free radical excreted from body

Anti-oxidants work together. When Vitamin E neutralises a lipid free radical, it becomes a free radical itself – and a pro-oxidant, unless neutralised ('refreshed') by a carotenoid. The carotenoid is oxidised in this reaction, and becomes a dangerous pro-oxidant in turn; one which can cause considerable tissue damage unless it is neutralised by Vitamin C.

Now the C becomes a radical – but a stable, and therefore a safe one, which is water soluble and can be excreted in the urine. Vitamin C can be regarded as the foundation of the anti-oxidant systems.

To help you choose a supplement that will best provide an comprehensive anti-oxidant shield and a strong immune system, I will summarise, as we progress, my conclusions on which nutrients you need, at what levels and in which form, in boxes headed 'Look for' – like the one in the next page.

In order for you to quickly check what foods – or spices and herbs – you should emphasise in your diet, we have highlighted these in side boxes headed 'Include' – like the one on page 67.

LOOK FOR ...

a supplement that
combines Vitamins A, C
and E with a flavonoid
complex, eg grapeseed
or bilberry extract, plus
the trace minerals
needed by
oxidant enzymes, ie
manganese – 4mg
zinc – 10mg
copper – 2mg
selenium – 120mcg

Minerals in chelate form
are claimed to be best
absorbed.

In this form the minerals
are bound chemically to
amino acids.

LOOK FOR ...

a supplement with
at least 500mg of Vitamin
C in time-release form.

Across Europe the
average intake of Vitamin
C is only 57mg.

Neanderthal Diet

Analysis of the
Neanderthal diet
suggests that our
ancestors evolved on
400-500mg of
Vitamin C a day.

How much?

SODAs (Suggested Optimal Daily Amounts) may well represent the best dosage levels found in the American subjects who were investigated, but are they genuinely optimal doses for humans in general? Are they safe? Could one run into problems with anti-oxidant overdose?

There are so many anti-oxidant nutrients that it would take hundreds of trials to be absolutely definitive about the best doses and combinations of anti-oxidants for short-term health. Industry is unlikely to fund such trials.

And to discover the best doses/combinations to increase life-long health and life span would require generations of scientists, and an equal number of generations of human guinea pigs.

The problem is that anyone eating a varied diet is consuming hundreds of different anti-oxidant compounds, and for many of these there is not enough data to recommend optimal dosage ranges, let alone specific optimal doses. There are, however, guidelines which cover a handful of the more established compounds and the following are best guesses for general preventative regimes.

Vitamin C – 500mg/day in two doses, morning and night or time release (natural or synthetic)

In the guinea pig (one of the few animals other than humans which cannot make its own Vitamin C), oxidative damage to the liver is prevented at a dose some 20-40 times larger than the tiny dose that prevents scurvy[57]. In human terms, this works out at 500-1000mg/day. Other clinicians have found that 500mg in the morning, and 500mg at night, keeps blood levels of C high enough to ensure that a little spills out into every urine sample, implying good anti-oxidant cover around the clock.

Larger doses are seldom needed, but appear to be safe; at doses of up to 5g (5,000mg)/day there is no increased oxalate in the urine[64], and probably no increased risk of kidney stones[232]. Nevertheless, I recommend anyone taking large doses of Vitamin C to drink plenty of fluids.

TOP VITAMIN C FOODS

Yellow pepper	341mg	in 1 medium fruit	Strawberries	85mg	in 1 cup
Papaya	188mg	in 1 medium fruit	Broccoli	58mg	in ½ cup
Guava	165mg	in 1 medium fruit	Brussels sprouts	48mg	in ½ cup
Orange juice	97mg	in 8oz	Potato	26mg	in 1 medium
Grapefruit	94mg	in 8oz	Tomato	24mg	in 1 medium
Kiwi fruit	75mg	in 1 medium fruit			

NB Canned fruits have much lower levels of Vitamin C.

Beta carotene – 10-15mg/day – mixed, natural source carotenoids are best[239] – always combine with Vitamin C

This dose puts you in the top few per cent of the population, a group which appears to be at reduced risk of oral and colon cancers, coronary artery disease and cataracts. Larger doses are generally safe: 500 patients with skin conditions took 180-300mg beta carotene/day for 10 years, without adverse effects[63]. However, smokers and others at risk of lung cancer must be cautious with beta carotene (see Chapter 13, Cancer).

It is best to combine beta carotene with other carotenoids: 6mg lycopene and 6mg lutein per day is a reasonable level, and beta carotene should always be taken with Vitamin C.

LOOK FOR ...

a mixed carotenoid supplement with at least 10mg of beta-carotene, plus additional carotenoids including alpha carotene, lutein, cryptoxanthin, zeaxanthin, lycopene.

The average intake of beta-carotene is only 1-2mg/day[247].

! Smokers should be cautious of beta carotene supplements (see Chapters 12 & 13)

TOP BETA CAROTENE FOODS

100g of carrot contains approximately 5-8mg of beta carotene in only 35 calories. Foods high in beta carotene are:

Carrots	Sweet potato	Squash
Spinach	Kale	Apricots
Peach	Red pepper	Broccoli

Vitamin E – 400IU (265mg)/day – natural source is best[251, 156]

The retrospective American Physicians Trial and other data suggest this is an optimal dose for coronary disease[110, 274]. It should be natural E: the natural form contains only one isomer, D-alpha, whereas synthetic E contains eight.

Why natural Vitamin E? Because whereas D-alpha inhibits the proliferation of smooth muscle cells in blood vessel walls (a highly

LOOK FOR ...

a supplement with 400IU (265mg) of **natural** Vitamin E per day.

The average intake of Vitamin E is just 15IU (10mg) a day[246].

Micro-nutrients aren't medicines

Recent intervention studies with Vitamin E have been disappointing. This indicates that micro-nutrients should not be used as single agents (like drugs), but integrated into nutritional support programmes.

desirable anti-coronary effect), some of the other isomers in synthetic E block this property, and could therefore be cardiotoxic[58].

Very high doses of E are probably not generally useful and may be potentially harmful[236, 157] if used without other anti-oxidants. They may also inhibit the absorption of beta carotene[59] and Vitamin K.

Go for the larger doses!

Some people absorb vitamins less well than others – so go for the larger doses[207,208]. They can all be safely taken together[144, 145, 206, 231].

TOP VITAMIN E FOODS

Wheatgerm oil	20mg	in 1 tbs	Peanuts	25mg	in 1 oz
Sunflower seeds	14mg	in 1 oz	Sunflower oil	6mg	in 1 tbs
Hazel nuts	7mg	in 1 oz	Almonds	7mg	in 1 oz

To get the level of Vitamin E (266mg per day or 400IU) that studies show is cardio-protective (a 50% reduction in risk according to the America Health Care Workers Study) you would need to eat about a kilo(!) of almonds at a whopping 5,000 calories. OR swallow 13 tablespoons of wheatgerm oil (at 1,600 calories)!

The only practical solution is a supplement.

Ensure it's natural – the d-alpha-tocopherol version. Vitamin E works in combination with Vitamin C, selenium and carotenoids.

The Pot of Life

The Indian Ayurveda medical tradition uses a medicine called Amrit Kalash, which translates as 'Pot of Life'.

Amrit Kalash has been used for centuries to improve general health and to extend life, as its name suggests. It comes close to being a dose-finding (although uncontrolled) experiment with long-term anti-oxidants in a large human population.

A glance at the list of fruit and vegetable ingredients reveals that it must contain a rich mix of anti-oxidants. Samples of the syrup and the tablets (Amrit Kalash comes in two parts) have been analysed in various laboratories and contain moderately high levels of anti-oxidants, including Vitamins C and E, and a wide range of carotenoids and flavonoids. It also contains other compounds which boost levels of the body's anti-oxidant enzymes.

The overall effect on anyone consuming Amrit Kalash is a significant increase in anti-oxidant status, and an equally significant decrease in free radicals in the body.

The levels of anti-oxidants in Amrit Kalash are some way above the anti-oxidant RDAs and underline the inadequacy and timidity of current government nutritional guidelines.

It is possible that even the doses in Amrit Kalash may be on the low side in terms of what we need for optimal health today. They were designed for people eating a predominantly vegetarian diet, and who were therefore consuming more anti-oxidant compounds than we do.

In addition, Amrit Kalash was designed for people living in a pre-industrial age. They probably breathed cleaner air than ours, and were exposed to fewer sources of free radicals than we are.

'New' anti-oxidants

Glutathione

Glutathione is not a micro-nutrient: we make it ourselves, inside the body's cells where it is probably the most important anti-oxidant and detoxifying agent. The energy to make this vital compound comes from the mitochondria; if these are impaired, the resulting decline in glutathione leaves our cells vulnerable to free radical damage and death.

With age, the mitochondria become less efficient and levels of glutathione fall. The mitochondria accumulate more free radical damage[105] and produce less energy. Levels of glutathione fall still further, forming a vicious circle that is probably a central part of the ageing process.

All the evidence suggests that maintaining high glutathione levels might be a very good thing[75, 76]. Boosting glutathione levels in mosquitoes, for example, increases their life span by up to 40 per cent. This strategy appears to be quite safe. Doses of up to 250mg per kg of body weight per day of glutathione have been given to animals with no ill effects. This approximates to 15g a day in a human: the doses used in clinical studies so far are considerably lower, at 300-600mg a day.

Glutathione is a small molecule which can be absorbed from the gut, although not much enters the cells[83]. However, it could have positive effects by interacting with the cell surface. It has been suggested that in this way glutathione may boost the immune system[83], sex hormone production and cognitive enhancement. Some clinicians claim it may also reduce the production of inflammatory substances, which would benefit arthritis and asthma.

Glutathione given as a drug, however, doesn't increase levels of glutathione inside the cells. Drug companies have developed synthetic versions with some success[106, 216, 217]. Alternatively, try the glutathione analogue, alpha-lipoic acid, plus Co-enzyme Q10, mixed carotenoids and a wide-spectrum anti-oxidant preparation.

Yet again we come back to the idea of anti-oxidant combinations. Glutathione is a major anti-oxidant inside our cells;

INCLUDE ...

Fresh fruits, vegetables and whole grains provide many of the vital anti-oxidants.

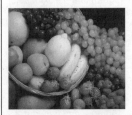

In addition you should drink (in moderation!), red wine, rather than white, or green tea.

Wine, thyme, ginger, garlic, ginseng, liquorice, chilli, ginkgo, paprika, cocoa, green tea and turmeric all contain powerful anti-oxidants that will reduce your 'rancidity index'[72-74, 204, 240, 241, 285]. These ingredients are explored further in Chapter 6, Flavonoids & Isoflavones.

THE DEFENCE BOOSTERS : **Anti-oxidants**

Vitamin C is crucial in plasma and in the extracellular fluids that bathe our cells; Vitamin E is essential in the cell membranes between the two fluid compartments. All three anti-oxidants are mutually supportive, and we need all three – plus Co-enzyme Q10, flavonoids and carotenoids, our own anti-oxidant enzymes, and a range of other anti-oxidant compounds.

HIGH IS HEALTHY

The exception to the general rule that glutathione levels fall with age is in the very healthy elderly, who appear to combine slowed biological ageing with unusually high levels of glutathione[75, 76]. A (small) American study of 33 people over 60 found that those with the highest levels of glutathione were the healthiest[75]. They had lower blood pressure, lower cholesterol levels, were less likely to be overweight, and rated themselves as healthier than average.

At the opposite end of the scale, those with chronic disease conditions such as heart disease, arthritis and diabetes had lower than normal levels of glutathione. Dramatically reduced glutathione levels are also found in acute respiratory distress syndrome (ARDS), which has a 50 per cent mortality rate[215]; and in HIV infection, where glutathione depletion worsens as the disease progresses to AIDS. Both conditions respond well to the synthetic glutathione precursor Procysteine[106, 216, 217].

Melatonin

Melatonin is one of the most recently 'discovered' major anti-oxidants. Long known as the 'dark hormone', melatonin is released by the pineal gland, located at the base of the brain, during the hours of darkness.

This relatively small molecule is now emerging as an important anti-oxidant[198, 203]. It is a very potent quencher of free radicals, doing the jobs of both Vitamin C and Vitamin E in the types of free radicals it neutralises. It is active outside the cell, in the cell membranes and, like glutathione, inside the cell itself. It has been shown to be equally effective in protecting against cataracts caused by glutathione depletion and against DNA damage caused by free radicals[205]. Few compounds have such a broad spectrum of anti-oxidant activity, or such an extensive ability to protect against free radical damage. So what is its relevance to our health?

Curcumin – the 'hot' new supplement

Curcumin, found in the spice turmeric, is a potent anti-inflammatory and anti-oxidant[69].

It also boosts levels of the anti-oxidant enzyme glutathione peroxidase, which protects against free radicals in the eye and other tissues[240]; and reduces protein cross-linkage, thereby slowing the ageing process.

Curcumin at about 100-150mg a day would not only improve your anti-oxidant status, but is likely to ease joint stiffness.

To obtain 100mg curcumin, you'll need a 400-800mg turmeric supplement.

Melatonin

Where melatonin can be sold over the counter, it usually comes in 2mg tablets.

Take melatonin in the evening, as it makes you feel drowsy. Frequent flyers find that melatonin capsules help them to recover from jet lag more quickly[279-282].

Firstly, it emphasises the positive aspects of a good night's sleep, in a dark room, to maximise melatonin production. Exposure to light blocks melatonin synthesis, which is why insomnia is associated with reduced melatonin. This may also explain why recent surveys show that chronic insomnia is linked to a somewhat decreased life expectancy.

Secondly, the ability to synthesise melatonin decreases with age. This is yet another cause of the increased vulnerability to free radical damage found in old age, and which is an important part of the ageing process. This could explain the health benefits (including longevity) which have been ascribed by Indian mystics to drinking their own morning urine, which contains high levels of melatonin. Most people, however, prefer to take their melatonin in tablets!

Anti-oxidants as healers

Coronary Artery Disease

The current theory of coronary artery disease centres on the oxidisation of LDL (low-density lipoprotein) cholesterol particles in the blood. The resulting lipid and cholesterol oxidation products attack the artery walls, increase the risk of clotting[80] and raise blood pressure[25, 26] – all of which increases the risk of heart attacks.

Many anti-oxidants help protect LDL cholesterol from oxidation. When supplements of selenium and the Vitamins C and E are given to human volunteers, their cholesterol becomes more resistant to oxidation[22, 23, 28, 95, 193]. Vitamin E has been shown to reduce the risk of heart attacks by half or more in three recent trials[109, 110, 201], and to reduce the progression of atheroma (furring of the arteries)[121] in ways which are now well understood[253]. So should we all be taking Vitamin E?

Yes, but not on its own. Under certain conditions, Vitamin E can accelerate the oxidation of LDL cholesterol[111, 158] unless there is enough Vitamin C (or flavonoids) around to protect the Vitamin E itself from being oxidised[165]. (See the E-C Cycle on page 63.)

Anti-cancer too?

Melatonin has anti-cancer effects in a variety of models[276-278]. The human implications are not yet clear.

Night milk

'Night milk', from cows milked at night, contains high melatonin levels and has long been reputed to have beneficial properties[200].

LOOK FOR ...

a supplement that includes selenium as selenium-enriched yeast at 120mcg a day.

Junk food warning

Fatty meals make your arteries malfunction – a key early step towards atheroma formation. This effect can be inhibited by a combination of Vitamins E (800IU) and C or by pycnogenol[12, 126, 127, 275] (flavonoids extracted from pine bark).

THE DEFENCE BOOSTERS : **Anti-oxidants**

This is probably one of the main cardioprotective roles of Vitamin C. However, Vitamin C also helps to maintain the lining of the arteries[242, 245] and reduces levels of clotting factors in the blood[122]. It used to be thought that Vitamin C could increase levels of the 'good' HDL (high-density lipoprotein) cholesterol, but this now looks unlikely[30].

All this means that Vitamin E should really be taken with Vitamin C, Co-enzyme Q10 (which appears to be a critical anti-oxidant in LDL), and the metal trace elements manganese, zinc and copper which are necessary for the anti-oxidant enzymes to function properly – because all these anti-oxidant defence systems work together[112, 113, 230].

This sort of combination will undoubtedly help to prevent LDL oxidation in the plasma and slow the migration of oxidised cholesterol from the plasma into the artery walls.

In anyone over the age of 20, however, some oxidised LDL cholesterol is already inside the artery walls, and here we need different anti-oxidants to stop the disease process[114]. At this stage the flavonoids come into their own: these anti-oxidants are able to get into the arterial walls, and slow or stop the progression of atheroma there (see Chapter 6, Flavonoids & isoflavones). Beta carotene may be important too: it does not protect circulating LDL from oxidation[196, 197], but it prevents cells in the blood vessels' walls from further oxidising the LDL that is already there[94].

The evidence that anti-oxidants reduce the risk of coronary artery disease is overwhelming. Conversely, some eminent scientists now say that a poor anti-oxidant status is a better predictor of the risk of heart attacks than high cholesterol levels, blood pressure or any other of the known risk factors[27, 96, 107].

Oxidative damage also contributes to the late stage complications of diabetes, where the incidence of coronary artery disease, cataract, nephropathy (damage to the kidneys) and neuropathy (nerve damage) soar. The increased oxidative stress in these patients means they have more oxidised lipids[24] in their blood and abnormally low levels of anti-oxidants. Their Vitamin C levels are often so low that some late stage diabetics are close to suffering from scurvy[97]. High dose anti-oxidants are clearly indicated.

HEART ATTACKS CUT BY TWO THIRDS

In two studies, high dose Vitamin E (in supplement form) reduced the risk of heart attacks by around 40%[109, 110], but not in others. In a group of doctors with coronary artery disease who were given 50mg beta carotene per day, subsequent heart attacks were not reduced[29, 128].

In two different studies of non-smokers, it was found that in those whose diet contained the highest amounts of beta carotene, the risk of heart attacks was reduced by over 70 per cent, compared to the lowest beta carotene group[81, 229]. And in another major trial, it was shown that in people whose diet contained high amounts of flavonoids, the risk of fatal heart attacks was reduced by as much as 75 per cent, compared to the lowest flavonoid consumers[124].

These dietary studies are difficult to analyse. A diet rich in flavonoids, or in beta carotene, is also likely to be high in other plant compounds such as lutein, a powerful anti-oxidant which protects LDL cholesterol from oxidation up to ten times more effectively than Vitamin E[32, 33, 176], and lycopene which is also strongly cardio-protective[129].

This means that we cannot always be sure which anti-oxidant is the important one; but perhaps the methodological problems are less serious than they seem, because all the major anti-oxidants probably contribute to the reduction in risk[81].

The lesson, again, is that you need a **combination of nutrients for protection**.

Essential for eyes

Supplements of lutein and zeaxanthin build up the protective layer in the retina[227]. They protect the retina by absorbing damaging high frequency light, and neutralising free radicals.

They are in addition precursors for the visual pigments (the rhodopsins).

The increasing incidence of macular degeneration in younger people is probably the result of diets depleted in these carotenoids – and rich in 'empty calories'!

Blindness

Cataract and age-related macular degeneration (damage to the retina) are the two leading causes of blindness in the developed countries. In the USA, cataract surgery is the single largest item in the Medicare budget, costing some $3.2 billion per annum. Worldwide, cataracts blind 50 million people every year; and the tragedy is that much of this is preventable.

The risk of cataract is increased by oxidative stresses such as increased exposure to UV, which oxidises the normally transparent proteins in the lens of the eye, and possibly smoking. The risk is reduced by anti-oxidants such as Vitamins C and E, alpha-lipoic acid, turmeric and possibly beta carotene[36, 40, 61, 192, 240].

It is estimated that 30-50 per cent of all cases of cataract could be prevented by eating more anti-oxidants[34, 256, 300]. Add a supplement of riboflavin to boost the metabolism of glutathione, an important anti-oxidant in the eye[273]. For comprehensive cover, also add half an aspirin or a spoonful of turmeric, which protect lens proteins from destructive glycosylation reactions[125, 240]. (Glycosylation is the cross-linking of proteins.)

INCLUDE ...

Supplements of lutein and zeaxanthin. A diet rich in kale and spinach, which contain them, has been shown to thicken the layer of macular pigment in the eye. This provides anti-oxidant protection against free radical damage caused by light entering the eye[227].

Always combine with Vitamin C.

THE DEFENCE BOOSTERS : **Anti-oxidants**

Macular degeneration is the other major cause of deteriorating sight. Here again, oxidative damage is involved and anti-oxidants such as E, C and beta carotene are protective[35]. This is probably not the most effective combination of anti-oxidants, however. In primates, the main anti-oxidants in the retina are the carotenoids lutein and zeaxanthin[38, 39, 160-162]. The optimal strategy to preserve sight, even if it has started to fail, is almost certainly a combination of lutein and zeaxanthin, together with Vitamin C, riboflavin, lycopene, selenium and a turmeric supplement to boost the anti-oxidant enzyme glutathione peroxidase; and the flavonoids in bilberry, a herb traditionally used to treat visual complaints[37].

SYNTHETIC ANTI-OXIDANTS

For those who prefer a medical to a nutritional approach, the drug companies are developing new synthetic anti-oxidants. Synthetic selenium compounds are already in use (ie Ebselen), and are reportedly very effective; but some chemists believe that an even newer group of anti-oxidant compounds based on tellurium may do even better[70].

The problem with synthetics, however, is that we have never encountered them before, and the possibility of new adverse effects cannot be ruled out entirely. On a slightly less contentious note, a new stable, water-soluble and (so far) non-toxic anti-oxidant called fural glucitol, or 2,4-monofurfurilidensorbitol, is probably going to be a very popular ingredient in future 'cosmeceuticals'[71].

Parkinsonism

In Parkinsonism, toxic tetrahydroquinolones are found in the affected areas of the brain. These compounds are mitochondrial toxins and they cause a decrease in glutathione, an increase in free radical formation, and an increase in nerve membrane damage and death.

If a horse is unlucky enough to eat yellow star thistles, which contain compounds called sesquiterpene lactones, the same sort of things happen – and the horse develops a condition rather like Parkinsonism.

If the changes in mitochondrial function and anti-oxidant status are an important part of the disease process in Parkinsonism, a nutritional approach must be worth trying. This would include a wide spectrum anti-oxidant combination, plus Co-enzyme Q10 and beta carotene to try to improve mitochondrial function; cysteine and alpha-lipoic acid to help boost glutathione levels; and flavonoids to bind free iron, which is released when cells in the brain die and triggers the production of more free radicals[222, 223].

For flavonoids in this case read hawthorn flavonoids. These powerful anti-oxidants enter the brain (hawthorn is known to cause sedation) and probably enter and protect nerve cell membranes from oxidative damage. I would combine the above with thyme oil, or thymol, which has a similar effect[255]. There is some evidence that nitrous oxide (NO) radicals may be involved, so turmeric, together with beta carotene, or the even more effective carotenoid lycopene, is also worth incorporating in the programme[100, 101].

Finally, add Vitamin E to this multi-component regimen. Vitamin E alone is not very helpful in treating this condition[48, 49, 174, 175, 178, 214], but chronic Vitamin E depletion is linked to a form of brain damage in animals rather like the damage found in Parkinsonism[233]. In humans who cannot absorb Vitamin E, the risk of Parkinsonism also rises.

Something rather similar to Parkinsonism is found in patients given long-term anti-psychotic medication. They often develop a syndrome, called tardive dyskinesia (TD). Free radical damage is thought to be involved.

Some scientists report that large doses of Vitamin E help [43-45, 257], although the evidence is disputed[224]. E is an important anti-oxidant in the brain[49], but at least six months of high-dose supplementation are needed to pump up the levels to where they are needed[49-52, 235]. By that time, much of the nerve damage caused by the anti-psychotic drugs may have already occurred – so it might be better to co-prescribe anti-oxidants from the start.

Asthma

Cases of asthma are doubling every 10 years. This astonishing trend has generated much research into possible causes of the disease, such as atmospheric pollution, excessive hygiene in childhood, or exposure to the house dust mite – but no case has as yet been proven.

Some work links asthma to car exhaust fumes; diesel fumes in

Try turmeric

Turmeric's active ingredient, curcumin, blocks the production of NO radicals.

Saving 100,000 lives a year

The US National Center for Health Statistics calculates that if every adult in the US took an extra 500mg of Vitamin C a day, it would cut heart disease deaths by 100,000 a year!

The equivalent UK figure is probably 25,000.

A year's supply of Vitamin C costs about £30. A by-pass operation costs about £25,000.

Worth trying

Some brave clinicians should prescribe thyme oil with anti-psychotic agents, to see whether TD can be prevented.

THE DEFENCE BOOSTERS : **Anti-oxidants**

particular have been shown to lead to the formation of dangerous NO (nitrous oxide) radicals and anti-oxidant depletion[104]. This can't be the whole story, however, because although Stockholm has much cleaner air than London, their asthma problem is just as bad.

Nutritional factors have a part to play; recent surveys show that children in the Mediterranean countries are relatively unlikely to get asthma[228]. Decreased anti-oxidant consumption may well make asthmas more likely. Vitamin C is important in protecting the lungs from oxidative damage: a high C intake is linked to better lung function, even in smokers and in patients suffering from chronic obstructive lung disease[82].

Fish oil reduces inflammation of the airways in **high** doses (8-10g/day); but must always be combined with anti-oxidants, preferably Vitamins E and C and flavonoids (see box opposite).

These will reduce the formation of LOPs (Lipid Oxidation Products), which may contribute to the inflammation of the lungs (see Chapter 8, Essential oils) which underlies asthma.

A high magnesium intake is linked to improved lung function[52], and some clinicians have found magnesium aerosols useful in relaxing the airways of their asthmatic patients[53].

Arthritis

Low anti-oxidant consumption is a risk factor for developing arthritis[54]. Some anti-oxidants such as beta carotene reduce symptoms in animal models of arthritis[55]. Other anti-oxidants, such as those found in ginger[72], reduce joint swelling and pain in clinical trials[56], but these flavonoid compounds have specific anti-inflammatory properties. (See also Chapter 10, Amino sugars)

Tumour necrosis factor alpha (TNF-alpha) is important in inflammatory conditions such as asthma, Crohn's disease and arthritis, and anti-TNF antibodies have been used with some success in clinical trials of arthritis[129, 136, 137]. The success, however, was tempered; patients who made antibodies to the anti-TNF antibodies developed allergy-type responses.

The nutritional approach may offer a more durable solution. The spice turmeric contains curcumin, a powerful inhibitor of TNF-alpha[69]. In my experience, a combination of turmeric and ginger, which blocks the key inflammatory enzymes, has powerful anti-arthritic properties; when combined with high dose (ie 8-10g a day) fish or hemp oil, plus 1200mg per day of Vitamin E[258] and 1-2g of Vitamin C.

Skin and stomach ulcers

Free radicals are involved in the destruction of tissue that leads to ulcers of the skin[220] and digestive tract[218, 219, 221]. Smoking, which decreases our anti-oxidant defences, is a risk factor; conversely anti-oxidants can treat these condtions[218, 220] and, if used prophylactically, may prevent them. The flavonoids may be particularly useful here (see Chapters 6, Flavonoids & isoflavones, and 10, Amino sugars).

Is anti-oxidant poisoning possible?

Anti-oxidants are not panaceas, and should not be used indiscriminately. Nor should anyone imagine that because large doses of anti-oxidants are good, larger ones are necessarily better. However, despite theoretical concerns that very high doses of anti-oxidants might cause toxicity, immuno-suppression, pro-oxidative damage or even increase the risk of cancer, there are few cases where anti-oxidants have been shown to cause harm.

1 Direct Toxicity

The majority of anti-oxidant micro-nutrients are safe even in very large doses, and very much safer than most medical drugs[249]. With the few micro-nutrients which are potentially hazardous in overdose, we generally have mechanisms to regulate intake and tissue levels. If the body has enough zinc, for example, it reduces the amount of zinc it absorbs from the gut, thereby keeping body levels in the right range[5]. The same is probably usually true for copper[6].

Of all the trace metal anti-oxidants, selenium has the worst reputation for toxicity. But let's keep that in perspective. The recommended daily intake of selenium is around 100-200mcg, depending on lifestyle factors. Doses 30 times higher have been used to treat various conditions without adverse effects. The toxic dose of many selenium compounds is around 40

Toxic Pre-eclampsia

Toxic Pre-eclampsia, which can occur near the end of pregnancy is dangerous for mother and baby. The condition is linked with low anti-oxidant status[138-143]. In one major trial, Vitamins C and E reduced the incidence by 76%![144]

No overnight miracle

Some of the nutrients recommended take time to affect your anti-oxidant status.

It can take up to six months for Vitamin E levels to build up, for example.

Selenium needs

A high intake of poly-unsaturated oils increases selenium requirements, as do smoking, exposure to heavy metals such as mercury and lead, and a diet deficient in other anti-oxidants[172, 173, 180-185].

times the recommended daily dose[102, 103, 186-191]. By way of comparison, the toxic (even lethal) dose of a familiar medicine like paracetamol can be less than 10 times the therapeutic dose.

Vitamin E is very safe[65, 68, 74, 259-261]. However, high doses can reduce the ability of the blood to clot and, if given to patients with atherosclerosis, high blood pressure and lesions of the small blood vessels (ie smokers), may increase the risk of haemorrhagic stroke. This may have occurred in the Finnish ATBC study, cited elsewhere. Perhaps the trialists, who were all smokers, should have been primed beforehand with Vitamin C and Crataegus (hawthorn) flavonoids[259-261].

Vitamin A increases the incidence of certain birth defects at doses as low as 10,000 IU/day [195] (ie 4 x RDA), so should be used with caution by women of child-bearing age. Beta carotene is a safe substitute, but must always be combined with Vitamin C, and never with smoking (see Chapter 13, Cancer).

Selenium – Safety Data*	
	Dose (mcg/day)
Deficiency (Keshan)	10-20
Estimated safe/ adequate	50-200
Cancer protection	200-800
Max. acceptable intake	500
Highest national intake (Greenland)	1,280
Lowest observed adverse effect	>5000

*Swedish State Nutritional Agency

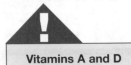

Vitamins A and D

Very high doses of Vitamins A or D can damage the liver.

2 Immuno-suppression

Our immune cells produce free radicals to help destroy certain kinds of disease-causing micro-organisms. For this reason some clinicians have suggested that anti-oxidant supplements could cause immuno-suppression.

Theoretically, extremely large doses of anti-oxidants taken during the start of an infection might make the infection worse. However, in practice anti-oxidants appear unlikely to cause immuno-suppression, except at implausibly large doses.

For most of us, anti-oxidant supplements are more likely to result in improved immune function[16, 17, 262-264]. Immune cells accumulate Vitamin C as and when they need it, and they need it whenever they're active in order to protect themselves from the free radicals they produce. When there isn't enough Vitamin C available, activated immune cells kill themselves with their own free radicals. The resultant immuno-suppression and free radical damage caused by the immune cell's death may lead to even greater tissue damage [17].

Anti-oxidants given late in the course of an illness, when the immune cells have quietened down, could help by reducing

Too little selenium is linked to low fertility

Selenium deficiency is extremely common in some countries[234]. In parts of China and Africa, selenium deficiency is linked to a particularly severe form of arthritis, cardiac damage, infertility, thyroid problems[7, 42], an increased risk of cancer and acute pancreatitis[250].

Selenium depletion is even more common. There are many countries such as Finland (where the soil is now routinely seeded with selenium salts), New Zealand and the UK where selenium levels are low enough to be a potentially significant cause of ill health[85-89].

The UK recommended daily intake of selenium is 60mcg/day for women, and 75 mcg/day for adult men.

However, levels of selenium in the British diet fell between 1978 and 1994, from 60mcg/day to around 30mcg[91]. This fall occurred when the UK stopped importing Canadian wheat and switched to home-produced varieties, grown on selenium-deficient soil[90].

As a result, selenium depletion is increasing, particularly in those who eat a lot of PUFAs, are exposed to heavy metals, or who have amalgam dental fillings[172-173].

The elderly are another high risk group, as they tend to have greater body loads of heavy metals, and are more likely to be depleted in selenium and the other essential anti-oxidant trace metals[10].

Signs of early selenium depletion are already emerging. Selenium is essential for fertility, and selenium deficiency leads to reduced fertility in all animal species studied[42].

If you give selenium supplements to infertile, selenium deficient animals, embryonic mortality falls, sperm motility improves, and conception rates increase.

In a recent study of Scottish men, selenium supplements increased their sperm motility considerably, indicating that they were selenium depleted before the supplementation programme started. When the supplements stopped, their sperm motility fell back to pre-treatment levels[8].

Selenium is not a cure-all for infertility. Low levels of Vitamins E and C also reduce fertility, and both of these vitamins should also be tried in cases of otherwise unexplained infertility[9, 237].

But too much may be dangerous.

Different forms of selenium have different levels of toxicity.

Selenite, selenate and seleno-methionine are the most toxic; but even here relatively minor problems, such as prolonged clotting time, only begin to appear at doses of 750mcg a day[186-188].

Excess selenium may become pro-oxidative[190-191] and may be linked to an increased cancer risk[189]. 150-200mcg/day is probably close to optimal.

Exercise and anti-oxidants

Exercise increases the formation of free radicals up to five-fold, so does this mean exercise is dangerous for your health? Actuarial tables reveal that in exercise, as in so many other things, moderation is the key.

People who take a moderate amount of exercise live, on average, longer than those who take no exercise. One Czech study showed, however, that former high-level professional athletes have a rather shorter life-span, and do no better than those who take no exercise at all[283, but see also 284].

It seems likely that these athletes' increased risk of cancer, heart disease and arthritis in their later years was related to their increased exposure to free radicals during prolonged periods of extremely intense physical exertion.

Muscle damage caused by free radicals occurs even in the most highly trained athletes[144, 145, 177]. With really heavy exertion, the level of free radical damage can lead to DNA damage, and contribute to immuno-suppression and an increased susceptibility to skin and upper respiratory tract infections[146-147].

For some reason men tend to be more badly affected than women; but in both sexes, anti-oxidant supplements such as Vitamins E and C, and Co-enzyme Q10 reduce muscle damage, with a resulting increase in stamina and a corresponding decrease in post-exercise pain and stiffness[148-153, 275]. These anti-oxidants also reduce inflammation of the airways[209].

Partly as a result of these findings, many professional athletes now rely on 'tanking', ie taking large doses of broad-spectrum anti-oxidants. This speeds up post-exercise recovery, reduces DNA damage and decreases the incidence of infection[146-147]. And just in case anyone thinks this is merely a placebo effect, identical benefits have been shown in rats![154-155]

The increased life span associated with moderate exercise is probably due to increased levels of anti-oxidant enzymes in the body. This enzyme boost is the body's way of adapting to the extra free radical load caused by increased oxygen demands during exercise.

The up-regulated enzymes work very efficiently and go on doing so even after the athlete leaves the track and goes home, leading to a significant reduction in free radicals in the body, and thereby slowing key aspects of the ageing process[156].

Athletes and sportspersons should remember that their increased anti-oxidant enzymes won't be able to work effectively if they are deficient in any of the vital trace metals needed to let anti-oxidants work efficiently.

Professional athletes in particular, should maintain an adequate intake of the anti-oxidant trace minerals, high doses of the anti-oxidant vitamins and the amino acid glutamine.

EXERCISE BOOSTS THE BODY'S PRODUCTION OF ANTI-OXIDANT ENZYMES!

You can increase the amount of anti-oxidant enzymes your body makes with moderate exercise. The minimum 'dose' of exercise to boost your anti-oxidant enzymes is probably around 20 minutes of aerobic activity three times a week (that's exercise sufficiently intensive to raise the pulse rate).

Professor Ken Cooper of Dallas University has shown that this is the minimum 'dose' of exercise which improves health status and life expectancy.

Twenty minutes three times a week tones the heart, lowers blood pressure, improves blood cholesterol ratios and reduces the blood's tendency to form clots.

The fact that moderate exercise also reduces the risk of cancer[156] probably means that this 'dose' of exercise is sufficient to trigger a compensatory increase in the level of anti-oxidant enzymes too.

SUMMARY

The Anti-oxidant Checklist

▶ Eat more fruit, vegetables, nuts and grains.

▶ Drink alcohol in moderation, preferably red wine.

▶ Take moderate amounts of exercise to boost your anti-oxidant enzyme levels – 20 minutes of exercise three times a week is the minimum.

▶ Get a good night's sleep in a dark room to boost your melatonin levels. Capsules are available in some countries.

▶ Most people would benefit from a daily supplement of Vitamins C (500mg), D, E (400IU OR 265mg), B group, Q10, mixed carotenoids (10-20mg) and alpha-lipoic acid.

▶ Mineral supplements of zinc, selenium, copper and manganese will ensure the anti-oxidant enzymes are working properly.

Supplement with iron only if iron deficiency has been diagnosed.

▶ Curcumin, thyme, rosemary, ginger, garlic, chilli, ginkgo, cocoa and green tea are all good anti-oxidant 'extras' [72-74, 241].

▶ If you smoke, exercise, sunbathe or are suffering from chronic inflammation or infection, you need extra anti-oxidants.

▶ Athletes should supplement with higher dose E, C, beta carotene and Q10 to reduce muscle damage.

To protect against and treat the following, incorporate these into your diet and supplement mix:

▶ Heart disease: selenium (100-200mcg), C, E, Q10 (90-270mg) and mixed carotenoids, grapeseed, hawthorn or bilberry flavonoids, betaine.

▶ Cataracts: C, E, alpha-lipoic acid, mixed carotenoids, riboflavin (B2) and turmeric

▶ Macular degeneration: Vitamins E and C, lutein, zeaxanthin, selenium, bilberry extract, lycopene and riboflavin (B2).

▶ Parkinson's disease: Full anti-oxidant combination, including Vitamins E and C, Q10, beta carotene, cysteine/alpha-lipoic acid, hawthorn extract, thyme oil.

▶ Asthma: Fish oil, Vitamins C and E, magnesium, turmeric, ginkgo, lecithin and/or betaine. Reduce poly-unsaturates in oils and spread.

▶ Arthritis: Vitamins C and E, ginger, fish or hemp oil. Experiment with turmeric – begin with 4 teaspoons a day building up to 2 tablespoons a day. (Turmeric oleoresin, if available, is easier to take.)

Chapter 6

Plant magic – flavonoids and isoflavones

The flavonoids are one of the most important groups of compounds derived from plants. Over 20,000 have now been identified since the early days when they were all lumped together as Vitamin P by the great Hungarian biochemist Szent Gyorgyi in 1936 (who also discovered Vitamin C).

Following Szent Gyorgyi's discovery, pharmaceutical companies brought out a range of medicines containing Vitamin P but, by the '60s, most had disappeared. As a natural compound, P could not be patented and because nobody knew exactly what P was, how best to measure it, or even whether P was a single compound or a group, the drug companies found it difficult to produce a reliable product.

Modern techniques have resolved these problems. The flavonoids have been identified and divided into approximately 12 sub-types, many of which have profound anti-oxidant activity.

Each of these groups is under intensive study. Interestingly enough, the results often mirror long-established folk medicine. For example, it has been discovered that one group of flavonoids especially good at mopping up damaging free radicals in the liver is found in particularly high levels in milk thistle[23], a herb traditionally used to treat liver disease.

Another type of flavonoid which quenches free radicals in the lining of arteries occurs in very high concentrations in hawthorn and yarrow[24-26], two plants which have long been used to treat cardiovascular disease.

These are not coincidences. Not all herbal remedies are effective but the tradition goes back thousands of years and is based on generations of experience. Very often, the herbal lore in different countries and even different continents turns out to rely on the same herbs and plants to treat the same diseases, and this again is no coincidence.

So it is not entirely surprising that when the tools of modern science are brought to bear on traditional herbal remedies, they uncover a wealth of valid medical information – information which is forming the basis for new, rational and often highly effective forms of preventative and curative medicine.

VITAMIN P

Vitamin P's Hungarian discoverer named it after Paprika (a rich source of this group of compounds and a staple in Hungarian cuisine); and Permeability, as the extract was effective in reducing bleeding and bruising.

In this respect Vitamin P seemed to resemble Vitamin C, and Szent Gyorgyi concluded that the two vitamins worked together in the body. Although his views subsequently fell from fashion, more recent work shows that he was broadly correct: at least one group of flavonoids, the leucoanthocyanidins, can save guinea pigs dying from scurvy by substituting for Vitamin C[52]. (Guinea pigs and humans need Vitamin C in their diet, all other mammalian species make their own.)

There are well-documented reports of scurvy in humans being cured by infusions of pine bark, a rich source of flavonoids. The same flavonoids, combined with Vitamin C, are highly effective in the treatment of cardiovascular conditions[53-56, 62-64, 78-82].

Where do flavonoids come from?

Flavonoids form a vital but, until very recently, sadly neglected part of human nutrition. The Western diet contains anything between 25 mg and 1g of flavonoids per day[1, 2, 3], and the level of your flavonoid intake is now considered by some to be a major factor in determining your risk of developing coronary artery disease[3], and cancer[4, 5].

Flavonoid sources

Flavonoids are found in fruits and vegetables like apples, prunes, citrus fruits, cabbage and lettuce, and particularly in the following foods (type of flavonoid in brackets):

- **Red and yellow onions, shallots** (quercitin)

- **Grapeseed, red wine, maritime pine bark, haws, flowers and bark of hawthorn, most parts of the yarrow, leaves and buds of hazel tree** (procyanidins)

- **Walnuts, blackberries, pecan nuts** (elagic acid)

- **Coffee** (caffeic acid)

- **Tomatoes** (chlorogenic acid)

- **Green tea, black tea** (catechins)

- **Rosemary** (carnosic acid)

Even if you don't know what flavonoids are, you are almost certainly already eating them. The question is whether you are eating enough of the right ones to stay healthy.

Flavonoids are found in a huge variety of edible plants, fruits and vegetables, including apples, prunes, citrus fruits, cabbage, lettuce, tomatoes and tea[6, 7]. But although they are so common, most of us are likely to be flavonoid depleted[3], thanks to changing eating habits. We're eating less than half the amount of fresh fruit we did at the turn of the century, and more processed fruit[99-101]. The highest concentrations of flavonoids in fruits and vegetables tend to be found in the skin and seeds[8] and industrial processing methods almost invariably discard these parts.

The flavonoids concentrate in the external tissues and core to defend the plant, and its DNA, against external threats. Many flavonoids are powerful anti-oxidants, and high concentrations of these compounds in the skin or peel of a plant protect it from free radical damage generated by UV in sunlight. Flavonoids also have potent anti-viral, anti-bacterial and anti-fungal properties, and the flavonoid 'ring' around the plant provides an important defence shield against pathogen attack.

Flavonoid depletion

What are the results of flavonoid depletion likely to be? We can begin to answer that question by reviewing all the therapeutic things that flavonoids do – and it's a long list.

Many flavonoids have anti-bacterial, anti-fungal, and anti-viral effects. Although they are designed as defence compounds for plants, fortunately for us they work against the micro-organisms that cause disease in humans too[9-11, 65-70, 86, 102]. For example, certain flavonoids are able to inhibit viruses such as HIV[12-20].

Many members of the flavonoid group have powerful anti-oxidant, anti-allergic and anti-cancer properties and boost the immune system.

Other flavonoids inhibit enzymes involved in inflammation, the breakdown of bone and cartilage, and vascular spasm[12-20]. They block the release of histamine, reduce inflammation, strengthen

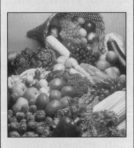

Wash, but don't throw away the skin

The highest concentration of flavonoids is found in the leaves, skin, peel or seeds of fruits and vegetables – which are mostly discarded in processing.

Flavonoids are part of the plant's own defence mechanism

Another reason for the high concentrations of flavonoids in the plant's outer parts is that many of these versatile compounds are brightly coloured, and are used by the plant to attract insects or birds for pollination and seed dispersal.

capillaries and slow the leakage of antibodies into the blood stream[103-106, 169, 170]. And finally, some flavonoids are thought to increase levels of anti-oxidant enzymes like SOD (Super-Oxide Dismutase)[188, 189].

The overall effect is anti-inflammatory – so you'd expect flavonoids to alleviate allergy symptoms and chronic inflammatory diseases such as arthritis, asthma, coronary artery disease and Alzheimer's. And there's a growing body of evidence that flavonoids do indeed have an important contribution to make in these areas.

STONE AGE FLAVONOID CONSUMPTION

During the period when homo sapiens evolved, our diet contained large amounts of flavonoids. I believe that the decline in our flavonoid intake, particularly in the last 50 years, is linked to the current increase in degenerative and inflammatory illness.

Our immune systems appear to have become unbalanced and this may be because vital dietary checks and inhibitors, like flavonoids, have been reduced. This would result in an increase in inflammatory illnesses such as asthma, coronary artery disease and arthritis; and is likely to be one of the main reasons why vegetarians live longer than omnivores[21, 215].

How the plant magic works

The key to the role of flavonoids is that many of them are extremely potent anti-oxidants[119] and anti-flammatory agents[12-20].

Different flavonoids work in different tissues of the body; some can enter the brain, for instance, whereas others appear to concentrate in the lining of blood vessels. This means that different flavonoids can be used to target different tissues[23-31]. For example, a flavonoid which is taken up by the lining of capillaries might be expected to be good for capillary function – and the ginkgo flavonoids, widely used to improve blood flow to the brain, hands and feet, do just this.

Many flavonoids neutralise free radicals, including the highly dangerous hydroxyl radical[37, 38]. One group is particularly good at quenching the radicals which cause liver damage[23] (these are the flavonoids found in milk thistle).

Genetic protectors

The flavonoids concentrated in the pips and seeds provide protection for the plant's precious genetic material.

Powerful blenders are now available which can liquidise fruit and vegetables, pips and all. Drunk immediately, this is a great way to give yourself a good dose of anti-oxidants, flavonoids and fibre!

Four types

There are four types of flavonoid anti-oxidant:

- **Type 1a – neutralise free radicals**[23,32-38,57]

- **Type 1b 'chain-breakers' – stop the cascade of lipid (fat) peroxidation**[39-43]

- **Type 2 – bind and neutralise free iron**[41, 44-46] **and copper**

- **Type 3 – neutralise free oxygen**[46, 47]

THE DEFENCE BOOSTERS : **Flavonoids & isoflavones**

Some flavonoids bind to dangerous free iron and copper in the body, thereby stopping free radical formation[41, 44-46]. Many are capable of locking up free oxygen[46, 47] and preventing the oxidation of ascorbic acid, thereby protecting Vitamin C in fruit, fruit juices, and in the body.

Quercitin

One flavonoid, quercitin, found in onions and apples may be one of the most cardio-protective substances yet discovered[48, 49, 224, 227]. The Zutphen Elderly Study[3] measured the flavonoid content of the diet of their subjects and discovered that the number of cardiac deaths in the group eating the most flavonoids was a quarter of the death rate in the group which ate the least flavonoids. And quercitin accounted for two-thirds of the total flavonoid intake.

In fact, all mortality rates were lower in the high flavonoid group, even when other dietary anti-oxidants such as Vitamins C and E were ruled out.

Since Zutphen, two more trials have found that quercitin (a powerful anti-oxidant and anti-inflammatory agent[48, 49, 224]) is cardio-protective[225-226].

There was some controversy over whether quercitin is absorbed from the gut, because little is found in the bloodstream[50]. Recent work shows that quercitin and related compounds are absorbed[223, 234, 235, 245, 246] and concentrated[193-205] elsewhere in the body[51, 83].

There's other evidence that flavonoids are absorbed. Tannins, for example, which consist of long chains of flavonoids linked together, protect against stroke in hypertensive animals[65]. Tannins are found in, eg tea, wine, quince and persimmons.

Or try eating a good helping of beetroot. The purple pigment in beets consists of flavonoids which, when eaten, are absorbed from the gut and excreted in the urine – a colourful fact you can check for yourself![210] Combine beets with rhubarb or spinach at the same meal to get the most spectacular results[247].

Procyanidins

Procyanidins are an extremely promising group of flavonoids. They are well absorbed from the gut[55, 264], and are already used (in the form of pycnogenol and grapeseed extracts) to treat arthritic conditions, because of their ability to quench free radicals and stop the breakdown of synovial (lubricating) fluid inside inflamed joints.

These flavonoids also target blood vessels and, once there, protect the connective tissue in the artery walls by exerting a powerful anti-oxidant, anti-inflammatory and anti-permeability effect. They also block enzymes which have a destructive effect on the connective tissues (see Chapter 14, Heart disease)[58, 59, 74-76].

These protective actions mean the high procyanidin content of black grapes (and red wine) is probably one of the main factors underlying the so-called French paradox. The French eat a high fat diet, yet are relatively immune from heart disease[60]. There are probably several factors involved, including the widespread use of olive oil, but there is evidence that consumption of two to four glasses of red wine a day reduces the risk of a heart attack by an astonishing 40 per cent[107, 176-180].

Hawthorn and yarrow plants, both exceptionally rich in procyanidins, have long been used to treat angina and circulatory problems[24-26, 61]. Hawthorn is reported to alleviate the pains of angina within a month or two of treatment which, if due to 'defurring' of the arteries, is breathtakingly fast. I know of serial angiograms, taken in a South African hospital, which apparently demonstrate that atheroma can indeed be made to shrink within a period of months[111, 112]. The fact that hawthorn also strengthens the heart beat[228], which would tend to make angina worse, supports the anti-atheroma claims – see Chapter 14, Heart disease.

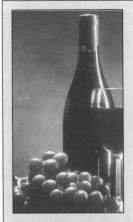

2-4 glasses of red wine a day may reduce heart attacks by 40 per cent – (see the Wine List on page 234).

Angina?

Try a hawthorn or yarrow supplement. These have been reported to alleviate pain in 1-2 months.

RED WINE

Moderate amounts of alcohol reduce blood platelet stickiness[108, 181]. In addition, flavonoids in red wine and in grape juice are powerful and specific inhibitors of platelet clotting[182-185, 212].

Red wine (but not white wine) produces a significant rise in the anti-oxidant capacity of the blood plasma[114, 187], lasting for up to four hours. This is related to its ability to stop LDL cholesterol being oxidised[109, 110]. In addition, red wine (but not white wine) is reported to increase levels of the 'good' HDL cholesterol[187] – and its valuable protective enzyme, paraoxonase.

Flavonoids used in medicine in Europe

- **Grape and wine extracts, which contain procyanidins, are being used to treat circulatory disorders, ulcers, dental caries, and to provide radiation protection**

- **Pycnogenol (also contains procyanidins) is used to treat varicose veins, diabetic retinopathy and heart disease**

- **Bilberry extracts are used in ophthalmology, and circulatory diseases**

- **Milk thistle extracts are given to aid liver function**

- **Cerebral vascular problems are widely treated with ginkgo**

cont. opposite

Using flavonoids to treat illness

Heart attacks

Anyone seriously concerned about reducing their risk of heart attacks should consider combining quercitin with a procyanidin product, eg grapeseed extract.

The two types of flavonoid, though similar, appear to block two distinct steps in the chain of events that leads to atheroma formation. Quercitin's main role is to protect lipids in the blood from oxidising; whereas the procyanidin's main role is to prevent oxidative damage from occurring in the blood vessel wall.

The procyanidins' ability to bind to and protect the fibres in the vessel walls (like collagen and elastin) from oxidative or enzyme attack helps to reduce the amount of damage to the walls. If there is already damage, the two flavonoids seem to stop the site becoming inflamed and slow the furring of the arteries[115- 118, 62-64, 216-222] (see Chapter 14, Heart disease).

Procyanidins are best used preventatively, but even after a heart attack they can help. Their phenomenal ability to scavenge free radicals means that a procyanidin product will reduce your risk of developing a life-threatening arrhythmia after the attack[113].

Drink to your health

I can heartily recommend a procyanidin flavonoid supplement like grapeseed or bilberry extract to most people, because although these compounds are very safe[96-98], and occur in many fruits and vegetables, we do not eat enough of them.

This is because they are mostly found in the rind, pips and seeds that we generally discard. Grape seeds, an excellent source of these compounds, are usually spat out or pass through the body. Quince, another rich source, is too astringent to eat uncooked and cooking destroys most of the procyanidins.

The only significant source of these compounds in most people's diet is red wine, which not only explains the French Paradox but also the fact that alcoholics who favour red wine tend to outlive those who drink beer or spirits[56].

Red wine, it seems, contains enough of these flavonoids to protect against some of the free radical damage that causes the cirrhosis and pancreatitis which kill many alcoholics [190-192].

A recent report in the British Medical Journal confirmed all my ideas about the health benefits of flavonoids. This trial showed that the more wine you drink, the lower your risk of death, not just from coronary artery disease but from all causes of death, including cancer[176, 179].

Danish scientists found that spirit drinkers were more likely to die than teetotallers, and beer drinkers as likely to die as non-drinkers, but in those who drank three to five glasses of wine each day, the risk of death from all causes was reduced by an amazing 52 per cent[176, 179].

This pattern had already been hinted at by others[107, 177, 178]; and is supported by the fact that, although alcohol consumption is stable in Denmark, a recent shift from beer and spirits to wine drinking has coincided with a fairly dramatic fall in deaths due to coronary artery disease[179, 180].

Although alcohol itself has some cardio-protective effects[181], it is the procyanidin flavonoids in wine that do most of the good[186], and these are predominantly found in red wine rather than white wine. If the Danes had looked at the health benefits of red wine in particular, they would have probably found even greater health benefits[182-184, 212].

Grape juice has some beneficial (ie anti-clotting) effects[185] but it's prepared aerobically (ie: it's exposed to the air during production), so some of the valuable flavonoid content is lost. Wine, on the other hand, is prepared anaerobically, (ie: in sealed containers where oxygen reactions don't take place) – and so the procyanidins are preserved.

As recently as 25 years ago, the medical establishment's view was that the flavonoids had no place in clinical medicine[174]. A quarter of a century is a long time in medicine. We can now see that this versatile group of plant compounds offers simple solutions to many of the major health problems of our time.

cont. from previous page

- **Hawthorn is particularly valuable in treating coronary artery disease and heart failure**

  Its flavonoids help to reduce atheroma[111,112]. They are also unique in increasing the strength of the heart muscle while decreasing the risk of arrhythmias[228,229]

  They also lower blood pressure by blocking Angiotensin Converting Enzyme, which is another strongly cardiac-protective factor[230]

What's in a name?

Procyanidins have several other names, including anthocyanidins, procyanidolic oligomers (PCOs), oligomeric procyanidins (OPCs), and pycnogenols.

Anti-cancer effect

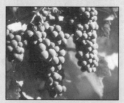

Red wine contains resveratrol, a flavonoid which raises levels of the 'good' HDL cholesterol and reduces platelet stickiness[182-184, 243].

Resveratrol also has a wide range of anti-cancer properties[233, 250], as does catechin, another red wine flavonoid.

The combination of the two, given in a red wine extract, increased life-span in cancer-prone mice by 50 percent or more[234].

But avoid too much alcohol!

Even with red wine, there's a point at which the flavonoid benefits are outweighed by the dangers of high alcohol intake.

The official (Dept. of Health) guidelines are 21 units (glasses) a week for men and 14 for women. If you want to take higher doses of flavonoids, switch to supplements.

WINE AND RADIATION

Procyanidins have been shown to protect animals from radiation, because they neutralise the free radicals formed by the radiation[71].

This strongly suggests that they could be used to protect against damage during radiotherapy. I recommend a half bottle of good red wine to anyone about to entrust themselves to the tender mercies of their local Radiology Department, combined with Vitamin E and GLA[72], together with C and Co-enzyme Q10.

This is no joke – Chernobyl victims were advised to drink Crimean red wine, which is known to have a very high procyanidin content[54]. Russian scientists are well aware of the radio-protective effects of procyanidins – their astronauts are routinely given an extract of green tea.

Other micro-nutrients also have radio-protective effects, including lycopene, a flavonoid found in tomatoes, which has been shown to reduce mouse mortality after radiation by an amazing 50 per cent[73].

Vascular problems

Because of the ability of procyanidins to keep blood vessels healthy, it's not surprising that reports have appeared describing improvements in varicose veins, oedema and haemorrhoids[78-80].

Anyone suffering from any of these should try a procyanidin product for at least two months, although in some cases improvement is noticeable in one month. Vitamin C should be taken with it, and in serious cases an additional glucosamine supplement (see Chapter 10, Amino sugars) is advisable.

Alternative sources of flavonoids which help blood vessels include ginkgo and horse chestnut seed extract. This was traditionally used in Germany to treat chronic venous problems and recently shown to be as effective as, or more effective than, wearing compression stockings[206-209].

Diabetes

In diabetes, the capillaries become especially fragile, and micro-bleeds in the capillaries supplying the retina are a common cause of blindness.

Pycnogenol, an extract from the bark of maritime pine consisting mainly of procyanidins, has been used for many years in France to prevent diabetic blindness. Studies show that it is safe[96-98] and it can be remarkably effective in stabilising and improving vision in diabetic patients[81, 82]. As above, Vitamin C and a glucosamine supplement are also recommended.

Another important cause of sight loss in diabetics is the growth of new blood vessels supplying the retina. The procyanidins block this effect, another reason why they are helpful in this condition.

Other flavonoids can help diabetics too. The cholesterol in the blood is more prone to oxidation than in non-diabetics[232], which is one reason why diabetics suffer more heart attacks. In a recent study, a flavonoid preparation (Diosmin) not only reduced the rate of cholesterol and lipid oxidation but also reduced the rate that proteins were damaged (cross-linked) by the excess blood sugar[175]. This would not only reduce blood vessel damage in the eye and elsewhere in the body, but also protect against cataracts and renal damage, where excess cross-linking is involved.

Skin care

Procyanidins are being incorporated into the latest cosmetics[55]. They form a protective shield around the collagen and elastin fibres which give skin its firmness and texture, and protect them against the enzymes which break down these fibres, and against free radical damage too[58, 59, 74-76].

It's early days, but procyanidin's anti-allergic, anti-inflammatory and anti-oxidant properties could constitute a major cosmetic break-through; especially when combined with other anti-ageing nutrients such as the amino sugars (see Chapter 18, Skin).

Dental care

Procyanidins target the bacteria which cause dental decay. The flavonoids seem to stop the bugs sticking to the teeth and to dental plaque. Some dental scientists are looking at these flavonoids as a way of slowing down tooth decay[212]. The anti-inflammatory effects may also help to control or minimise gingivitis (gum disease) which is responsible for more tooth loss than dental decay.

LOOK FOR ...

a supplement that includes a procyanidin complex, eg grapeseed or bilberry extract at a level of at least 100mg a day.

Citrus flavonoids have a role to play, but may not be as powerful as the procyanidins.

For treatment purposes, this procyanidin dose increases to 1000mg a day.

INCLUDE ...

Lots of fruit and vegetables with a high flavonoid content in your diet, ie prunes, dark cherries, blueberries, raisins and currants.

Prunes have one of the highest ORAC ratings of all, ie they have a proven capacity to absorb large numbers of damaging free radicals.

Athletic Injury

Whether it's a sprain, strain or muscle tear, an athletic injury is accompanied by inflammation. The procyanidins are particularly helpful here because of their profound anti-inflammatory actions. They inhibit many of the destructive enzymes involved in the inflammatory process[58, 59, 74-76]; and also inhibit the release of histamine and other important inflammatory mediators[77].

Athletes who wish to minimise the impact of any injury would be well advised to take a preventative dose of procyanidins, combined with a good amino sugar preparation (see Chapter 10, Amino sugars).

Osteoporosis

At least one flavonoid derivative, ipriflavone, has been shown to reverse the process of osteoporosis, and rebuild old bones (see Chapter 15, Bones).

The flavonoid-cancer story

Vegetarians live longer. They have less cancer and fewer heart attacks too[83, 84]. But you don't need to go the whole hog, because omnivores who eat above average amounts of fruit and vegetables can cut their risk of most cancers by 50 or even 75 per cent[85, 248].

We already know that Vitamins A, C, E and carotenoids, which are only found in fruit and vegetables, have anti-cancer properties, but the flavonoids may be even more promising.

Flavonoids boast an extensive array of anti-cancer effects which add up to an extremely impressive cancer defence package:

- Free radicals damage DNA. Many flavonoids are potent anti-oxidants which mop up large numbers of free radicals, and reduce the amount of DNA 'hits'. Free radicals also damage cell membranes. This damage might also lead to tumour formation, so once again anti-oxidants, like flavonoids, should help.

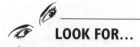

LOOK FOR...

Green tea extract in a supplement.

This polyphenol complex has good all-round protective power.

Tumours and flavonoids

Tumours can only grow if they can stimulate the growth of a new blood supply[156-168]. The flavonoids can block tumour growth by preventing the growth of new blood vessels[144-150].

- Some flavonoids bind to the histones around DNA, forming a shield around it[89].
- 'Free' iron atoms in the body can generate large amounts of free radicals. Various flavonoids bind to iron, and make it inert[41, 44-46].
- Flavonoids bind to some carcinogens very avidly, and neutralise them[87, 88]
- Many chemical carcinogens in the diet (or inhaled in cigarette and other smoke) are neutralised by enzymes which make them soluble so they can be excreted from the body.

  Some flavonoids stimulate the body to make more of these enzymes, with the result that some carcinogens are more rapidly detoxified, and excreted more efficiently[90, 242].
- Conversely, flavonoids reduce the activity of other enzymes which can make carcinogens more dangerous[90,242]
- Various flavonoids can boost the immune system. They enhance the action of the natural killer cells, and boost the body's own anti-cancer substances, interferon and interleukin-2[95].
- Flavonoids can block the start of tumour growth[91-93, 124]. Once a cancer has started, they can inhibit the invasiveness of cancer cells[94], and prevent the ingrowth of new blood vessels[236-240].
- Flavonoids can also force cancer cells to commit 'suicide'[250, 271].

These effects help to explain the up to four-fold reduction in cancer associated with higher consumption of fruit and vegetables mentioned earlier. It also helps explain the 20-fold difference in the risk of certain cancers between different countries.

If we knew exactly which fruits and which vegetables contained which flavonoids, and how best to combine them, it should be possible to cut the risk of many cancers by up to 90 per cent, perhaps even more.

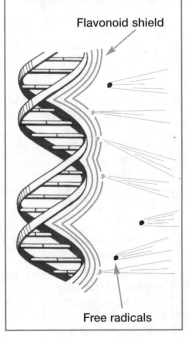

Flavonoid Shield

The DNA in your body cells is constantly under attack from free radicals.

Some flavonoids have an affinity for DNA and act as a protective shield against this attack, lowering the risk of damaging DNA and therefore cancer.

Flavonoid shield

Free radicals

Pycnogenol

Pycnogenol, an extract of pine bark rich in flavonoid compounds known as procyanidins, is used by many nutritional therapists.

Pycnogenol combines wide-spectrum efficacy with an excellent safety record[96-98], as does quercitin[58,59, 74-76, 121-123].

Not surprisingly, a great deal of nutritional research is concentrating on just this area. Some of the most active and best researched compounds include:

> quercitin – onions
>
> ellagic acid – walnuts, pecan nuts
>
> caffeic acid – coffee beans
>
> chlorogenic acid – tomatoes
>
> epigallocatechingallate – tea
>
> carnosic acid – rosemary
>
> genistein – soy

This is by no means an exhaustive list, but all of these have been shown to possess anti-cancer effects in cell culture and animal experiments. So a diet rich in all the above would make an excellent basis for a cancer-free lifestyle.

It should also include turmeric, which contains curcumin. Curcumin has extensive anti-mutagenic[126, 130], anti-carcinogenic[127], and anti-tumour powers[128, 130].

Curcumin also has an important role in any anti-arthritis nutritional plan – and it should be considered as an ingredient in any supplement that aims to protect joints.

Garlic should be on the menu too; the garlic compound diallyl sulphide has anti-cancer effects[129] (for more about anti-cancer diets, see Chapter 13, Cancer).

Beyond chemotherapy

The flavonoids have one final anti-cancer property that may be the most significant of all: their ability to slow cell migration. Inhibiting the movement of cells not only reduces tumour growth, but it also reduces the risk of metastasis – the spread of cancer to other parts of the body.

It forms the basis of a completely new approach to cancer that is certainly kinder, and probably more effective than anything we have seen before. The biotechnology industry is pumping millions of dollars into this area, but the nutritionists got there first – and so can you.

INCLUDE ...

Try to eat onions and cooked or processed tomatoes frequently and drink two cups of tea (preferably green) a day.

A couple of flavonoid-rich dishes would be tomato and onion pizza sprinkled with rosemary, or leek and potato soup, flavoured with black pepper and thyme, or mixed dark fruits.

For more enriched recipes, the *Health Defence Cook Book* is being planned.

How cancer spreads and how flavonoids can protect you.

1 The reason why our bodies keep their shape is that the cells in our organs and tissues are held together by a dense network of collagen, elastin and other fibres.

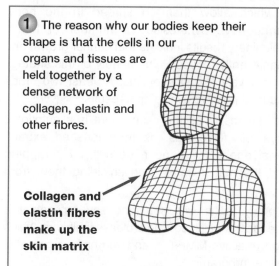

Collagen and elastin fibres make up the skin matrix

These fibres form a tough matrix outside the cells which prevents most cells from moving around too much. This "extra-cellular" matrix can be visualised as rather like netting.

2 Cancer cells secrete a comprehensive range of enzymes which they use to dissolve the matrix as they multiply and spread.

These enzymes are called the **M**atrix **M**etallo**p**roteases, or MMPs.

MMPs are so destructive that cancer cells cannot produce them internally, or they would blow themselves apart!

Instead they secrete MMP precursors which have a built-in 'safety catch'. When these precursors are safely out of the cell, a group of secondary enzymes strips away the safety catch and activates the MMPs.

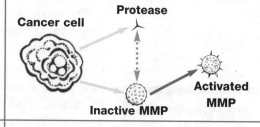

Cancer cell **Protease** **Inactive MMP** **Activated MMP**

3 The MMP enzymes begin to eat holes in the matrix to allow the cancer cells to spread[131-136, 151, 152].

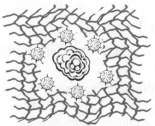

MMPs are crucial to cancer growth and spread; the more MMPs a cancer cell produces, the more malignant it becomes[133, 137-143].

4 Procyanidin flavonoids (eg bilberry or grapeseed extract) shield the matrix fibres and protect against MMPs[58, 59, 74-76,94].

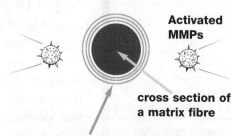

Activated MMPs

cross section of a matrix fibre

Procyanidin flavonoids wrapped around and protecting the matrix fibre

Refer to page 213 for a six step Defensive Plan against Cancer.

Cancer cells secrete enzymes commonly known as MMPs (see page 93) which allow them to spread in the body. Biotechnology firms have synthesised a number of MMP-inhibitors, and preliminary results indicate that cancer growth and spread can be significantly reduced. The beauty of this strategy is that there are relatively few side effects. At least two drugs have already produced positive clinical trial results[154, 155].

But as so often seems to be the case, there is a nutritional equivalent. Procyanidin flavonoids, as in grapeseed extract, reduce the invasiveness of cancer cells[94] by wrapping themselves round the matrix fibres, and shielding them from MMPs[58, 59, 74-76].

Combine the procyanidins with soy (and soy nutrients like genistein) and other beans which contain protease inhibitors, which block the formation of active MMPs[125], and you have a powerful nutritional anti-cancer programme.

The illustrations on page 93 show how cancer cells attack the structure of body tissue – and how flavonoids can create a protective shield.

A combination of beans and peas, together with procyanidin flavonoids, should give significant protection against the spread of cancer. For maximum effect they should be taken with genistein and lycopene (and possibly shark cartilage), both of which appear to inhibit cancer in other, complementary ways (see Chapter 13, Cancer).

Soy – protein without the fat

According to popular belief, animal proteins are complete while plant proteins are incomplete.

This is one reason why Western governments put so much stress on animal protein production, and it is also one of the reasons why we suffer from so much heart disease, cancer and osteoporosis.

Sadly, the whole nutritional (and environmental) disaster is based on a mistake. The useful protein content of foods is not simply a question of quantity, but also digestibility. The most up-to-date method of assessing this is the Protein Digestibility Corrected Amino Acid Score (PDCAAS), as used by the World Health Organisation[251]. On this scale, soy scores 1, the highest rating possible – the same as animal proteins and better than any other plant food[252, 288-290].

Soy's oil content is also interesting. There is very little saturated fat, and no cholesterol. About eight per cent of soy oil is linolenic acid[253], one of the Omega 3 fatty acids otherwise found in fish. This suggests that soy oil may help to reduce the risk of heart disease if taken with vitamin supplements (see page 127).

But soy can do so much more for our health.

Soy and cancer

About one in 11 British women will develop breast cancer at some time in their lives. In Japan, the figure is as low as 1 in 65. The cancer detectives, the epidemiologists, have studied the problem intensively[268]. And many believe two dietary factors play a crucial role – selenium and soy.

The Japanese diet contains more of the anti-oxidant mineral selenium than the typical Western one does, and that's thought to protect against breast cancer. There is evidence that a high intake of soy products might also be protective.

A wealth of new research has revealed that soy beans not only have an unequalled nutritional profile, they are also the most important single source of dietary anti-carcinogens.

At a 1989 National Cancer Institute meeting in Washington, a panel of international experts identified no fewer than six families of anti-cancer compounds in soy beans[254]. Each one of these appears to be able to reduce the risk of cancer on its own. In combination, their synergistic anti-cancer effects[255] are likely to be considerable. This unusual combination of anti-cancer nutrients undoubtedly helps to account for the very low rate of many cancers in countries where soy is widely eaten.

Oddly enough, some of the anti-cancer nutrients have been known for many years. But because they inhibit certain metabolic processes, they were labelled anti-nutrients, or low-grade toxins.

> **The anti-cancer food**
>
> No less than six anti-cancer compounds have been found in soy beans – and where soy is widely eaten, many cancers are rarer.
>
> Selenium and soy appear to be two factors which give Japan a far lower rate of breast cancer than the UK.

Now it appears that these anti-nutrients may be soy's crowning glory.

Here are the six anti-cancer elements in soy beans.

- **Protease inhibitors (lectins)** – which block genes which promote cancer

Soy beans contain growth-inhibiting substances called protease inhibitors, which act to reduce the spread of cancer (see Chapter 13, Cancer).

Recent work has demonstrated that protease inhibitors also block the action of a number of genes which cause cancer. Most protease inhibitors are destroyed by cooking, but there is evidence that enough survive to confer a significant protective effect[262, 277, 302-304].

- **Phytate** – can act as an anti-oxidant

The second anti-cancer ingredient is phytate, generally regarded as another anti-nutrient because it binds iron. But in certain conditions this is a good thing, as excess (free) iron in the body is a potent source of free radicals, and a potential carcinogen.

When phytate binds iron, it is effectively acting as an anti-oxidant. This helps to explain why phytate is a powerful inhibitor of colon cancer[263], where free iron is one of the key causative factors. (I don't recommend phytate for everyone, however. Iron deficiency anaemia is still widespread, particularly among women of child-bearing age, and too much phytate could worsen an existing anaemia.)

- **Phytosterols** – protect against carcinogenic bile acids

Third up are the phytosterols, the plant equivalents of cholesterol. They are poorly absorbed and remain in the gut, where they are thought to protect against the harmful effects of certain (secondary) bile acids. These bile acids are formed from cholesterol and have mutagenic and carcinogenic properties. This may be why some phytosterols are capable of reducing the incidence of colon cancer by as much as 50 per cent.[264]

Experimental evidence that soy inhibits cancer

Lab experiments have shown that soy's protease inhibitors reduce the incidence of cancer in the breast, skin and bladder[256], and in the colon[257], lung[258], pancreas[259], mouth[260] and oesophagus[261].

Full of beans

Increase your intake of both legumes (beans) and soy bean products.

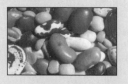

They appear not only to protect against cancer, but also help slow its spread[268].

- **Saponins** – anti-mutation, anti-oxidants

Fourth on the list are the saponins, anti-oxidants[265] which protect against free radical damage. Lab tests have shown that saponins prevent mutations that can lead to cancer[266].

- **Phenolic compounds** – protect DNA

Fifth are a group of phenolic compounds. These too possess anti-oxidant activity, and are thought to protect DNA from attack by certain categories of carcinogen[267].

Isoflavones – most potent of all

The above is an impressive array of anti-carcinogens, but I have left the sixth and best till last. Soy beans are extremely rich in a sub-group of the phenolics known as isoflavones, and these are among the most potent anti-carcinogens of all.

Isoflavones block oestrogen, a hormone linked to an increased risk of breast and other hormone-dependent cancers. They act rather like Tamoxifen, a drug widely used to treat and prevent breast cancer.

When small amounts of soy are fed to animals, their rate of breast cancer falls by nearly 50 per cent[269], as does the incidence of prostate cancer[270]. In this last case, the isoflavones appear to be acting as testosterone blockers; not altogether surprising, as the molecules of oestrogen and testosterone are very similar.

Men who think that soy is just for women should think again; considering the high rate of prostate cancer in the West, it seems that men have just as much to gain from adding soy to their diet.

Prostate cancer, like breast cancer, is usually hormone-dependent. But whereas breast cancer is encouraged by oestrogen, prostate cancer is often driven by testosterone. Isoflavones which block testosterone reduce the tendency for prostate cancers to grow. (See also Lycopene in Chapter 13, Cancer.)

Bad genes

There are known genetic risk factors for breast and prostate cancer. But they are not nearly common enough to account for the epidemic of both these diseases.

International evidence

In soy-eating countries like Korea, the rate of breast cancer is between a sixth and a tenth of the rate in the West. The rate of prostate cancer is about 1/15th[268].

In the developed Western nations, where the rate of cancer has risen 10 per cent in the last decade, soy is still a relatively minor item in the diet.

A key anti-cancer ingredient

An isoflavone called genistein not only inhibits cancer cells – it can force them to turn back into normal cells [271-273].

LOOK FOR ...

a supplement that includes genistein (and other isoflavones).

40mg of a genistein/daidzein/ glycitin combination would be my recommendation.

It gets you to approximately the daily isoflavone intake of the Koreans – where the rate of breast and prostrate cancer is far lower than in the UK.

Prostate Cancer

Japanese men have just as many prostate cancers in situ (small and localised) as do American men – but they have fewer cases of clinical cancer. If they emigrate and switch to an American diet their prostate cancers rapidly emerge.

This is probably because they are no longer being held in check by the protective elements in the Japanese diet, such as the anti-cancer compounds in soy.

REDUCING BREAST CANCER

Because of their ability to mimic and block the effects of oestrogen, isoflavones are often called phyto-estrogens. A major risk factor for breast cancer is thought to be the amount of oestrogen a woman is exposed to over her lifetime, which is related to the number of menstrual cycles she has experienced.

Anything that reduces the number of cycles, such as late start of menstruation, early menopause or multiple pregnancies, lowers the risk of breast cancer. The phyto-estrogens in soy slow down the menstrual cycle, lengthening it by up to six days, and so reduce the total number of cycles.

Amazing genistein

King of the isoflavones, and subject of well over 300 research papers to date, is genistein. Genistein has little effect on normal cells – but it is a powerful inhibitor of nearly every cancer cell type examined so far[271].

Its anti-cancer effects are wide because its mode of action is so profound: it inhibits several of the products of oncogenes, genes which cause cancer[272].

But genistein doesn't just inhibit and kill cancer cells. Remarkably, it also causes cancer cells to revert to normal cells[273]. This is an absolutely crucial anti-cancer property, and a very unusual one: called 'redifferentiation'.

If that were all that genistein did, it would be a miracle in itself. But genistein has another amazing trick up its sleeve. It inhibits the growth of new blood vessels, as shark cartilage extract does[274] and should therefore be able to starve cancers even after they have begun to grow (see also Chapter 13, Cancer).

CHOKING OFF CANCER

Growing cancers are dependent on new blood vessels to supply oxygen and nutrients and take away waste products. New blood vessels are fragile, break down and need to be constantly replaced. Any substance that prevents the growth of new blood vessels should theoretically leave a tumour without a blood supply, choking it to death.

This is a relatively new area of research, but there is good evidence from various trials that angiostats, as they are called, can work. The only side effect is some interruption of the menstrual cycle, which is quite logical when you think what angiostats do.

Soy and the heart

Soy protects against heart disease as well.

One of the most insidious aspects of coronary artery disease (CAD) is that it is a hidden disease. For most people, the first sign that anything is wrong is the first heart attack. The great majority of survivors are left with a permanently damaged heart and a long-term risk of complications.

Even advanced cases of CAD are often not diagnosed in time. An American investigation called the Sudden Death Study, discovered that an astonishing one in four people who died suddenly of a heart attack had seen their doctor in the week before they died. But they had not been diagnosed accurately, and had not been hospitalised[284].

This is why with coronary artery disease, as in so many other diseases, prevention is better than cure.

Diet is the key. A diet rich in animal fats and low in anti-oxidants and fish oil is a fast route to a heart attack, as is smoking. And so is high blood cholesterol.

Most of us have a cholesterol level that is higher than 'normal'. According to Drs Brown and Goldstein, who won a Nobel Prize for their work on cholesterol, the normal level is between 100 and 150 mg/dl[276]. This is the level found in people who eat a low fat, high fibre diet, and who have a low risk of heart disease.

But there is more than one form of cholesterol. LDL cholesterol is potentially harmful, as it is the form of cholesterol which is released by the liver, and distributed to all the cells in the body, including the cells in the artery walls.

HDL cholesterol, on the other hand, is a good thing. HDL particles remove cholesterol from the body cells, and take it back to the liver. They remove cholesterol from artery walls, which is one reason why high levels of HDL are cardio-protective.

This is where we come back to soy. Soy should be a part of any cardio-protective diet, because it reduces cholesterol absorption from the gut, and increases cholesterol excretion[299-301]. The overall effect is a lowering of LDL cholesterol by up to 30 per cent, and a simultaneous increase in HDL cholesterol by up to 15 per cent[280, 291-298].

WARNING

Our arteries don't just start clogging in later years – in the West the earliest signs of atheroma have been found in young adults and even children, thanks to a diet high in animal fats and low in anti-oxidants and fish oil. However ...

In most Western countries, heart disease is the major killer, responsible for approximately 50 in every 100 deaths.

Coronary artery disease is insignificant in Crete, Iceland and Japan, even in the elderly.

In China, a mere six deaths in a hundred are caused by heart disease[275].

The difference is diet.

LDL cholesterol is not all bad

LDL cholesterol is essential for transporting lipid-soluble anti-oxidants in the bloodstream. It only becomes dangerous if there are insufficient anti-oxidants in the diet.

Soy's effect on the heart

Soy even helps in cases where blood cholesterol is way above normal. Italian doctors examined the cholesterol-lowering effects of soy in patients with hypercholesterolaemia – a genetic condition associated with extremely high blood levels of cholesterol and a very high risk of heart disease.

They found that adding soy to a low-fat diet dropped cholesterol levels by an impressive 26 per cent[282]. Because of these excellent results, the Italian National Health Service now provides soy in the form of textured vegetable protein free to all patients with hypercholesterolaemia.

Before we leave soy, we have to return once more to genistein. This compound, you'll remember, has a number of powerful anti-cancer effects. One of them, the ability to inhibit the growth of certain cell types, is also cardio-protective. As oxidised cholesterol begins to accumulate in the artery walls, and an atheroma forms, the artery responds by growing more smooth muscle cells in the affected areas.

As they grow, they contribute, along with the growing mass of cholesterol, to the gradual blocking of the vessel. Genistein blocks this smooth muscle response[283]. This presumably plays a role, together with the soy's cholesterol-lowering effect and anti-oxidant content, in reducing heart disease in those Far Eastern countries where soy is so widely eaten, and where coronary artery disease is so uncommon.

What should you drink with soy? We've already covered red wine, so I'll briefly review the benefits of tea – with, believe it or not, chocolate for dessert.

More tea, vicar?

Although some health food pundits say tea isn't such a good idea, they're wrong[311, 312].

The cup that cheers is a rich source of flavonoid anti-oxidants. Green tea contains up to 30 per cent by weight of flavonoids, and black tea is nearly as good.

How much soy?

Adding soy to the diet has cut levels of those with ultra-high cholesterol by a quarter. And the good news is you don't have to eat soy at every meal to achieve the desired effect.

A mere 50gm of soy protein (approximately one 2 oz serving) daily will do the trick[281].

Or eat a 4 oz serving every two days.

Textured vegetable protein (soy) is a good source for cholesterol lowering. However, this form of soy has no anti-cancer properties.

Quorn has similar cholesterol-lowering effects[285-287].

More HDL benefits

HDL has anti-oxidant properties, and can protect the 'bad' LDL cholesterol from oxidation – another reason to aim for high HDL cholesterol levels.

The most important flavonoids in tea are a group of extremely potent anti-oxidants based on the catechin molecule; catechin itself, epicatechin, epigallocatechin, and epigallocatechingallate (EGCG)[313].

EGCG is among the best of this lot and Nestlé researchers have already developed methods of increasing and standardising levels of EGCG in a new range of teas, which may be launched as the first products in what could eventually be a whole range of 'functional foods'[314, 315].

Where will tea be in this brave new world of functional foods? It's early days, but there is increasing experimental evidence that tea (especially green tea) may have a role in preventing some cancers, especially skin, gastric and bladder cancer[316-318, 325].

Japan has a far higher rate of gastric cancer than the UK, probably due to their high intake of pickled foods, but there is one area, Shizuoka, where gastric cancer is rare. The inhabitants of Shizuoka are famous for their tea drinking, and this is thought to be the key protective dietary factor.

Cardiologists have discovered that EGCG in tea has other beneficial effects, including lowering blood cholesterol[319, 320], and possibly reducing blood pressure[324], and the tendency for platelets to form clots. This suggests that tea may reduce the risk of coronary artery disease, and heart attacks.

Intriguingly, chocolate contains flavonoids (known as 'cocoa red') which are similar to those found in red wine[334, 335] and is also therefore likely to be cardio-protective[331, 332, 336].

More tea, dentist?

There is evidence that tea may help prevent tooth decay!

Tea leaves are a good source of fluoride and one British study went so far as to suggest that heavy tea drinking would supply enough fluoride to reduce the risk of dental decay in children[321] if you could get them to drink it ...

The flavonoids in tea appear to amplify the protective effects of fluoride[322], and reduce the build-up of plaque[323].

The Japanese already use green-tea-enhanced toothpaste and chewing gum to fight dental decay.

Choco-holics rejoice!

A survey published in 1998 found that chocolate eaters, like wine drinkers, lived longer[336]. This is almost certainly because dark chocolate, with a high cocoa solid content, like wine, is an excellent source of flavonoids[335].

THE BRITISH PARADOX

Tea has only a third of red wine's anti-oxidant capacity, but because its anti-oxidant molecules are smaller than those in red wine, they are more quickly absorbed and cause a larger increase in plasma anti-oxidant levels than does wine.

The good effects fade within an hour or so[120, 172, 173, 183], but both green and black tea are thought to protect against heart attacks[213, 214].

Do drink your tea black; milk neutralises the flavonoids[231], which may explain why there is no British paradox.

SUMMARY

Flavonoids

▶ Get more flavonoid-rich foods into your diet – prunes, strawberries, bilberries, apples, citrus fruits, raisins, raspberries, blackberries and particularly red and yellow onions and shallots; walnuts; pecan nuts and tomatoes.

▶ Switch from beer, spirits or white wine to red wine.

▶ An anti-cancer diet should include onions, walnuts, pecans, tomatoes, tea, coffee, rosemary, turmeric, and garlic. Also ...

▶ Increase your intake of legumes (beans) and soya bean products. They may not only protect against cancer, but also help slow its spread.

▶ The flavonoids in (dark) chocolate are also protective.

▶ Tea and especially green tea contains flavonoids called catechins that are cancer and cardio-protective.

▶ Consider flavonoid-rich supplements – especially grapeseed, bilberry, ginkgo, pycnogenol, yarrow, hawthorn or hazel.

Isoflavones

▶ Soy contains six of the most powerful anti-cancer ingredients that we know of.

▶ Most powerful of all is genistein – which you can now take as a supplement.

40-50mg a day gives you a level roughly equivalent to the daily intake in countries like Korea, where levels of breast and prostate cancer are a fraction of Western Europe.

▶ Soy products also have a role to play in preventing heart disease, because they can lower LDL cholesterol and increase HDL cholesterol.

- A new type of fibre will help protect against food poisoning, bowel problems, and colon and liver cancer

- This 'pre-biotic' fibre is found chiefly in vegetables like artichokes, leeks and onions

- Fruit and veg kept in storage for a long time – like some supermarket produce – lose their pre-biotic value

- Pre-biotics help 'good' bacteria in the gut to grow – crowding out disease-causing bugs

- Breast-fed babies have 95 per cent 'good' bacteria

- Older people have more bad bacteria – these can be reduced with pre-biotics

- If you're low on pre-biotics, you're vulnerable to all kinds of gastro-intestinal problems

- A daily bowl of onion soup can help colitis

- A healthy gut absorbs calcium better – reducing the risk of brittle bones

- A daily dose of pre-biotics could help reduce heart disease and tooth decay!

Chapter 7

Gut reactions – the power of fibre

Ever since Dr Kellogg launched his breakfast cereals, a daily intake of dietary fibre has been considered a good thing.

We know that it helps to prevent constipation, haemorrhoids, diverticulosis and varicose veins. We know, too, that some fibres can help to smooth out blood sugar levels in diabetes. And although the experts are still not in complete agreement, there is a reasonable amount of evidence that increasing the fibre in our diet will help to reduce the risk of heart disease, bowel cancer, and possibly even breast cancer.

But there is a problem with fibre which has caused a great deal of confusion and disagreement, among scientists as well as among the public. Until very recently, nobody could agree on what fibre actually was.

It's now generally agreed that there are at least six types of fibre – more according to some experts – which all have different properties, are handled differently in the body, and which all make a different contribution to our health. Some work within the gut; others have important effects elsewhere in the body.

I won't go into all the sub-types of fibre, as it gets rather complicated, but the main point is that, until recently, only two types were used in medicine. These are the insoluble fibres which occur in bran, for example, and which are used to treat constipation. Then there are the soluble fibres in gums such as guar gum, which are used to slow down the absorption of sugar from the gut in diabetics. Both these fibre types are hardly broken down in the gut at all, and pass through the body basically unchanged.

But the emphasis is now switching to another type of fibre that is broken down in the body. This may seem a strange concept, because you probably think of dietary fibre as being indigestible – and you'd be correct. These new fibres are resistant to our digestive enzymes, but they are broken down by enzymes produced by bacteria that live in the colon. These fibres are known as non-digestible oligosaccharides or pre-biotics[19, 47, 136].

A new kind of fibre

The large bowel, which is where the majority of gastrointestinal cancers occur, is full of four to five hundred different species of bacteria, known in medical language as 'flora'. Some of these can cause serious illness, while others are associated with positive health.

Ever since the beginning of this century, doctors have experimented with different diets in an attempt to modify the gastrointestinal flora, and push it in a 'healthy' direction (without much success).

There are at least two types of health-promoting bacteria, the lactobacilli and the bifidobacteria[6-11,42-44,82,83]. Some of these are found in live yoghurt, and various scientists and nutritionists have used yoghurt to try to change the flora of the lower bowel.

However, the bacteria have a limited shelf-life, even when freeze-dried, and many of them are unable to survive the acid conditions in the stomach. Even if the bacteria do arrive in the colon, they have to compete with the dense population of hostile bacteria that are already there.

Yoghurt

Eating live yoghurt can boost the number of 'good' bacteria in your gut for a while – but pre-biotics are more effective, and the effects last longer[65, 67].

The highest concentrations of pre-biotics are found in:

- **Chicory root**
- **Jerusalem artichoke**
- **Leeks**
- **Onions**
- **Salsify**
- **Wheat**
- **Bananas**
- **Oats**

As long as you eat a daily helping of live yoghurt, some lactobacilli and bifidobacteria remain in the gut, but they disappear almost immediately when the yoghurt diet stops[65].

Pre-biotics have none of these disadvantages. They are stable, safe (they are found in many staple foods), and they have a longer-lasting effect on the gut's flora[67]. They encourage the growth of 'healthy' bacteria, and put a check on other bacteria which can cause disease by overgrowth or by producing toxins[48].

We'll consider two of the main types of natural pre-biotic – inulin and oligo-fructose. The general rule is that the fresher the vegetable, the higher its inulin content. When plants such as onions are stored for long periods of time, and particularly in cold or cool storage, their pre-biotic content declines dramatically[1-3].

Because most of us buy our fruit and vegetables from supermarkets where the foods may have been in cold storage for months, this could mean that your pre-biotic intake is actually very low[116].

A low intake of pre-biotics leads to increased numbers of disease-causing bacteria in the gut – which could be the cause of many gastrointestinal and other health complaints[6-11, 42-44, 82, 83].

Safe

Pre-biotics are very safe. A bowl of French onion soup contains around 6-18g of the pre-biotic inulin. In the name of science, clinicians have injected themselves with ten times this dose of inulin, with no ill effects[81].

Vegetables stored for a long time are low in pre-biotics.

Antibiotics

Some antibiotics cause problems by killing too many of the gut bacteria.

The French remedy, live yoghurt, is relatively ineffective, but a pre-biotic can help return the gut flora to normal.

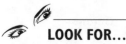

LOOK FOR...

A daily oligosaccharide supplement of about 6-10g.

There are now commercial sources which can be mixed with orange juice or sprinkled on cereal. It's sweetish and pleasant tasting.

WHAT ARE PRE-BIOTICS?

The two main pre-biotics are the non-digestible oligosaccharides (NDOs) inulin and oligofructose. These are the plant equivalent of fat – plants accumulate them when there is plenty of solar energy available, and use them as fuel when the skies are dark or overcast.

Inulin and oligo-fructose are both made up of chains of fructose (fruit sugar) molecules, and are similar to starch, a more familiar and digestible plant storage compound found in potatoes and cereals.

The richest plant sources of inulin and oligo-fructose are chicory root, which has a long history of medicinal use[4, 5], and Jerusalem artichoke. Then, in descending order, there are leeks, onions, salsify, wheat, bananas and other fruits, grains and vegetables.

Because inulin occurs in so many foodstuffs everyone eats some of it – probably around 1-4g in the USA, and 3-11g a day in Europe[3].

Another pre-biotic, beta glucan, is found in oats – and reduces (LDL) cholesterol levels.

How pre-biotics work

Unlike most sugars and starches, pre-biotics cannot be digested and they pass into the colon intact. Once there, they act as a growth enhancer for the health-promoting lactobacilli and bifidobacteria.

As the 'good' bacteria multiply, they secrete enzymes which break down pre-biotics into acids such as acetic and butyric acid. These inhibit the growth of disease-causing bacteria[31, 52, 53]. The 'good' bacteria also secrete antibiotic substances which restrain the 'unhealthy' bugs, including most of those responsible for food poisoning[10, 11, 18, 30, 54-56].

As a result, the balance of the flora of the gut tips in a healthy direction[10, 15-17, 32, 51, 57]. The flourishing lactobacilli and bifidobacteria in the gut join gastric acid, the digestive enzymes and the immune system in 'crowding' out disease-causing bacteria. You'll benefit from improved intestinal 'regularity'[66] and an increased resistance to food poisoning[62, 64].

> **Stress and stomach upsets**
>
> Stress causes a sharp fall in gastrointestinal secretions, and large changes in the colonic flora, including a dramatic reduction in the lactobacilli and bifidobacteria[139-140].
>
> Stress is also an immuno-suppressent; and these two factors explain why stressed individuals are more vulnerable to stomach upsets and food poisoning.

How pre-biotics tilt the balance in favour of 'good' bacteria

Introducing pre-biotics (shown as hexagonal long chains) provides food for the 'good bugs'.

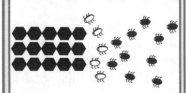

The harmful bacteria (shown black) cannot digest the pre-biotics

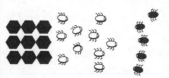

The 'good bugs' (shown white) can digest the pre-biotics and now start multiplying

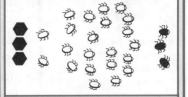

Finally the good bugs crowd out (and kill) the harmful intestinal bacteria

---

Babies and pre-biotics

Bifidobacteria are particularly important in the new-born, whose immune defences are not yet fully working. Breast milk contains substances which promote the growth of bifidobacteria, which is why these bacteria represent up to 95 per cent of the bacteria in the gut of breast-fed infants, but a mere 25 per cent in bottle-fed infants. This explains why breast-fed babies are more resistant to stomach upsets and diarrhoea[59-61]. Recent studies show that live yoghurt cultures fed to infants significantly reduce their risk of contracting diarrhoea[84, 112]; and speed recovery if given as a treatment for diarrhoea[93].

As we age, the proportion of bifidobacteria and lactobacilli gradually falls. This is one reason why we become more prone to gastrointestinal upsets and it is probably also linked to the age-related increase in the risk of bowel cancer[58] and other illnesses[113].

Cancer protection

The cancer story is a complicated one, and many dietary factors (as well as genetic factors) contribute to the overall risk.

There is evidence, however, that bifidobacteria and pre-biotics protect against colon and other cancers[33-36, 92].

Bifidobacteria's anti-cancer effects are probably linked to the acids they produce in the gut, which include butyric acid[46]. Butyric acid is essential for the health and normal growth of the cells that line the colon[49, 50, 70].

Butyric acid has quite dramatic effects on these colon cells: it slows down abnormal colon cell growth, makes cancer cells less cancerous[79] and helps to kill established cancers[132,133]. It may be no coincidence that the bacteria that produce butyric acid concentrate in the upper colon, which is relatively immune to cancer[57]. But pre-biotics have other anti-cancer effects.

The risk of colon cancer is increased by a diet high in animal fats – a diet which causes more bile to be secreted. Unhealthy gut bacteria convert bile acids into cancer-causing compounds which increase the risk of liver cancer[114].

Pre-biotics reduce the disease-causing bacteria in the gut, and the amount of cancer-causing compounds they produce[15, 44, 115, 131], which could well have a protective effect.

Finally, as the bifids grow they bind free iron[134], thereby reducing levels of free radicals in the colon[139]. This must be another cancer-preventing property.

COLITIS

In ulcerative colitis, levels of butyric acid are very low in the affected areas of the gut[101, 102]. This probably indicates that levels of bifidobacteria are low.

Considering the importance of butyrate to the health of colon cells, it's not surprising that butyric acid infusions improve patients' symptoms[103, 104].

Colitis sufferers can increase their intake of inulin with a small but gradually increasing daily dose of onion soup (or as a supplement). This will increase the numbers of bifidobacteria, and the amount of butyrate that these friendly bacteria produce.

Fibre for the whole body

Heart

Read the contents' list on a carton of yoghurt and you'll see it contains significant amounts of thiamin, riboflavin and other vitamins. This is because the lactobacilli and bifidobacteria make B vitamins, and are probably the major species of bacteria in the colon which do this[128].

B depletion is surprisingly common in the developed countries[105-109], and low B levels are a major risk factor for coronary artery disease[110-111]. So pre-biotics, by increasing the good bacteria in the gut and B vitamin levels, will be cardio-protective by lowering homocysteine, and simultaneously raising HDL levels[38-42, 68, 71, 72, 76-78].

This is one way in which oats and inulin contribute to a healthy heart; although LDL cholesterol reduction also plays a role.

Short chain = heart + colon health

Short chain pre-biotics (ie FOS) are rapidly fermented, stimulating the production of bifidobacteria (bifidogenesis) in the proximal colon. As they grow they bind the bile acids present in this part of the gut and remove them from the body[121]. This lowers LDL cholesterol levels [19,26-29, 37,42-44,82,83, 99,113,121-123] and confers additional cardio-protection. The combination of bifidogenesis and bile acid binding is also likely to be cancer protective[141-143], especially if FOS is combined with longer chain pre-biotics.

Pre-biotics and breast cancer

Pre-biotics may help to prevent cancer elsewhere in the body[115]. They reduce the incidence of mammary cancer in rats[82] by altering the way in which oestrogen is metabolised by bacteria in the bowel.

Five more good things about pre-biotics

- **They encourage bifidobacteria to grow, producing acids which smooth out blood sugar levels**

- **These acids may discourage the body from laying down fat**[12-14, 25]

- **Oligofructose is a low calorie sweetener – at 1.25 calories per gram it's less than a third of sugar**[20]

- **Oligofructose and inulin cause less tooth decay than sugar, and are safe for diabetics**

- **Pre-biotics may stimulate the immune system, either directly or via the bifidobacteria**[137].

Long chain = colon health

Longer chain pre-biotics (ie inulin) are slowly fermented, stimulating bifidogenesis further down the gut in the lower colon and rectum. This is the main site of bowel cancer, and bifidogenesis here (with the resulting local production of butyric acid, etc) probably confers significant protection important against this type of tumour.

Bones

Bifidobacteria produce Vitamin K, which is essential for bone growth and repair (See Chapter 15, Bones). At the same time, they help with the absorption of calcium and magnesium from food[21-24, 69]. These are two powerful anti-osteoporosis effects.

Contrary to previous medical opinion, calcium is now known to be absorbed in the colon. One of the reasons why calcium in milk is better absorbed than from chalk-type supplements is because milk contains substances which promote bifidobacteria, which in turn boost the absorption of the calcium in the colon.

Vaginal and urinary tract infections

Bifidobacteria are an important part of the normal bacterial population of the vagina. The acids and antibiotics they produce make it hard for other micro-organisms to thrive[117-119]. When the balance of bacteria in the vagina is disturbed, thrush, bacterial vaginosis or urinary tract infections can follow.

Live yoghurt, which can contain either bifidobacteria or lactobacilli, has traditionally been used as a treatment for thrush, but it is messy and not very effective. More scientifically, pessaries containing lactobacilli have been shown to reduce urinary tract infections by as much as 80 per cent[120]. An oligo-fructose pessary, which would encourage the growth of lactobacilli, is a simpler solution, and could be used both as a treatment and as a preventative measure for women prone to bouts of candida, bacterial vaginosis or UTI.

It may also have some protective effect against sexually transmitted diseases such as chlamydia, gonorrhoea, syphilis, and even HIV[118].

Teeth and gums

There is evidence from a Finnish lab that oligosaccharides can help protect your teeth. After eating live yoghurt, the population of bifidobacteria in the mouth increases, and remains high for a few days[98].

This almost certainly helps to crowd out the other species of bacteria which cause dental decay and gum disease. So buffered pastilles containing oligosaccharide may help to keep your teeth intact (see also Chapter 9, Co-enzyme Q10).

The mouth is an important reservoir of potentially disease-causing bacteria, many of which are resistant to antibiotics. A pre-biotic-loaded chewing gum is therefore an interesting approach not just to tooth decay but also to other infections. For example, the bacterium which causes peptic ulcers, helicobacter pylori, lives in the mouth. Oligofructose pastilles or gum could keep it in check,[100,127] and reduce the risk of peptic ulcers in high risk groups such as smokers.

Many bacteriologists believe that oral bacteria can escape from the mouth to cause infection after operations, meningitis, upper respiratory tract infections and septicaemias[125]. By reducing the disease-causing bacteria in the mouth, pre-biotic pastilles should protect against these infections. They should also contain buffers and xylitol to minimise dental decay[138].

LIVE YOGHURT

Early this century, the great Russian scientist, Eli Metchnikoff, published his theory that eating live yoghurt was the way to achieving long life.

Although this idea was based on keen observation, his views were dismissed by the establishment because Metchnikoff could not explain how his theory might work.

Now we can see a plausible way in which eating live yoghurt could reduce the risk of a number of serious disease conditions, his theory no longer seems quite so absurd.

Should I take a pre-biotic supplement?

Yes, if you are:

- **Prone to stomach upsets**

- **Travelling to an area where gastro-intestinal illness is common**[94-97]

- **Suffer from gastroenteritis, Crohn's Disease or ulcerative colitis**[75]**. Combine pre-biotics with amino sugars and/or glutamine**

- **Taking antibiotics. Pre-biotics may reduce the diarrhoea often caused by antibiotics and help to re-establish a healthy gut**[85]

- **Prone to attacks of thrush or bacterial vaginosis. A pre-biotic pessary will encourage the growth of healthy bacteria in the vagina and crowd out the nastier types of micro-organisms**

Old-fashioned fibre

We shouldn't forget the more familiar insoluble dietary fibres such as bran, which pass through the entire gut unchanged, and used to be called roughage. Here too, the scientists have uncovered a possible anti-cancer effect – and again, the bacteria that live in the gut play an important role.

Even so-called indigestible fibre is broken down, to some extent, by bacterial enzymes. Part of the fibre is broken down to release compounds which have considerable anti-oxidant properties[86-88]. These are thought to scavenge dangerous radicals, which have been linked to gastrointestinal and other cancers[89-91].

So while the recently discovered soluble fibres are important, a regular intake of the old-fashioned kind of roughage is a good idea as well for anyone concerned with staying healthier, for longer.

Indigestible fibres and anti-oxidants

Foods with a high content of indigestible fibre are also high in anti-oxidants[144]. These are:

High fibre cereals
Wholegrain wheat
Wholegrain oats
Wholemeal bread

White bread has only half the anti-oxidants of wholemeal bread.

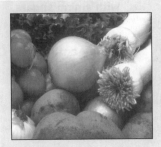

STAY POPULAR!

The only downside of the pre-biotics is that, in some people, they may cause flatulence and, if very large amounts are taken, diarrhoea.

In this respect, inulin is less likely to cause problems than oligofructose. If you react badly to onion soup or vichyssoise (made of leeks), which both contain large amounts of inulin, you can probably still take pre-biotics – but start with small doses. Any initial problems generally soon subside, once the new colonic regime becomes established.

Processed food problems

1   Many processed foods contain sulphate and sulphide preservatives.

2   Recent research has shown that certain 'hostile' bacteria in the gut turn sulphur compounds to hydrogen sulphide, which is toxic, and linked to colitis and irritable bowel syndrome.

3   Not everyone has these hostile bacteria but in those that do, sulphur compounds in the diet stimulate the growth of these bacteria, which produce more hydrogen sulphide and increase the symptoms[124].

4   Hydrogen sulphide also appears to block the production of butyrate – the acid which promotes healthy cells in the colon – and so could be a cancer risk. This is another reason to cut down on processed foods.

5   **Don't** cut down on foods which naturally contain sulphur compounds (brassica, such as cabbage, broccoli and Brussels sprouts). These vegetables contain many health-enhancing compounds and are protective against cancer.

SUMMARY

Fibre providers

▶ Include pre-biotic rich foods like leeks, onions, oats and bananas in your diet.

▶ Make sure your fruit and veg is as fresh as possible.

▶ Alternatively, take daily a pre-biotic supplement. Ideally combine a rapid-acting short chain pre-biotic (ie FOS) with a slower-acting pre-biotic (ie inulin or beta glucans). You could combine these with a proven probiotic such as LC1 from Nestlé to create a 'symbiotic'.

▶ The combination of a pre-biotic and a pro-biotic is known as a 'symbiotic'.

▶ Maintain your intake of roughage, ie bran products, fruit or vegetables.

▶ Anyone with arthritis or other auto-immune conditions should use pre-biotics with caution.

▶ Where possible, babies should be breast-fed to protect them against stomach upsets.

▶ Formula milk should be fortified with a pre-biotic to make it more like breast milk.

▶ Infants with stomach upsets can be given live yoghurt.

- The surge in heart disease, asthma and arthritis is partly due to the unbalanced mix of fats in the modern diet

- Trans-fats in processed foods may cause more heart disease than saturated fats

- Natural polyunsaturates in fish, nuts and grains are essential to health – too few increases the risk of heart disease, arthritis, sterility and senility.

- High-dose PUFAs (in refined oils) are not recommended. Unless accompanied by anti-oxidants, they form toxic breakdown products in the body.

- Until Westernisation, Eskimos were practically immune to heart disease – thanks to the fish they ate

- Oily fish like salmon, herring, mackerel and tuna contain valuable Omega 3 oils, which keep arteries healthy, lower damaging cholesterol and reduce the risk of clots

- Large doses of Omega 3 can cut the risk of a heart attack by 30 per cent

Chapter 8

Essential Oils – the facts about fat

For years we have been tyrannised by food fads dressed up as science. The idea that fat is dangerous, for example, has created an entire low-fat industry, a generation of low-fat gurus, and a rash of low-fat, low-brow books.

We were told that saturated fats cause heart disease – and many of us changed our diets in a way that we thought would protect our hearts. But now it seems as if much of this was a waste of time.

The early idea that saturated fat intake was the most important cause of coronary artery disease is no longer popular. The so-called Seven Countries Trial, which started the low-fat ball rolling, has been effectively discredited. Death from coronary artery disease has been falling since around 1968-1970, which was well before saturated fat intakes began to decline. In Japan, the rate of coronary artery disease is falling even though people are eating more saturated fat[106].

Too much saturated fat is still not a good thing, but the latest thinking is rather more complex than the early 'fat = bad' equation. It involves LOPs, COPs, anti-oxidants and more. But don't despair – it's not as complicated as that, and once you've grasped the essentials, avoiding heart attacks is relatively plain sailing.

Subtle differences in the molecular structures of fatty acids determine their melting point and their effect on our health.

Saturated Fats SAFAs	Poly-Unsaturated Fats PUFAs	Mono-Unsaturated Fats MUFAs
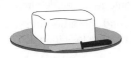	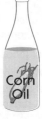	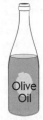
Saturated Fatty Acids are solid at room temperature, eg: butter and lard. These are typical fats.	Poly-Unsaturated Fatty Acids are liquid at room temperature, eg: corn oil and sunflower oil.	Mono-Unsaturated Fatty Acids are also liquid at room temperature, eg: olive oil, hemp oil, and flaxseed oil.

The edible fats and oils, known collectively as fatty acids, are basically similar compounds. Oils, however, melt at lower temperatures than fats, and at room temperature oils are liquid and fats are solid.

Fatty acids (fats and oils) are a rich source of calories, which can either be 'burned' to produce energy, or stored as fat for lean times ahead. They are also incorporated into cell membranes and other tissues, where they have an important structural role.

Finally, fatty acids are metabolised into compounds called eicosanoids. Fats and oils produce quite different eicosanoids: broadly speaking, **fats** form eicosanoids which **increase inflammation,** and **oils** produce eicosanoids which **reduce inflammation**.

This difference is important to know, because many chronic diseases are basically inflammatory conditions. These include arthritis (inflammation of the joints), eczema (inflammation of the skin), asthma (inflammation of the lungs) and coronary artery disease (inflammation of the arteries).

Your risk of these conditions is affected by your genetic make-up, tobacco consumption and the amount of anti-oxidants in your diet; but the fats and oils we consume are also important.

The Fat Facts

The shorthand for the different types of fats is:

Saturated fats – SAFAs (**SA**turated **F**atty **A**cids)

Poly-unsaturates = PUFAs (**P**oly-**U**nsaturated **F**atty **A**cids)

Mono-unsaturates = MUFAs (**M**ono-**U**nsaturated **F**atty **A**cids)

SAFAs tend to be solid at room temperature and are termed 'fats'.

MUFAs and PUFAs are liquid and are called 'oils'.

Watch out for 'hidden' fats

All fats found in food contain a mixture of SAFAs, MUFAs and PUFAs, ie Saturated, Mono-unsaturated and Poly-unsaturated.

But the proportions in different foods vary considerably.

SAFAs are primarily animal fats, and are found in meat and dairy produce – coconut oil is the only vegetable oil which contains large amounts of SAFAs.

Three good sources of MUFAs are olive oil, rapeseed oil and peanut oil.

The essential PUFAs are Omega-3, found in oily fish, and Omega-6 found in plant oils such as evening primrose oil and walnut oil.

Eggs are the odd ones out. They contain SAFAs, but in the form of phospholipids. These increase HDL, the 'good' cholesterol.

Watch out for 'hidden' fats. It's easy to monitor how much butter, oil, or bacon fat you're eating, but less easy to check the fat content of foods like eggs and cheese which are naturally rich in fat.

Most deceptive are foods which have fat added during processing. Manufacturers don't like to throw away the fat they remove from reduced-fat products, so in many cases they simply conceal it in biscuits, cakes, quiches and a wide range of other standard processed foods.

Below is a checklist of foods showing the percentage of calories from fat.

To check the fat content of foods not listed, read the label and use the calories/gram formula below. If the calories from fat are less than 30% of the total calories, this is a reasonable balance.

Less than 10%	Most fruits, veg, baked or boiled potato, fat-free milk
Over **10%**	Bread
Over **20%**	Crackers, crab meat, lean fish
Over **30%**	Chicken, cottage cheese, tuna fish, low fat milk
Over **40%**	Whole milk, cake, chips
Over **50%**	Ice cream, steak
Over **60%**	Crisps, ham, eggs
Over **70%**	Cheddar cheese, bacon, most nuts inc. peanuts
Over **80%**	Cream cheese, salad dressing, chocolate
Over **90%**	Butter, margarine, cooking oils, cream

The fats in fatty foods

	Total fat per 100g	Saturated Fat	Mono- unsaturated	Poly- unsaturated
OLIVE OIL	100g	14g	70g	11g
BUTTER	82g	54g	21g	3g
MARGARINE	82g	16g	21g	(Inc. trans) 41g
CHEDDAR	34g	22g	10g	1g
AVOCADO	20g	4g	12g	2g
EGGS	11g	3g	5g	1g
WHOLE MILK	3g	2g	1g	0g

McCance and Widdowson. *The Composition of Food*, Fifth Edition, Royal Society of Chemistry and Ministry of Agriculture Fisheries and Food

Calories per gram	
Fat	9 cals
Protein	4 cals
Carbohydrate	4 cals
Alcohol	7 cals

Stone Age body, 20th-century fats

During the hundreds of thousands of years it took us to make the long evolutionary trek from ape to man, our ancestors ate a predominantly vegetarian diet based on shellfish, fruits, vegetables, grains and nuts, with occasional fish and game.

This Stone Age diet contained high levels of mono- and poly-unsaturated oils, with relatively little saturated fat. (Wild game is lean compared with farmed meat, and contains more PUFAs.) Our bodies were designed to run on this sort of fatty acid mix, which produces a healthy balance of eicosanoids.

The fatty acid composition of our diets today is very different. In the developed nations, most fatty acids in the diet are saturated fats contained in meat, dairy products and processed foods. Most of us are eating too few vegetables and fish and not enough oils and anti-oxidants.

As a result of this disproportionate intake of saturated fats, the balance has been upset. Anti-inflammatory eicosanoids have been reduced, leaving the inflammatory compounds unchecked – contributing to an epidemic of chronic inflammatory diseases like heart disease, arthritis and asthma.

The obvious remedy is to redress the balance. To do this we can either change our diet, and/or supplement it. If we were to reduce our intake of saturated animal fats and increase our intake of MUFAs and PUFAs by eating more fish and vegetable foods, we would all be a lot healthier. (The environment would benefit too.)

Eating more PUFAs means more anti-inflammatory eicosanoids are produced, and less pro-inflammatory compounds. This is why fish oil, for example, is used to treat arthritis and to protect against coronary artery disease; and why evening primrose oil (taken orally) can reduce the severity of eczema and other inflammatory skin disorders[113, 115].

To achieve these gains you need quite large doses of PUFAs – typically 6-10g a day or more.

Beware the label

The solution to not eating enough poly-unsaturated oils does not, sadly, lie in eating more processed poly-unsaturated spreads and oils.

These can cause problems because the anti-oxidants which occur naturally alongside poly-unsaturates in unprocessed foods like nuts and grains have all been removed.

Instead, eat more nuts and grains – which contain MUFAs, PUFAs *and* anti-oxidants.

More fatty benefits

Fats and oils have other important effects. Saturated fats raise the levels of 'bad', ie LDL, cholesterol in the blood[37, 38]. Fish oil, on the other hand, slows the formation of LDL cholesterol, reducing the risk of heart attacks.

The medical profession found it hard to believe that a simple switch from fats to oils could have significant health benefits, but the sheer weight of all the clinical trials which have shown positive health benefits has begun to change their opinion. The evidence is particularly good in the area of coronary artery disease; and the PUFAs are rapidly gaining a role in even conventional circles.

The essential oils

Not all PUFAs (poly-unsaturated fatty acids) are the same. Some of them are more important than others, and a few are so important they are termed, collectively, the Essential PUFAs.

There are two families of essential poly-unsaturated fatty acids, Omega 6 and Omega 3, both of which are oils. These oils are vital for the functioning of every cell in our bodies, and yet our bodies cannot make them. We have to obtain them from our diet, and in that sense they are similar to vitamins[26].

Once the oils have been absorbed from our food, our enzymes make all the other Omega 3 and 6 PUFAs our cells and systems need[24].

Saturated Fats ...

decrease the number of LDL receptors in the liver. This reduces the liver's ability to remove LDL from the blood and leads to raised LDL levels[37, 38], and an increased risk of coronary artery disease[33, 34].

Fish oil reduces LDL (and triglycerides)[5, 35, 36], reducing the risk of heart attacks.

More PUFAs

A lack of the essential PUFAs in the diet leads to deficiency symptoms such as dry skin, and an increased risk of heart disease, sterility and arthritis.

HEART DISEASE RISK CAN BE CUT BY 33% WITH PUFAS

PUFAs encourage the formation of compounds which lower blood pressure, reduce blood platelet stickiness, improve capillary function and reduce inflammation[12]. In addition, the Omega 3s reduce the levels of 'bad' plasma cholesterol[10], and inhibit the formation of plaque in artery walls[9].

Fish are no better than we are at making Omega 3 oils; fish in the wild get their Omega 3s from marine algae, which live in the cold Arctic waters.

Farmed fish only contain EPA and DHA if they have been fed on fish scraps which themselves contained Omega 3.

At least two USA companies intend to bring an algae-based Omega 3 oil to the market once safety tests[17, 18] have been completed.

How your body uses Omega 6 and Omega 3

OMEGA 6

1 The process begins when you eat foods containing linoleic acid (LA) found in flax, hemp, walnut, linseed, safflower, sunflower, soy oils.

2 Our enzymes slowly turn the linoleic acid into gamma linolenic acid (GLA).

3 The problem is that saturated fats in our diet slow down the process, causing a bottleneck and insufficient GLA is available.

4 The solution is to *by-pass* the process and take GLA directly as a supplement.

It's found in oils such as evening primrose oil, borage (starflower) and blackcurrant seed oil.

Linoleic acid

Saturated fats cause a bottle-neck

GLA

OMEGA 3

1 The process begins when you eat food containing linolenic acid (LNA) found in oily fish, flax, hemp, pumpkin seeds, soya beans and walnuts

2 Our enzymes slowly turn the linolenic acid into eicosapentanoeic acid (EPA) and docosa-hexaenoic acid (DHA)

3 Once again the problem is that bottlenecks can result in insufficient EPA and DHA being available.

4 The *short-cut* is to take EPA and DHA directly from oily fish like salmon, trout, herring and mackerel or from Omega 3 supplements.

Linolenic acid

bottle-neck

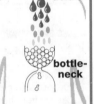

EPA DHA

Note: Hempseed oil, flaxseed oil or soy oil can be the start point for **both** processes. These plant oils contain Omega 3 but usually at a lower level than fish oils[11]. A recommended dose for a general supplement would be at 2-3g a day, rising to 10-15g a day to treat an existing case of heart disease or arthritis[6].

Check labels carefully. A 1000mg capsule of fish oil does **not** contain 1000mg of Omega 3. The Omega 3 content may be 300mg or less. The level of Omega 3 as a general supplement should start at 400-500mg a day.

PUFAs cut risks of heart disease

The best documented clinical use of PUFAs is in the prevention and treatment of heart disease. It is well-known that a high intake of animal fats increases the risk of heart attacks, while vegetarian or fish-based diets, which contain Omega 6 or 3 respectively, reduce the risk.

This explains why fish-eating folk like the Eskimos don't have heart attacks. Fish oil doesn't make us quite as immune to heart attacks as the Eskimos are (or used to be before the introduction of processed foods), because the effects of the PUFAs in fish oil are reduced by the large amounts of saturated fats we eat, but nonetheless the benefits are significant.

In the American MRFIT trial, the risk of heart disease was cut by around a third in men who consumed more oily fish; and similar results have been obtained in at least four other large European studies[43-46, 98] – see also pages 131-137.

Quite apart from its cardio-protective properties, fish oil is also able to damp down an over-active immune system[63-67]. This would explain why Eskimos are not only singularly free from heart disease, but eczema and arthritis as well; findings which have recently been duplicated in clinical studies[104, 105]. The immuno-regulatory effects of fish oil are currently being used in treating allergies and improving the success rate of organ grafts.

Research into Omega 6 PUFAs in nuts and grains has been overshadowed by the Omega 3 work. There are a few studies, however, which indicate that Omega 6s may also be cardio-protective.

In a trial reported in the British Medical Journal, 400 heart attack patients were put on either a Western diet (which contained meat, eggs and butter), or a vegetarian diet, which contained nut and vegetable oils. The veggies did considerably better, with significantly fewer cardiac problems and fewer fatal heart attacks than their meat-eating colleagues[1, 8].

In the same year the New England Journal of Medicine reported that snacking on walnuts, a rich source of Omega 3 and 6 PUFAs and MUFAs, reduced total cholesterol levels, and improved the HDL/LDL cholesterol ratio in normal men[116].

Omega 3

In small doses, Omega 3 makes the heart less vulnerable to dangerous arrhythmias after a heart attack. At higher doses, the other cardiac benefits emerge and heart attacks themselves becomes less frequent.

Reminder!

Omega 3 = PUFAs (poly-unsaturated oils) usually from fish sources.

Omega 6 = PUFAs from vegetable sources.

Think of "Omega 3 – from the sea".

Capsules are better

If you take a fish oil supplement, avoid bottled oils; fish oils in capsules are safer.

For enhanced cardio-protection, combine with garlic and other anti-oxidants, such as Vitamins C and E, and take with food for better absorption.

Further work has shown that almonds are just as good at lowering LDL cholesterol as walnuts[107], and should be just as cardio-protective. The best bet may still be fish, however, as fish eaters appear to have lower blood pressure, and lower cholesterol levels than vegetarians[6, 11]

The overall health benefits of a dietary shift may include not only healthier hearts, but better-balanced immune systems as well.

PUFAs FOR PEPTIC ULCERS?

There are additional, unexpected benefits linked to going back to our nutritional roots, and eating a high PUFA diet. There is some evidence, for example, that this could protect against peptic ulcers. Peptic ulcers are caused by a bacterium called Helicobacter pylori. When there are plenty of PUFAs around, H pylori absorbs them into its cell membranes. This makes the membranes more permeable, and the bacterium becomes more vulnerable to attack by the gastric juices[99].

This strongly implies that a diet rich in nuts, cereals and fish, and low in animal fats, could reduce the risk of infection with H pylori – and might even be able to eradicate it, if used together with other nutritional components (see Chapter 7, Pre-biotic fibre). In Central Europe, flaxseed soup was traditionally used to treat stomach ulcers.

The right mix

PUFAs are a powerful force for good health but, as with other powerful agents, they should not be taken indiscriminately. The ratio of the various PUFAs in the diet is important[17, 27, 30], and the fact that in most mammals' cells the level of Omega 6 (from vegetable sources) is three to four times higher than the Omega 3 content (from fish sources), gives us a pointer as to what we should aim for.

The Japanese diet was traditionally the other way round – three times higher in Omega 3 than Omega 6. The fact that Japanese mortality rates have fallen since the '50s, when the diet first began to shift towards a more Western style and incorporate more vegetable oils, is thought by some to be linked to their increased intake of Omega 6 PUFAs.

Balance

The first step to a better balance of fats in the diet is cutting down on butter, lard, milk, cheese and poly-unsaturated vegetable oils.

Although some vegetable oils contain linolenic acid, which is slowly converted in the body to Omega 3s, the overall effect of most vegetable oils is to reduce the synthesis of Omega 3s.

Saturated animal fats are not entirely unhealthy. There are essential saturated fatty acids too, such as myristic acid[23], and perhaps 20 others.

All of these are found in the tissues and many of them have essential and specific roles in metabolism, cell-to-cell interactions, and in modulating immune responses[22].

The Western diet, however, is skewed in the opposite direction. The ratio of Omega 6 (vegetable oil derived) to Omega 3 (fish oils) in our diet is about 6 to 1[16] – and that's almost certainly too high[11, 14, 17].

As a final piece of evidence of the importance of the PUFA ratio, consider the composition of human milk. The proportion of Omega 6 and Omega 3 in the diet of vegetarian and fish-eating communities is wildly different but the PUFA content of breast milk is identical – between 2:1 and 3:1[21]. It's a reflection of the most basic nutritional needs of the growing child[26, 28, 29].

LOOK FOR ...

a fish oil supplement containing 500mg of Omega 3 a day.

This will provide about 300mg of EPA and 200mg of DHA.

LOW FAT FOODS? MAYBE!

Low or reduced fat claims on food labels are almost meaningless, and have never been legally defined. In many cases it appears to be little more than a marketing exercise. Check the contents list on the label, remembering that fat has more than twice as many calories per gram as protein or carbohydrate.

Beef and dairy products, such as cheese and butter, contain more saturated fats than pork and poultry, which contain slightly more PUFAs.

This is why nutritionists recommend switching from red meat to white meat. However, game meats are healthier than farmed meat because they contain far less fat and the fat they do contain has a higher percentage of PUFAs[8].

Take care

If you eat a lot of poly-unsaturated products, or if you take PUFA supplements like evening primrose oil or fish oil, you must also take a good anti-oxidant combination.

But if your poly-unsaturates come from a vegetarian diet rich in nuts and grains, don't worry too much, as these foods contain their own anti-oxidants.

What next?

How much should we modify our intake of fats and oils to achieve optimum health?

The current recommendations from the health experts suggest we eat less saturated fats and more mono-unsaturated oils and Omega 3, while maintaining our consumption of Omega 6 vegetable oils[69, 85]. There are several very simple steps we can all take to achieve this nutritional balance, and better health.

1 Cut down on meat and dairy produce, and/or change where possible to genuinely low-fat products.

2 Eat more oily fish.

3 Eat more olives and olive oil products

4 Switch from sunflower oils to hemp, flax or linseed oil products. The composition of hemp oil or flax oil is as close to

nutritional perfection as a vegetable oil can get, containing Omega 6 and 3 fats in a near optimal 3.5:1 ratio[72].

Virgin hemp oil has a green colour due to its chlorophyll content, tastes like sunflower oil, and is good for all uses except frying. To extend its shelf life, squeeze a Vitamin E capsule into the bottle.

The dangers of processed PUFAs

To get the maximum benefit from the new diet, and to avoid the possible dangers, we have to look very seriously at anti-oxidants.

The problem with poly-unsaturated fatty acids (PUFAs) is that they are very prone to going rancid, or oxidising. It's fine to eat a high PUFA diet if the PUFAs are in unprocessed foods such as nuts and grains, because these foods contain their own anti-oxidants, such as Vitamin E, carotenoids and flavonoids. Without these they would go rancid, and the seeds, grains and nuts would not survive long enough to propagate the species. But if your intake of PUFAs is in the form of refined poly-unsaturated oils and spreads, you could be in trouble.

These processed foods have had the naturally occurring anti-oxidants stripped away, and are therefore highly prone to being oxidised. This has two potentially very serious effects.

Firstly, the PUFAs form lipid oxidation products[91] (LOPs). LOPs are extremely toxic: they literally rip holes in the lining of the arteries[48] and are therefore a substantial risk factor for heart disease[16]. Secondly, as the PUFAs oxidise they soak up anti-oxidants in the body[90], leaving an excess of free radicals and causing accelerated ageing[209].

The end result is an increase in the risk and severity of chronic degenerative diseases from heart disease to cancer to asthma.

At the Royal Prince Alfred Hospital in Sydney, Australia, epidemiologists have linked the huge increase in childhood asthma with a five-fold increase in margarine consumption since the War. Their theory is that the increased PUFA content in the diet has led to an increase in inflammatory and toxic LOPs, which leave the airways raw, and trigger the asthma[31,32].

Why are allergies on the increase?

One reason for the huge increase in allergic conditions may be too little Omega 3 and too much Omega 6[31, 32]; together with too few flavonoids and other anti-oxidants.

The increase in childhood asthma could be linked to the increase in processed PUFAs (eg from margarine) in the diet since World War 2 – and the related decline in phospholipid intake (see pages 73-74).

Overweight?

Anti-oxidants are particularly important if you are overweight.

The so-called Metabolic Syndrome is probably a form of pre-diabetes: symptoms include putting on weight, experiencing cravings for sweet foods, and getting spells of cold, tiredness and irritability.

The rate of PUFA oxidation is raised in this condition[93], so a good anti-oxidant combination is strongly recommended.

Keep oil cool

PUFA oils stored where they are subjected to light and heat will form LOPs. Keep them in the fridge.

Bad COPs

When animal fats (including lard and butter) containing cholesterol are heated, this forms cholesterol oxidation products (COPs), which are as harmful as LOPS.

Don't overheat these fats, don't re-use, and don't cook in iron pans or woks, as this increases COP formation.

More bad news for smokers

Smokers produce significant amounts of COPs and LOPs in their bodies, and should definitely take anti-oxidant supplements which reduce COPs and LOPs formation[55].

The Australian work, although provocative, has not yet been substantiated. But we can be sure that the common combination of eating too many poly-unsaturated spreads and oils and not enough anti-oxidants, leaves us with cholesterol which is very prone to being oxidised[112], dangerously high levels of LOPs[89, 91, 93] and dangerously low levels of anti-oxidants[90].

The only way to prevent this unhealthy scenario is to supplement with anti-oxidants[88, 90, 94, 112]. But which ones? Vitamin E on its own is relatively ineffective[7, 19, 91, 113]. The best approach seems to be to concentrate on anti-oxidant combinations. A combination of E, C, beta carotene and flavonoids is extremely effective at stopping the oxidation process, and has been patented by Nestlé[19]. Vitamin E combined with garlic and ginkgo, both of which contain complex mixtures of anti-oxidants, may be even more effective[92].

HEART DISEASE EPIDEMIC

Heat processed powdered egg, widely consumed in the '40s, was a rich source of COPs, and was probably an important factor in coronary artery disease deaths in the '50s and '60s. But we also have to consider the increase in the consumption of trans-fats which occurred rather earlier on, and which fits the beginning of the rise in heart disease in the West.

Nor should we forget the arrival of mass motor transport. Petrol and especially diesel exhausts produce enormous amounts of free radicals, which when inhaled lead to anti-oxidant depletion[53, 54].

The increasing popularity of cigarette smoking after World War 1, and the reduced consumption of fresh fruit and vegetables also play a part.

The recent fall in coronary artery disease in the professional classes is almost certainly caused by decreased smoking, and increased fruit, vegetable and supplement intake.

Bad COPs, bad LOPs

Anti-oxidant supplements can prevent COPs (Cholesterol Oxidation Products formed when animal fats are heated) and LOPs from being formed in your body. They won't protect you, however, against LOPs or COPs in your food.

LOPs and COPs are created by bad cooking and storage techniques. Once ingested, they are quickly absorbed into the blood stream[47, 49] and are among the most dangerous items on the menu, and certainly the worst for your heart.

COPs are produced in certain types of food processing. Particularly high levels of COPs are found in powdered egg. Few people eat powdered egg now, but it was a staple during World War 2, and was probably a major contributing factor to the epidemic of heart disease which peaked some 10-15 years later.

Major sources of LOPs are poly-unsaturated oils and margarines which are stored for too long, or under the wrong conditions, or over-heated during cooking.

Oils should be stored in dark glass containers, and preferably in the fridge. Margarines should also be kept in the fridge. Tubs of the stuff left lying around soon develop a translucent ring around the edge where the fat has melted and re-set, a sure sign that LOPs are being formed, ie the fat is being oxidised.

Some manufacturers add anti-oxidants such as Vitamin E to their products to prevent them from oxidising (going rancid). This helps to some extent, but has no protective effect whatsoever during cooking as Vitamin E breaks down when heated.

So what can we do to minimise our exposure to these highly cardiotoxic compounds? Tiny amounts of COPs and LOPs are formed in the body but the bulk are found in our food, and are already oxidised before we eat them, so anti-oxidant supplements offer no protection at all. The solution lies in modifying our food storage and cooking techniques (see the Cook Guide on the next page).

How to cook eggs

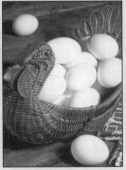

Fresh eggs contain cholesterol but no COPs and can be eaten with impunity.

Their phospholipid content boosts levels of HDL, the 'good' cholesterol.

Different cooking techniques produce different amounts of COPs, in ascending order:

1 Poaching or soft boiling   **-**

2 Hard boiling   **+/-**

3 Frying   **+** limit

4 Heat processing to produce dried egg.   **+++** avoid

N.B. Modern freeze-drying methods do not increase COPs levels and are inherently safer.

COPS AND LOPS AND CORONARY ARTERY DISEASE

There are three basic stages in the development of coronary artery disease: damage to the artery wall, the build-up of atheroma, and the formation of blood clots. COPs and LOPs help all three stages along the way[47, 113-115]:

- They are toxic to cells in general, and the cells lining the arteries in particular[48].
- They increase levels of LDL cholesterol.
- They increase platelet stickiness, which increases the tendency to form clots.

The Anti-COPs/LOPs Cook Guide

- Cooking with animal fats which contain cholesterol, such as lard or butter, produces COPs. Use as little as possible, and never re-use it.

- Don't fry with poly-unsaturates, these produce LOPs even at normal frying conditions[87], and should **never** be re-used.

- Deep-frying, where the oil not only forms dangerous amounts of oxidation products but is also generally re-used, especially in commercial establishments, should be off limits altogether.

- When cooking, do not overheat the oil: if it's smoking, it's too hot.

- Don't fry in iron cookware, as the traces of iron that leach into the oil increase the formation of LOPs and/or COPs many times over.

- Wherever possible, cook with mono-unsaturates such as olive, peanut or rapeseed oil. These form no COPs and relatively small amounts of LOPs[34], although re-use should still be avoided.

To make your cooking oils safer:

- Store them in dark glass, in the fridge. Glass is better than cans, as there is some concern that iron in the walls of metal cans could leach into the oil and accelerate the oxidative process.

- Add grapeseed or green tea extract (available from some health food suppliers) to the oil before using.

Both extracts contain catechins and catechin gallates, powerful heat-stable anti-oxidants which inhibit COPs and LOPs formation during the cooking process.

- If you like herbs in your cooking, rosemary or rosemary extract has been shown to prevent the formation of COPs and LOPs in frying trials[39, 109-111].

Grind the rosemary in olive oil, and then use the same oil for frying. If you don't like rosemary, then sage, thyme and oregano are almost as good[39].

Fried or grilled meats such as hamburgers are particularly bad, because the minced meat leaks iron (from blood) during the cooking. The iron is a powerful oxidant and increases the amount of COPs produced many times. Fast food companies would not accept that they are selling cardiotoxic food, but the evidence against them is strong.

You can make safer burgers simply by adding barley bran and wild rice to your hamburger mix. This adds fibre and improves the texture and the taste.

Furthermore, the wild rice contains powerful antioxidant compounds which reduce COPs and LOPs formation almost to zero, and the bran locks on to free iron, which also reduces oxidation.

It's a modification that the burger chains should look at. It could save many thousands of lives.

Secret danger in 'healthy' spreads?

Anti-oxidants are anti-COPS

The COPs-LOPs story is yet another reason why a high intake of anti-oxidants correlates with higher levels of health.

Most of us have heard a lot about vitamins and minerals, and yet our knowledge about fats and oils, for the most part, is pretty hazy. It's a nutritional scandal, as dietary fats are just as important to health as vitamins and minerals.

We know that too much saturated fat isn't a good thing, but did you know that ultra-low fat diets can lead to health problems by causing deficiencies of the fat-soluble vitamins and have been linked to serious birth defects?

Or that trans-fatty acids in some poly-unsaturated margarines – sold as 'healthier' alternatives to butter – may actually increase the risk of heart disease, and probably certain cancers?

It's true that poly-unsaturated fatty acids can be good for you, but what the food manufacturers don't tell you is that PUFAs come in two forms: **cis**, which occur naturally and are essential to health, and **trans**, which are neither of those things. Unfortunately the body cannot discriminate between the two, so trans-fats in the diet are incorporated into cell membranes and tissues where cis-fats should be. Once there, they impair various aspects of cell function.

Trans-fats compete with normal fats in the body for enzymes. They replace normal fats and oils, with unknown consequences in eicosanoid formation, and cell membranes and functions[75, 78].

Because of their ability to substitute for normal fats, trans-fats raise levels of 'bad' LDL cholesterol in the blood, lower levels of 'good' HDL cholesterol, increase levels of triglycerides (a particularly important risk factor in women), and increase levels of lipoprotein (a hereditary risk factor for coronary artery disease that is otherwise little affected by diet[79, 80, 108]).

The resulting health problems are thought to include a loss of skin pliability, impaired brain and nervous function, an increased tendency to asthma and rheumatoid arthritis, and an elevated risk of coronary artery disease.

It is amazing that in most countries, with the exception of Scandinavia, little has been done to remove these pernicious fats from the food chain.

The links between trans-fat consumption and heart disease are particularly strong[73, 74].

In one early study, people dying of CAD (Coronary Artery Disease) were found to have higher levels of trans-fats in their bodies than in people who had died from other causes[81]. This was not conclusive evidence, but it was highly suggestive; and then other trials began to show similar findings.

In one recent clinical trial, 748 men between the ages of 43 and 85 were studied to assess the effects of trans-fats on blood lipids. The doctors discovered that trans-fats not only had an

Impaired cell membranes

Fatty acids, built into phospholipids, form the bulk of cell membranes (see Chapter 17, A healthy brain). The altered structure of trans-fats disrupts normal cell membrane structure (causing irregularities known as 'packing defects').

The best vegetable oils

Go for cold-pressed vegetable oils with the highest Vitamin E/ PUFA ratio.

Safflower, cottonseed, olive and sunflower oils are best.

Corn and peanut oils are intermediate.

Soy oil and rapeseed oils are worst in this respect. Soy oil contains a version of Vitamin E called gamma tocopherol which our bodies are unable to utilise. So, if you use a lot of soy oil, consider an additional Vitamin E supplement.

For cooking, keep to mono-unsaturates such as olive oil.

adverse effect on blood lipid (ie fat) levels and ratios, but also increased the risk of a heart attack[14].

The following year, in a separate and very major study, a team of researchers at Harvard who had been studying 85,000 nurses for eight years, published results which confirmed the earlier findings. The data showed unequivocally that the nurses who ate margarine with high levels of trans-fats were at a higher risk of developing heart disease than those who ate butter[15].

The best evidence we have shows that an above average consumption of trans-fats nearly doubles the risk of a heart attack in men, and increases it by 60 per cent in women[82, 83] – causing more than 30,000 deaths per year in the USA alone[84].

Trans-fats may harm the unborn as well. They cross the placenta and are incorporated into foetal tissue, concentrating in the developing central nervous system. Unsurprisingly, an increased consumption of trans-fats in pregnant women has been linked to premature births, and low-birth-weight infants with a high risk of brain damage[86].

Too many processed foods are made with trans-fats. To avoid them, check on the label for 'vegetable fat', or 'partially hydrogenated vegetable oil'. Anyone who eats a lot of processed foods is at risk: vegetarians who eat basic foods do well, but vegetarians who eat a lot of convenience foods and hence a lot of trans vegetable fats, are especially vulnerable.

Why on earth should the manufacturers spend so much time and money changing perfectly healthy cis-PUFAs into unhealthy trans-PUFAs? Simple – the trans-fat forms are more suited to margarines, keep for longer and have better 'spreadability'. But what a price to pay!

(Small amounts of some trans-fats occur naturally in animal fats – but these are not the same as the trans-fats produced by industry, and don't appear to be as cardio-toxic.)

ULTRA-LOW-FAT DIETS

An ultra-low-fat diet not only leads to skin lesions and other problems but, if the dieter becomes pregnant, also increases the risk of foetal and paediatric complications including cerebral palsy. This is because, as the foetus grows, the developing brain and nervous system requires large amounts of PUFAs. A deficiency in the maternal diet can interfere with the normal growth of the baby's brain.

In addition, a very low-fat diet will reduce the amount of fat-soluble micro-nutrients (Vitamins A, D, E and K, and the carotenoids) absorbed from the diet. All these nutrients have, among other things, anti-oxidant properties.

I do not recommend ultra low-fat diets, even for coronary artery disease patients; there are more elegant alternatives (see Chapters 5, Anti-oxidants, and 6, Flavonoids & isoflavones).

No 1 for heart attacks

British men and women are at the top of the international heart attack league tables, although Eastern Europe is currently catching up.

The harsh reality behind these statistics is that one in every three British men, and one in every four women, die of coronary artery disease (CAD). And the tragedy is that it's largely preventable.

Trans Spotting

The trans-fat story starts just before World War 1. There was a glut of cheap vegetable and fish oils, difficult to sell and to store because they quickly went rancid.

Scientists and industrialists looked for ways to improve the keeping qualities of the oils, and in 1912 the process of hydrogenation was launched on an unsuspecting world.

By boiling the oils at high temperatures for hours on end, under hydrogen gas and in the presence of a nickel catalyst, the oils turned to fats. They solidified, becoming easier to store and less prone to turning rancid, and they took the market by storm.

In Europe it was predominantly fish oils that were boiled down into margarine, and in the USA they mostly used vegetable oils, but the end product was pretty similar. The public lapped it up. And a mere eight years later, in 1920, coronary artery disease really started to take off.

The consumption of trans-fats increased during the first half of the century, and then stabilised[107], a pattern which runs very much in parallel with the Coronary Artery Disease epidemic.

Today, trans-fats constitute about five per cent of dietary fat in the USA[75]. In processed foods such as cookies, pastries and french fries, trans-fats are generally over 10 per cent of the total fat content.

In margarines, the trans-fat content is often over 10 per cent, and in some brands may be as high as 60 per cent[76, 77]. Manufacturers are beginning to catch on and newer brands are better in this respect.

Fats and ageing

As we get older, our tissues deteriorate as they steadily lose PUFAs from their cell membranes[56, 57]. Most PUFA loss is due to oxidation[58], and anti-oxidants exert many of their health benefits by slowing down this degenerative process[59].

The central nervous system (including the brain) contains particularly high levels of PUFAs, in the membranes of nerve cells or neurones. As we get older PUFA oxidation in the brain and damage to nerve cell membranes contributes to brain cell death, memory loss, and eventually senile dementia (See Chapter 17, A healthy brain).

The products of PUFA oxidation include LOPs, which as we saw earlier are highly toxic, and lipofucsin, the so-called brown age pigment. The rate at which lipofucsin builds up increases if the diet is deficient in anti-oxidants[97]. Lipofucsin in the skin forms 'age spots', which are unsightly but harmless. When it accumulates inside nerve cells, however, it slows them down and eventually kills them.

Anti-oxidants which enter the brain and concentrate in the nerve cell membranes and prevent PUFA oxidation should protect against premature brain cell death. The latest data strongly suggests that they do.

Age spots

Centrophenoxine, a powerful anti-oxidant drug which concentrates in lipids, removes lipofucsin deposits[100, 101]. It erases age spots and is reported to improve mental function in elderly rats – and humans too[102, 103].

A question of thyme

Some fascinating work has been done on the oil found in the herb thyme at the Scottish Agricultural College in Auchincruive, Ayr. Thyme oil contains thymol, a powerful anti-oxidant, which has the useful property of concentrating in the membranes of the nerve cells in the brain.

Thyme oil has another complementary effect; it boosts levels in the body of glutathione peroxidase, an anti-oxidant enzyme involved in preventing PUFA oxidation.

The Scottish group fed thyme oil to mice and found that its dual effect led to a significant reduction in oxidative damage. The bodies and brains of the mice retained the PUFA composition of young animals, even into old age[60].

INCLUDE ...

Thyme, clove, nutmeg and pepper oils in your cooking.

Research shows they protect poly-unsaturated fats in the body and the brain.

The brains of the thyme-travelled mice showed significantly fewer signs of ageing, and had retained a higher number of viable nerve cells than the brains of untreated mice. This suggests that the inexorable loss of brain cells which accompanies human ageing could also be stopped, or at least slowed, by thyme oil.

If you don't like the taste or scent of thyme, there's a reasonably wide choice of alternative herbs and spices. The Scottish team showed that PUFA levels in aged mice can be almost equally well preserved with clove, nutmeg and pepper oils[62].

The Eskimo diet

In some countries, heart disease is uncommon, even rare. The Eskimos, for example, don't have a word in their language for a heart attack. In one study a Danish doctor examined 2,400 Eskimos and found, remarkably, only three of them with any signs of heart disease[150].

So what is the Eskimo secret? It's simple. Like us, the Eskimos are what they eat. After extensive research, cardiologists concluded that it is the Eskimos' eating pattern which makes them so immune to coronary artery disease. Many nutritionists recommend a so-called Eskimo diet to reduce our appalling incidence of heart attacks. But does anybody know what the Eskimos really eat? And if they did, would the Western palate be able to cope with it?

Before the arrival of modern processed foods, the Eskimo diet consisted largely of fish, shellfish and sea mammals such as seals, whales and walrus. And although they inhabited terrain known as 'the largest deepfreeze in the world', their diet was strictly seasonal.

Throughout the long winter the average Eskimo would chew his or her way through a couple of pounds of seal meat and blubber every day. Come the spring, and the salmon run would provide a welcome change of diet, together with varied shellfish – two to three pounds of salmon a day, even more during periods of heavy activity, was not unusual. Later in the year mackerel,

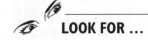

LOOK FOR ...

Thyme oil as a nutritional supplement as you get older.

It's a powerful anti-oxidant and may help to maintain brain function.

Toxic fish

Dangerous organic pollutants including pesticides and coolants are dumped at sea, and permeate the food chain from algae to fish to seals – where they are implicated in causing recent mass kills.

Choose, if you can, fish oils certified free from these toxins.

Fish oil reduces:

At low doses

- **Electrical instability of the heart muscle**

At higher doses

- **Inflammation of the artery walls**

- **The risk of blood clots**

- **LDL (the bad) cholesterol**

- **Blood triglyceride levels**

This combination reduces your risk of a fatal heart attack.

herring and cod would appear on the menu and, here again, a consumption of two or three pounds of fish per day was by no means untypical.

In the summer there might be assorted berries and roots, but the bulk of the Eskimo's food came from the sea. And because the marine food chain starts with plankton, which is a rich source of Omega 3 fatty acids, the Eskimo ate a large amount of these oils.

This is in complete contrast to the Western diet, which contains a great deal of saturated fat and only tiny amounts of Omega 3. But following an authentic Eskimo diet would be extremely difficult. Even if you could persuade your local supermarket to stock it, you might not be so keen on chewing under-cooked seal fat every day of the week.

Fortunately, there's an alternative. The seal gets its Omega 3 oils from the fish it eats, such as salmon, herring, anchovies, mackerel and tuna – and so can you.

A real chance of avoiding heart disease?

Does it work? In a word, yes. This particular nutritional topic has been intensively studied, yielding enough scientific evidence to convince even the most hardened sceptic.

Numerous studies have revealed that large doses of fish oil block many of the steps in the pathological sequence of events that culminates in a heart attack.

To begin with, the PUFAs (poly-unsaturated fatty acids) in fish oil reduce inflammation in the body[161, 162, 203]. Inflammation in the artery walls is one of the earliest steps in the formation of atheroma. Fish oil calms the arteries down, and reduces any inflammatory changes there. This is probably one way fish oil reduces the amount of LDL cholesterol (the 'bad cholesterol') entering the artery wall[162] – an integral and early step in the formation of atheroma.

Fish oil also reduces platelet stickiness, which inhibits clotting[163-165, 183, 201, 208], rather like aspirin does. This reduces the risk of thrombosis, which is generally the last link in the chain that leads to the heart attack.

Fish oil's ability to inhibit both the beginning and the end of the process that culminates in the heart attack begins to explain the Eskimo's good health, but there is more.

Fish oil reduces the level of LDL, the 'bad' cholesterol in the blood[174, 175], which is desirable in men. It also lowers triglycerides[166, 167], which is important particularly for women, for whom high triglyceride levels increase the risk of heart disease as much as five times[158]. At the same time, fish oil increases levels of HDL, the 'good' cholesterol which lowers the risk of a heart attack[184].

In addition, fish oils tend to prevent the constriction of small arteries, which again reduces the risk of blood clots forming[168, 197, 198]. This opening up of the small arteries, together with the cholesterol-lowering effect, probably explains why fish oil can lower the blood pressure by a small but significant amount, particularly in patients with hypertension and/or coronary artery disease[169, 190-195]. It also explains why so many patients say that fish oil alleviates their angina.

Finally, and at even quite small doses, fish oil reduces the tendency of the heart to develop an arrhythmia (irregular heartbeat)[170], a common cause of death after heart attacks.

Fish on trial

There are at least six ways in which fish oils theoretically protect the heart; but do they work in practice? The answer is yes.

There has been one major trial in the UK, the so-called DART study. DART stands for Diet and Reinfarction Trial and, as the name suggests, the subjects were at above average risk because they had already had at least one heart attack.

This trial showed that oily fish, or fish oil capsules, reduced the risk of a second fatal heart attack by 29 per cent[152]. This is a very significant reduction, all the more so because the subjects all had damaged hearts and arteries.

Which raises the question, how effective could fish oil be in healthy subjects, whose cardiovascular systems are in relatively good shape?

30% Reduction in Heart Disease with Omega 3

A major British study found fish oil reduced the risk of a second attack in heart patients by nearly 30 per cent[152].

In an American trial of high risk men, large doses of Omega 3 cut the risk of heart attack by over 30 per cent[153].

... even in low doses

The protective effects of small doses of fish oil (ie in capsules) are due to its abilility to prevent heart arrhythmias.

Ginkgo too?

Anyone prone to clotting disorders, and most Europeans[204], should consider combining fish oil with ginkgo and Vitamin E.

Ginkgo or Vitamin E also prevent unwanted clot formation in a way which augments the effects of fish oil.

The Eskimo data suggests that if you take enough fish oil, you probably won't get heart disease at all. But what happens if you eat a Western diet, with added fish?

In 1973 some 13,000 American men at risk of developing coronary artery disease were recruited into the Multiple Risk Factor Intervention Trial (MRFIT). (They were thought to have an elevated risk of CAD because they either smoked, had a high cholesterol or blood pressure, or all three.)

The trial ran until 1982, and the results make interesting reading. The more Omega 3 oils in the diet, the lower the risk of coronary artery disease, cerebrovascular disease and total mortality. The benefits were clearest in the highest dose group, who were consuming an average of 664mg Omega 3 a day. In this group, the risk of death from coronary artery disease was reduced by a little over a third[153].

A large Dutch study also concluded that eating more fish reduced the risk of heart attacks[154] and strokes[199]. Other studies have produced more or less identical findings[2, 3, 155, 156, 205-208].

Giving women priority

One of the problems with studies of coronary artery disease is that they concentrate almost exclusively on men. Women are conspicuous by their absence – which is a scandal, because this act of omission has led to lower standards of care for women.

It is only very recently, for example, that it has been shown that raised blood cholesterol (a risk factor in men) is not necessarily very important in women at all[157].

In women, raised triglycerides (another component of the blood lipid profile) are now considered to be much more important[158]. Fish oil, as we have seen, is particularly good at reducing blood triglycerides[166, 167].

This is a good reason for women to take fish oil or Omega 3 supplements, but there is more. Even though women are nearly as much at risk of CAD as men, the myth that women don't get CAD has prejudiced the medical profession to the extent that they do not give women such good care as men.

A woman with a cardiac problem is less likely to be diagnosed, less likely to be sent to a consultant, less likely to be given intensive care, and more likely, as a result, to do badly[159, 160]. That's another reason for women to pay special attention to preventative health care, and good cardio-protective nutrition.

Finally, for younger women, there is evidence that a fish oil supplement reduces the risk of developing the potentially dangerous increase in blood pressure that occurs in some pregnancies[181] and the risk of premature births[182].

Fish or supplements?

Governments and doctors alike have agreed that everyone should eat more oily fish[177, 178].

Nobody's going to eat an authentic Inuit (Eskimo) diet, but eating a good portion of oily fish three times a week will reduce the risk of coronary artery disease; not to the vanishingly low levels of the Inuit, but it will at least cut the Western risk of CAD by up to a third.

A simple change in eating habits should do the trick. Unfortunately, people don't work like that. Even people who have had a heart attack, and have been told to eat oily fish, don't generally do it for long. They won't modify their eating habits. They don't like the taste, they don't like the bones or they don't know how to cook it. They're worried about putting on weight, because the kilo of oily fish a week needed to get the recommended dose of 1- 2 grams a day of the vital Omega 3 oils knocks up over 4,000 calories.

A tiny minority of people – mostly in coastal communities – are genuinely allergic to fish.

There is also concern about levels of heavy metals and other contaminants such as PCBs and organo-phosphates in fish. Our unappealing habit of dumping industrial waste at sea has polluted many fishing sites to the point where measurable amounts of heavy metals and organic contaminants are commonly found in the catch.

Some governmental advisers have suggested, off the record, that fish should not be eaten more than twice a week.

This means that for many people, fish oil capsules are a preferred alternative. Whole fish contains certain nutrients that fish oil capsules miss out, such as iodine and selenium, but a good fish oil (or flax or hemp oil) supplement ensures that you get enough of the Omega 3 oils to reduce your risk of CAD.

LOOK FOR ...

an Omega 3 capsule in the form of free fatty acids or triglycerides, rather than ethyl esters.

Oily fish

Oily fish are better than fish oil, because they contain other good things – such as iodine, selenium and astaxanthin. This little-known carotenoid is a powerful anti-oxidant and anti-cancer agent. Derived from red algae, it is the red in red salmon, crayfish and flamingoes' legs.

Cod liver oil

Cod liver oil is the top selling supplement. But its benefits are not as clear as fish oil capsules.

First, fish oil capsules deliver far more Omega 3 by weight.

Secondly, a reputable brand of Omega 3 is less likely to be contaminated by heavy metal and other pollutants from ocean dumping.

And thirdly, cod liver oil contains Vitamins A and D – which can cause problems in overdose.

Sun factor

High doses of fish oil protect against sunburn[203]; and should be combined with Vitamins C and E and mixed carotenoids.

Asthma

Some asthmatics respond positively to fish oil[41].

FISH OIL MUST BE COMBINED WITH ANTI-OXIDANTS

Because poly-unsaturated oils are so prone to oxidation, it is very important to combine them with an anti-oxidant preparation, especially if you smoke.

Otherwise, you are likely to increase the load of PUFA radicals and oxidation products in your body, which are actually harmful to the arteries[171-173]. This may explain the disappointing results of a recent trial which found that fish oil supplements on their own have little effect on preventing atheroma formation[200].

The ideal anti-oxidant combination should contain

- Vitamin E (400IU/day)
- Vitamin C (500-1000mg)
- Mixed carotenoids (10-20mg)
- Mixed flavonoids (100-500mg)
- Co-enzyme Q10 (30-120 mg/day)

Co-enzyme Q10 is particularly recommended. Apart from its other benefits (see Chapter 9, Co-enzyme Q10), it is very good at preventing the increase in free radicals otherwise caused by fish oil supplements[196].

Helps osteoporosis, arthritis and smokers too!

Taken in large amounts (8-10g a day) fish oil can be also used as part of a nutritional programme to prevent osteoporosis. It has various effects on the body's ability to handle calcium. It has been shown to enhance new bone growth[179], and reduce the loss of calcium after the menopause[180] (see Chapter 15, Bones). **Lower doses of fish oil are ineffective.**

In addition, the anti-inflammatory properties of fish oil can play a very useful role in the treatment of arthritis. Increasing the amount of oily fish in the diet, or taking fish oil supplements, has been shown to reduce pain and stiffness in inflamed joints[40, 188, 189, 202, 206].

Other diseases where an anti-inflammatory effect is very helpful include the tobacco-related lung diseases, which are caused by the flood of inflammatory free radicals in cigarette smoke.

Eating more oily fish improves lung function, even in smokers[185, 186]. Another study found that smokers who ate a lot of oily fish cut their risk of developing chronic bronchitis and emphysema by two thirds and one third respectively[187].

Fish oil facts

What makes a good fish oil? The type of fish is irrelevant. All that matters is the content of the two key Omega 3 oils: eicosapentaenoic acid (EPA) and docosahexaenoic acid (DHA).

Not all brands of fish oil are equal in this respect: some have little medicinal value, with very low levels of EPA and DHA, and are the same grade of fish oil used in some parts of Scandinavia to run central heating plants!

- Check the small print and the EPA and DHA content. You need at least 500mg of Omega 3 a day.

- Check the form of the Omega 3s: free fatty acids and triglycerides are the best absorbed, while the cheaper esters are not good in this respect.

- Check that the preparation is certified free from heavy metal contamination, and from Vitamins A and D. These two vitamins are fine in moderation, but overdose can cause serious health problems.

- Avoid bottled fish oil such as cod liver oils. Many cod liver oils are low grade and do not contain sufficient anti-oxidants.

If it smells fishy, it's gone off, and the oil has begun to oxidise. Oxidised or rancid oils don't do you any good at all, and have been linked to the type of damage to the arteries that leads to coronary artery disease[171-173].

- Go for fish oil in capsules, and make sure the manufacturer has included an anti-oxidant such as Vitamin E.

- Always take them with meals.

OTHER SOURCES OF EPA AND DHA

If a fish-based diet is too expensive or you are vegetarian, there are alternatives.

- Eat plenty of linseed, hempseed or their oils, and walnuts and pecans. These foods don't contain EPA and DHA, but they do contain linolenic acid (LNA), which the body uses to make EPA and DHA.

  It's a slow process, and can be blocked by high levels of the Omega 6 PUFAs – found in most poly-unsaturated oils and spreads. So keep these to a minimum and cut down on meat and dairy produce for the same reason.

- EPA/DHA supplements derived from commercially grown marine algae (see below) will be available in the near future.

- In years to come crops will be bred to yield corn oil, for instance, containing EPA, DHA, more GLA and even more exotic oils designed for specific health benefits[171, 176]. Not all GM crops are bad!

- Another alternative is stearadonic acid, an Omega 3 oil derived from the purple viper bugloss. This will be commercially available in the next few years.

Go wild!

Wild salmon feed on marine algae which contain Omega 3.

Farmed salmon frequently have a lower Omega 3 content as they are usually fed on food pellets that have a lower Omega 3 content.

SUMMARY

The Good Fat Guide

▶ Follow a Mediterranean-style diet – olive oil, vegetables, fish, herbs like thyme and rosemary – and less meat.

▶ Cut down on saturated fats (dairy products and red meat) which block the production of EPA and DHA.

▶ Eat more mono-unsaturated oils like olive oil, and more Omega 3 oils – fish oil, and walnut, sunflower and soya bean oils.

▶ Switch to wild game or free-range meat which has less saturated fat than farmed meat.

▶ Increase your Omega 3 PUFAs with herring, wild salmon and trout, mackerel and tuna around three times a week.

▶ Take a daily Omega 3 supplement with 400IU Vitamin E and 500mg Vitamin C, mixed carotenoids and flavonoids. Look for fish oil in capsules rather than bottled.

▶ The Omega 3 supplement should :
  • have high levels of EPA and DHA (500mg a day total)
  • provide Omega 3 in the form of free fatty acids or triglycerides
  • not contain Vitamins A or D
  • be certified free of heavy metal and organic contaminants
  • have a clear 'sell by' date.

▶ A good Omega 3 supplement reduces your risk of a heart attack.

▶ Keep oils, especially polyunsaturates, in dark glass, in the fridge.

▶ When cooking, don't overheat the oil. If it's smoking it's too hot. Don't use iron cookware with oils or fats. Don't re-use cooking oil.

▶ Add ginkgo if you're prone to clotting disorders. Add garlic, rosemary or thyme when cooking for additional benefits.

▶ Add grapeseed or green tea extract (available from health food suppliers) to oil before using for cooking – it stops COPs and LOPs forming.

▶ Grind rosemary, sage, thyme or oregano in olive oil, and use it for flavour and better keeping.

▶ Use one of the more 'peppery' olive oils. These contain powerful flavonoid anti-oxidants[42].

▶ Cut down on or avoid:
  • poly-unsaturated vegetable oils and spreads.
  • foods which contain hydrogenated vegetable oils or fats.
  • animal fats like butter and lard for frying.
  • deep-fried food from commercial establishments.

- A course of Q10 can improve your fitness – without moving a muscle

- Q10 deficiency leaves us feeling tired, and vulnerable to heart disease, infection and cancer

- This vitamin-like substance can boost an athlete's performance by up to 13 per cent

- In trials high dose Q10 significantly improved the condition of patients with heart failure, gum disease and certain types of cancer

Chapter 9

The Q Factor

In August '94, the first recorded health food robbery took place, in Drammen, Norway. A well-organised band of criminals broke into a factory owned by health supplement company Pharma Nord, and made off with 17,000 packs of Bio-Quinone Q10. Valuable equipment, confidential documents and even the office safe were left untouched: the thieves were only interested in Co-enzyme Q10, which almost became an alternative currency in Norway after it was launched in the spring of '93.

Norway is not unique in its love affair with Q10. In every country where Q10 is sold, it has done amazingly well. The general public take it because it is a remarkable energy booster. Cyclists, runners, cross-country skiers, hockey players and other athletes have found that Q10 increases stamina and improves performance.

Dentists use Q10 to clear up gingivitis, the gum disease that causes more tooth loss than dental decay. Heart specialists use it to treat heart failure, angina, hypertension, and to prevent the cardiotoxicity caused by certain anti-cancer drugs. Perhaps most remarkably of all, a team of specialists in Stockholm and Texas have used Q10, in conjunction with other nutrients, with great success to treat advanced breast cancer.

Doctors unfamiliar with Q10 find it difficult to understand how a single nutrient can have so many therapeutic effects. They dismiss it as a placebo. When yet another person comes into the surgery singing the praises of Q10, they see this as just simply an example of the public's gullibility.

Q10 – Ubiquinone

Q10 is technically a quinone. The molecule is structurally quite similar to Vitamin E and the carotenoids.

Q10 is found everywhere – hence its name *ubiquinone*. First extracted from the tobacco plant, and subsequently from beef heart, commercial production now starts from yeast.

However, once you know how Q10 works, and what it does at the cellular level, its wide range of clinical uses makes sense. It's harder to understand why it has taken so long for many in the medical profession to appreciate what Q10 could do for them – and their patients.

What is Q10?

Co-enzyme Q10 is often referred to as Vitamin Q, but although it is vital to life, and occurs in trace amounts in certain foods such as sardines, Q10 is not technically a vitamin because we can produce small amounts of it ourselves in the liver.

Unfortunately, the process requires at least six other vitamins and minerals – and most people are depleted in one or more of these. Heavy drinking and liver disease slow the making of Q10 even further. The final problem is that after the age of 40 or so, our ability to make Q10 declines[42, 43, 46, 108], and levels of Q10 in the diet are too low to compensate for this.

This is where our troubles begin, because Q10 has two main roles in the body, both of which are vital for our health. It is a potent anti-oxidant[23-28, 70,] and it is central to energy production[4, 29-33, 65].

Q10 the anti-oxidant

Q10 is a powerful anti-oxidant like Vitamin E. It protects the lipids in cell membranes[110, 116] and LDL cholesterol ('bad cholesterol') in the blood[34, 35] preventing them from going rancid. Rancid cholesterol is considered to be a major cause of heart disease, so Q10 protects against heart attacks.

Some studies show that Q10 is better at protecting LDL cholesterol than Vitamin E[36, 93-95] – and, according to the major '94 Harvard trial, Vitamin E can cut the risk of coronary artery disease by over 40 per cent. Q10 may be even better than Vitamin E[21-23, 77], and a combination of Q10, E, C and a few other micro-nutrients should make you more or less immune to heart disease!

Q10's ability to protect against free radicals should also reduce the risk of cancer. But that's only half the story …

Discovered in the 1960s

Co-enzyme Q10 was discovered in Britain over 30 years ago[3], and earned Professor Peter Mitchell the 1978 Nobel Prize for Chemistry.

His discovery was ignored by British industry, and developed by the Japanese and Americans.

Many hundreds of research projects and scientific publications later, the importance of this 'new' nutrient is becoming clear.

Super Oxide Dismutase (SOD)

Q10 may also stimulate the body to produce more SOD, a key anti-oxidant enzyme[85, 86].

Q10 the Energiser

… because Q10, unlike any other anti-oxidant, is part of the process that gives us energy.

This process takes place inside the mitochondria. The mitochondria are tiny, bean-shaped structures which are the power-houses of each cell. The process transfers energy from the food we eat to ATP, which fuels the cells.

If cells lack Q10, they can't produce enough ATP. When Q10 levels are low, nerve cells fire less efficiently, the tails of sperm beat less strongly[109], muscle fibres tire more easily and, perhaps most notably, the heart beats less powerfully[38, 57].

Low Q10 is considered by some specialists in this field to be a prime cause of heart failure and a significant contributing factor to hypertension.

An early sign of Q10 depletion is feeling tired and drained of energy. The end stage of Q10 depletion is, inevitably, death.

The combination of Q10's anti-oxidant and energy producing properties makes it important for the immune system too. This means that a lack of Q10 is associated not only with heart disease and low energy, but also with a decreased ability to fight infection and an increased risk of cancer[91]. In short, the body begins to show all the signs of ageing.

Q10 – an antidote to ageing?

Some researchers believe that many symptoms of ageing are linked to the age-related slow-down in Q10 production[105-107], and many recommend Q10 supplements as part of an anti-ageing therapy.

In one animal experiment, Q10 supplements extended the life span of mice by up to 45 per cent, although it had little effect on rats[106]. If humans respond like mice rather than rats, this could mean an additional 30 to 40 years of life.

If this seems far-fetched, take a look at how Q10 reduces the impact of the ageing process on our cells. It's called the Mitochondrial Theory of Ageing, and the evidence to support it is quite persuasive.

Energy Formation

Energy is transferred from the food we eat into ATP, the cells' basic energy storing molecules. This energy transfer is called oxidative phosphorylation, and takes place in the mitochondria.

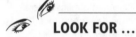

LOOK FOR …

a Q10 supplement in oil form (in a gel) at a level of at least 30mg a day – 90mg is preferable.

"The chances are 99% that free radicals are the basis for ageing."

Prof. Denham Harman, University of Nebraska Medical School

The Mitochondrial Theory of Ageing

1 The mitochondria are the cell's energy factories. It's where the main components in food are burned to create energy.

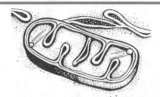

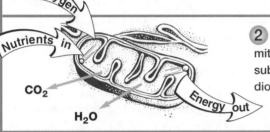

2 Nutrients are burned – with oxygen – in the mitochondria to produce energy in the form of a substance called ATP. The by-products are carbon dioxide (CO_2), water (H_2O), heat and free radicals.

3 Co-enzyme Q10 is needed for two important reasons.
1) It promotes the efficient production of energy (ATP) and,
2) It quenches the burst of free radicals that occurs when nutrients are oxidised, ie are burned in the presence of oxygen.
A healthy and young body will generate approximately 95% energy (ATP) and 5% free radicals within the mitochondria.

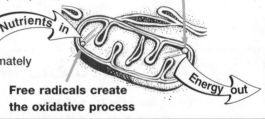

Q10 quenches and neutralises free radicals

Free radicals create the oxidative process

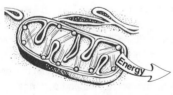

4 Without Q10 supplementation, the amount of Co-enzyme Q10 a person produces is reduced as they get older. The proportion of energy generated by the mitochondria drops to 75% and the proportion of free radicals rises to 25%. So, not only is less energy available, but more free radical damage occurs. The body cells are becoming less efficient[91,118].

5 Eventually this free radical damage means that the mitochondrial output of ATP energy is severely reduced. The cell switches to self-destruct and eventually dies. Ageing of the whole body would now be rapid. When enough cells self-destruct, organs fail and death results.

Anti-ageing strategies must include Co-enzyme Q10 and beta carotene supplements, as these nutrients – uniquely – protect mitochondria from within. Acetyl carnitine has also been shown to be protective but acts externally.

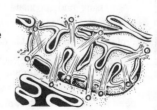

As mitochondria produce the energy their cells need, they also generate free radicals – which inflict accumulative damage on the mitochondrial structures. This is why elderly people have more damaged and less efficient mitochondria than younger people[80, 82]. This means that older people's cells don't function as well – tissues are slower to heal, for instance.

Q10 is an unusually interesting potential antidote. This is because Q10 increases the amount of energy that elderly, damaged mitochondria can produce[44]. And thanks to Q10's anti-oxidant qualities, it can cope with the additional free radicals this produces and protect mitochondria from further damage[45, 47-49, 87, 104].

It will be some time (perhaps another 20 years or so) before we have definitive evidence for Q10's ability to extend human life. But, in the meantime, there are very definite short-term gains that you can experience for yourself with Q10 supplements.

The most obvious of these is the increase in energy which appears at levels of 30 to 100 mg a day.

Beta carotene

Q10 should be combined with beta carotene. Beta carotene concentrates in the inner mitochondrial membranes, where the low oxygen levels enable it to play an anti-oxidant and damage-limiting role[155].

Q10 and heart disease

In 1993, at the 8th International Symposium on Q10, doctors from around the world reported using Q10 to treat angina, hypertension and heart failure.

In some cases heart failure patients improved from being bedridden to walking out of the hospital. A significant minority were able to stop taking all their medications[6, 7, 50-53, 97-99].

These extraordinary results confirmed predictions made a quarter of a century before, by scientists who found low Q10 in the hearts of patients who died of heart failure and speculated that Q10 replacement therapy might be an answer[66].

Professor Svend Aage Mortensen, who heads the Danish heart transplant programme, told the stunned meeting about his terminally ill patients. These invalids, who were waiting either to die or for a new heart to become available, responded so well to Q10 that several were able to come off the surgery waiting list – a world first.

Professor Karl Folkers, only the fourth person to receive the prestigious American Achievement Award in Preventative Medicine, told me: "Just as scurvy is a deficiency of Vitamin C, so is heart failure due to a deficiency of Q10. The studies all show that the lower the Q10 content, the worse the heart performs.

"There are other factors too, but Q10 is critical. When you give Q10 to a patient with heart failure[71], or even to elderly subjects with healthy hearts[72], you get a clear-cut and positive response.

"The studies show that as many as 97 per cent of the adult population is low in Q10. And if you look at the figures for heart disease, you can see the end result."

The no-exercise fitness programme

Could you improve your stamina, raise your energy levels and strengthen your heart without taking any exercise at all? It sounds unlikely, but, if for whatever reason levels of Q10 in your body are low, Q10 supplements can make a noticeable difference.

Research shows that Q10 supplements boost mitochondrial function, providing the body's cells (including the muscle cells) with more energy.

Professor Vanfraechem is senior researcher at the Laboratoire de L'Effort at the Free University of Brussels. He knew that Co-enzyme Q10 can be extremely helpful in heart failure by strengthening the heart, and guessed it might have a similar effect in healthy people.

The guinea pigs were medical students who were healthy but unfit. Professor Vanfraechem gave them Co-enzyme Q10 for eight weeks. It improved their physical fitness and strengthened their heartbeat by up to 20 per cent – the sort of improvement normally only found after an intensive course of exercise.

At Kobe University in Japan, Dr Hiroshi Yamabe and Dr Hisashi Fukuzaki carried out similar experiments with middle-aged women complaining of low energy levels and constant tiredness. After three months of treatment with 60mg Q10 a day, they improved their fitness by over 30 per cent. And, just as important, they felt much less tired[12].

Q10 and heart patients

Q10's combination of anti-oxidant and bio-energetic properties reduces oxidation injury to the heart.

In a recent trial, patients given Q10 before heart bypass grafts had less oxidative damage and fewer ventricular arrhythmia – irregular heart beats after surgery[81].

In another study, Q10 given to heart attack patients improved their symptoms and outcome very significantly[141].

ATHLETIC FANS

Q10 has gained a host of athletic converts. Sam Wright plays for the UK women's hockey team that won a bronze medal at the 1992 Olympics. "Last year I went down with a virus, and I was totally fatigued.

"I changed my diet and exercise programme, and I started taking Q10. Since then I've been really well, the fittest I've been for a long time.

"About half the squad are taking it, and we all want to go on with it as part of our training. There isn't too much difference between the top teams in the world, but if we get a bit extra from the Q10, that could make the difference between bronze and gold."

Jonathan Edwards, World and Olympic Triple Jump Champion, also swears by Q10 and takes it as part of his nutritional programme.

ME Patients

There are anecdotal reports of ME patients responding positively to high dose Q10, often given with an Omega 3 oil preparation.

Athletic use

If Q10 can improve physical performance by a third in untrained subjects, what might it do for athletes? At the University of Bologna, a team of scientists has been studying just this. Dr Pier Fiorella took a group of top runners and gave half of them Q10 for 40 days. Then the runners were sent on endurance trials.

The Q10 group outperformed the control group by 13 per cent[13]. In top level athletics this is a considerable gain – enough to put an also-ran onto the winning rostrum. The Q10 athletes also showed less sign of the muscle damage that usually follows endurance events[14], showing they would be able to train harder and recover more quickly between races.

Other researchers have published similar findings: even in well-nourished and apparently healthy subjects, supplements have been shown to increase Q10 levels in the muscles, and boost exercise capacity accordingly[58, 59]. In contrast, there has been only one negative report to date[92].

In the early days some athletes were suspicious of Q10, thinking that it might be a new form of doping. In fact, it's more like fluid replacement during a race. We manufacture Q10 in our bodies and during periods of intensive exercise blood levels of Q10 drop, possibly because it is being taken up by the muscles.

A Q10 supplement merely returns levels to normal[60-64]. Taking Q10 to improve performance is not so different to eating a specialised sports diet. If you could swallow three pounds of sardines a day you'd get an effective dose of Q10 the natural way. So it would be hard to make Q10 illegal.

The problem is that for dietary and other reasons we can't always make enough of it and, when levels of Q10 begin to fall, tiredness, loss of energy and performance follow. Taking a supplement to top up the levels of Q10 in the body is rather like taking extra Vitamin C – and just as safe.

Legal

Q10 levels often fall in athletes. Taking Q10 supplements merely returns them to normal[60-64].

On a cholesterol-lowering drug?

Anyone taking a statin (a cholesterol-lowering drug) should take a Q10 supplement. These drugs block the enzyme that makes cholesterol – but the same enzyme also makes Q10.

Patients taking these drugs tend to have very low Q10 levels[96], with all the risks that this implies. Q10 supplements repair the deficit[79], and are strongly recommended in these cases.

Oral health

Q10 for gum disease

The oral cavity is teeming with bacteria, many of which are potential causes of disease. It is only our immune systems, and oral hygiene, that keep them at bay.

But in many of us the bacteria are winning. Forty to 80 per cent of adults have some degree of gum disease – and gum disease is the biggest cause of tooth loss.

Good brushing and flossing techniques are important, but there is evidence that if you're deficient in Q10, brushing and flossing make little difference[67].

This is why the trials of Q10 in the treatment of gum disease are so interesting, because in the battle between the bacteria and the immune system, Q10 can tip the balance in our favour.

Sadly, the trials that suggest that Q10 supplements may help[10, 11, 15-20, 67, 69] are small and poorly designed – so they cannot be regarded as conclusive.

One problem is that the doses of Q10 used were too small. To achieve high and sustained levels of Q10 in the intracrevicular fluids (in the pockets around the roots of the teeth) requires at least 90mg Q10/day. At this dose Q10 kills the disease-causing anaerobic bacteria by oxidising them – in the same way as the antibiotic metronidazole.

Toothpaste containing 1% Q10 achieves very high levels of Q10 at the roots of the teeth, but only very briefly. A combination, however, of 90mg Q10/day PLUS Q10 toothpaste daily or twice daily should be highly effective at treating gum disease and holding it in check.

Xylitol for tooth decay

The most widely eaten functional food in the UK is Wrigleys Extra chewing gum. This valuable product contains xylitol, a sugar derived from birch bark. Not only does it taste pleasant, it also 'starves' the bacteria which cause dental decay, so that they die off and are replaced by less damaging bacteria.

Xylitol has also been shown to bind to calcium present in the saliva, forming xylitol-calcium complexes which are believed to increase the uptake of calcium into the tooth.

The end result is a very significant reduction in dental decay[142-145]. The changed bacterial populations in the mouth and throat also confer protection against middle ear infections[146].

Stop Press
In early 2000, Wrigleys (USA) instructed Wrigleys (UK) to remove the xylitol from Extra chewing gum. A bad case of corporate mismanagement – and bad news for British teeth.

Cranberries and green tea

Cranberries help, too. New work suggests that the flavonoids in cranberries prevent disease-causing bacteria sticking to the teeth and gums, and relieve symptoms – just as they do for urinary tract infections.

Finally, green tea – the flavonoids in green tea seem to be as active as those in cranberry (see Chapter 6, Flavonoids & isoflavones).

Green tea is now a major component in functional chewing gums in Japan. How long before it appears in your toothpaste?

Q10 and the cancer connection

Because Q10 is essential for cell energetics, a lack of Q10 leads to impaired cellular function – including the immune cells which form a crucial line of defence against cancer. Conversely, Q10 supplements improve immune function in animals, particularly in elderly animals where Q10 levels are reduced; and give significant protection against cancer[147-149]. Could this have clinical implications?

Professor Karl Folkers, one of the pioneers of Q10 research, found that Q10 levels in blood of cancer patients in Sweden and the USA were uniformly lower than in the controls[75, 150, 151]. He then started an open study, giving high dose Q10 and multi-nutrient support to a small number – 32 – of high risk breast cancer patients. This study does not meet the standards of current oncology trials, and the results are not scientifically safe. Nevertheless, they make fascinating reading[152-154].

All patients were given routine chemotherapy, radiotherapy and surgery. By now, according to the statistics, about nine of them should have died. There have been three deaths, for non-cancer-related reasons. The other 29 women report significant improvements in their condition. They use fewer painkillers, there have been no cases of cancer spread, and six cases of partial or complete cancer remission.

Cancer specialist Dr Knud Lockwood has treated over 200 cases of breast cancer every year for the last 35 years. "I have never before seen spontaneous regression of the type of breast cancers we treated in this trial", he said. "I call this a breakthrough. The fact that the patients feel so well on this treatment is a major bonus, and a huge improvement over conventional therapy."

If Q10 does have an anti-cancer effect, improved immune function may well be involved, but there are other possible modes of action. Cytokines (cellular 'messengers') are essential for some tumours' survival, and may be made by the cancer cells themselves. In one group of myeloma patients, high dose Q10 reduced levels of the cytokine TNF alpha to below detectable levels[2]. This implies that high dose Q10 may be effective in treating other diseases where TNF alpha is involved, including rheumatoid arthritis, asthma and ulcerative colitis.

Although similar results have been reported in the USA[90], leading cancer specialists are taking a cautious line. The finding that levels of Q10 are low in cancer patients is intriguing, but that doesn't necessarily mean that supplementing with Q10 will treat an established cancer. More work is needed.

Sven Moesgaard, the nutritionist who designed the programme, says, "We analysed the entire world literature on the anti-cancer effects of all the vitamins and minerals, and assembled a broad-based nutritional package based on that search.

"According to our patients, and the trial results, which I must emphasise are preliminary results, we think it works. But it's true that we need more data. The pilot trial raises a lot of questions, and we want to follow this up with a much larger study."

The Copenhagen patients have no doubts about the outcome. "When I was asked to join the trial I was hesitant," says Patient C, a 70-year old widow. "But I feel so well on the supplements, better than I've felt for years; whereas other cancer patients I know who just get the ordinary treatments have a terrible time.

"All women with breast cancer should have this treatment. Now the doctors tell me that my cancer has completely disappeared. I call it a miracle."

The future for Q10

There have been, and still are, Q10 sceptics. Their first argument was that Q10 could not be absorbed. Well-designed studies have disproved this: Q10 is absorbed[37-39, 88], if it is given in the optimal formulation.

(It should be pre-dissolved in soy oil in a soft gel, which must be impervious to light as Q10 degrades in sunlight. Q10 is insoluble in water; so Q10 in tablet or powder form is less well absorbed.)

The next concern was that taking Q10 supplements might suppress the body's own Q10 production. However, after stopping a 12-month course of high dose Q10 supplements, volunteers' blood levels of Q10 fell back to pre-treatment levels – but no further[78].

The third objection was that Q10 supplements wouldn't get to the mitochondria and other sites where it is needed. This too has been refuted[88]. People suffering from certain rare diseases, where mitochondrial function is very poor, have been successfully treated with Q10 supplements which boosted mitochondrial function[40, 41, 100-103].

This is no surprise – Q10 is made in the liver, and transported in the blood (in LDL cholesterol) to every tissue in the body. It is concentrated inside the mitochondria, so every cell must have a mechanism for absorbing Q10 from the blood. Q10 supplements presumably pass through the liver, enter the bloodstream and are taken up by the body's cells as required.

Additional clinical research is slow. Eisai in Tokyo has the world monopoly on production and, although it has a massive re-investment programme, it sees no need to fund clinical trials to achieve a product licence for Q10, as they are selling everything they can produce.

Most Q10 research is done by independent clinicians who have given it to their patients, seen it work, and then written up the results for a small scientific journal. Nevertheless there have been positive results in trial after trial, in country after country.

Not a cheap option

Q10 is not cheap. For that reason many Q10 products on sale in health food shops and chemists contain too little Q10 to have any effect.

The dose generally used by scientists and athletes is 60-100mg a day, but Q10 is so safe that you can experiment with higher doses.

Heart patients have been maintained for years on doses of over 300 mg/day without side effects[54-56, 68].

I recommend a minimum dose of 30mg a day, rising to 300mg to treat specific conditions. At the entry (30mg) level it costs about 20p a day or £6 a month.

SUMMARY

Guidelines

▶ Look for Q10 which is pre-dissolved in soy oil in dark gel capsules. Take it with food.

▶ Athletes commonly take 100-300mg of Q10 a day – heart patients take up to 300mg. A good start point for athletes would be 90-100mg a day.

▶ For increased physical performance, try combining Q10 with creatine, carnitine and carbohydrates[83-121].

▶ Q10 can become pro-oxidant after intensive exercise[138]. Athletes should also take Vitamins C and E and flavonoids to prevent this.

▶ If you're taking a cholesterol-lowering drug, take Q10 – as many of these drugs slow the body's own Q10 production.

▶ For mitochondrial protection, combine Q10 (min. 30mg a day) with beta carotene (at around 10mg a day)[84] and acetyl carnitine (250-750mg a day).

▶ Eat more broccoli, cabbage and Brussels sprouts – they up-regulate anti-oxidant enzymes which stabilise Q10[74, 115].

▶ A supplement containing mixed carotenoids, copper, zinc and manganese will also help make the most of extra Q10 in the body[119,120].

▶ To treat gum disease, a dose of at least 90mg is recommended, together with a Q10 toothpaste if you can find one.

> The body is constantly renewing itself. To do this it needs amino sugars – the basic building blocks of soft tissues

> Infection and certain inflammatory diseases break down tissue faster than the body can regenerate it

> The rate of regeneration slows with ageing

> Taking amino sugar supplements helps the body speed its natural healing

> Amino sugars could provide kinder treatments for arthritis and irritable bowel diseases, and help protect the skin from the impact of ageing

Chapter 10

Amino Sugars – the regeneration game

Amoebas and flatworms can regenerate almost their entire bodies. Octopi and salamanders can re-grow missing limbs. Many lizards can, if needed, shed their tail and grow another later on.

How do humans rate on the regenerative scale? We can't re-grow missing limbs, but our powers of self-healing are still quite impressive.

Even if 90 per cent of the liver is lost or damaged, the remaining 10 per cent will grow and expand until it replaces the original. If a kidney is lost, the other kidney grows to compensate. Blood vessels, bones, ligaments, even nerves can all mend. After surgery or injury, cut or torn muscle, gut and skin will, if all goes well, repair themselves.

The capacity for self-repair is strongest in the young. If a foetus in the womb is operated on, it heals quickly and without scarring. But after that, it's downhill all the way.

As youth gives way to middle and then old age, our ability to heal and mend slows down from a sprint to a walk, and finally a crawl. Most people assume that this slow-down is an unavoidable part of the ageing process, but they're largely wrong.

Just as with the immune system (where the run-down that comes with age can be reversed with well-designed supplements), recent work shows that healing rates can be accelerated, often dramatically, by improved nutrition.

Healing benefits

In the last few years, spurred on by the need to cut medical costs, hospital groups have found that post-operative healing is improved, complications reduced, and recuperation speeded by general nutritional programmes[1, 70-72].

But this is just the beginning, because these nutritional programmes are far from optimal. They are merely multi-vitamin and mineral preparations, similar to the commercial products stocked in health food stores. Supplements designed specifically to support the healing process would give better results.

In medicine, improved tissue healing means shortened recovery times after surgery, and a new approach to chronic health problems such as Irritable Bowel Disease, arthritis and psoriasis.

In the world of sports and athletics, faster healing after injury promises to save or extend careers, and minimise expensive down-time. And in the world of nutritional cosmetics, improved tissue protection and regeneration holds the promise of extended youthfulness (see Chapter 6, Flavonoids & isoflavones).

> **A nutritional approach to cutting healthcare costs**
>
> Faster healing cuts medical costs, aids chronic diseases, helps sports professionals recover from injury, and keeps skin looking younger, longer.

Cut and paste

The exciting new science of tissue regeneration emerged in the late '60s, when experimenters looked for ways to speed wound healing.

Working initially with rats, but then with humans, scientists achieved positive results with a paste made of ground cartilage and later shrimp shell. When this was applied to open surgical wounds, tissue regeneration was significantly improved; healing was faster and the scar was stronger[2].

Cartilage and shrimp shell both contain large molecules called GAGs, which consist of long chains of a smaller molecule, the amino sugar glucosamine.

Shrimp shell turned out to be even better at tissue regeneration than cartilage – and so did pure glucosamine obtained from fungi[3]. At this point the scientists realised that the tissue regenerator was glucosamine itself, and the rest of the puzzle fell into place.

> **GAGs and PGs**
>
> **GAG** = Glycosaminoglycan
>
> **PG** = Proteoglycan
>
> These macro-molecules have important structural properties and form part of the extra cellular matrix.

WHAT AMINO SUGARS DO

1 The extra-cellular matrix is a mesh of micro-fibres that gives your skin firmness and supports muscles, ligaments, blood vessels and inner organs. Although it is constantly being broken down, it is also constantly being repaired.

A problem arises if the rate of breakdown exceeds the rate of repair. Then skin (and other connective tissues such as cartilage) lose their structure. This shows up as ageing skin, or thinning cartilage – as in osteoarthritis.

2 To prevent this deterioration you must increase the rate at which the matrix is repaired. And that largely depends on the rate at which your body can produce the amino sugar glucosamine.

Glucosamine is formed when glucose (blood sugar) and the amino acid glutamine are combined by the enzyme glucosamine synthetase.

Glucose (sugar)

Glutamine (amino acid)

Glucosamine synthetase ⟶ Glucosamine (amino sugar)

3 Glucosamine molecules link up to form polymers such as GAGs and PGs. These together with two protein micro-fibres, collagen and elastin, make up the extra-cellular matrix.

Amino sugars produce

Polymers (eg GAGs PGs)

Amino acids produce

Proteins (eg collagen, elastin)

These combine to form the extra-cellular matrix

4 The production of amino sugars is important because they also form part of the glycocalyx, a thin layer of tissue which lines and protects the digestive, respiratory and genito-urinary tracts.

Amino sugars also produce GAGs which make up the lubricating fluids that cushion our joints, fill the eyeball and plump the skin.

5 **The problem** is that, with age, the enzyme glucosamine synthetase becomes less effective, which slows the rate of matrix repair. This is why healing is slower in the elderly.

Glucose   Glutamine

Glucosamine synthetase

Reduced production with age ⟶

Glucosamine supplement

Glucosamine

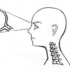

The solution is to bypass the bottleneck with glucosamine supplements, and thus accelerate matrix repair and tissue healing in skin, cartilage and other connective tissues.

The body's building blocks

Amino sugars are among the most important building blocks in the body.

Dr Frances Burton, an expert in amino sugars at the University of British Columbia, expresses it beautifully: "Amino sugars make up the structure of all tissues, on the surface of cells and in the spaces in between them; forming the substance which binds cells together, the membranes which envelop them and the protective layers which cover them."

Macro-molecules built up from amino sugars, called GAGs and PGs, together with the proteins called collagen and elastin, make up the framework for all our tissues. Combined in different proportions, they make tissues soft, slippery, squashy, stretchy or strong. They give our bodies shape, organisation, definition and function[4-7].

GAGs and collagen make up tendons, ligaments, heart valves, skin and finger-nails. Combined with another protein, elastin, they make cartilage in joints and the discs in the spine.

All of these macro-molecules are constantly being broken down and replaced as part of the body's on-going general maintenance programme.

How fast this happens is crucial in maintaining the strength and elasticity of every tissue in the body. However, there is one major problem.

The foundation stone

All the GAG and PG macro-molecules are built up from a single amino sugar – the glucosamine which is the basis of shrimp shell and cartilage. The rate at which glucosamine itself is made is controlled by a single enzyme. So right here is a potential bottleneck and limit to growth, and to tissue regeneration and repair[8]. If you don't produce enough glucosamine your extra-cellular matrix will start to break down.

The older we get, the slower the rate of tissue repair. One of the reasons for this is because, with age, levels of the vital enzyme that controls glucosamine production fall. Older people

---

A New You

The entire human skeleton is renewed every 10 years or so. This means we all need good tissue regeneration rates to keep us healthy.

Glucosamine speeds regeneration. As long as your rate of repair keeps up with the rate of tissue loss, your bones and tissues stay healthy.

Glucosamine

Glucosamine is made by combining one molecule of glucose (blood sugar), with one of glutamine (an amino acid).

This reaction is catalysed by the enzyme glucosamine synthetase[8].

De-stressing

Nutrition is important, but it's not everything. Psychological stress is another factor that slows down wound healing[63].

A de-stressing technique should be considered by anyone wishing to accelerate the healing process.

LOOK FOR ...

a glucosamine supplement of 500mg a day for prevention; 1-2g a day
for treatment
combine with
100mcg Vitamin K
10mg manganese
500mg betaine and
500mg curcumin
(the active ingredient in turmeric)
for best results.

Vitamin K is essential for the synthesis of matrix GLA protein and is vital for cartilage and bone production[11].

Glucosamine hydrochloride is cheaper and better than glucosamine sulphate, being less likely to cause gastro-intestinal problems.

simply can't produce amino sugars quickly enough – unless they get round the bottleneck by taking glucosamine supplements.

There is plenty of anecdotal evidence that glucosamine given to older patients can make a huge difference. It reportedly brings their rate of tissue repair and healing back up to the levels of youthful middle age, or better. Glucosamine supplements have been shown in some studies to increase the rate of tissue healing by a staggering 170 per cent[9, 10].

You might think that if you're not actively growing, or recovering from injury or surgery, the rate of tissue repair doesn't matter. But all the tissues of the body are constantly being repaired and recycled. Some work on a rapid cycle, like skin and blood. Some, like cartilage and bone, regenerate slowly. In fact, the entire body is renewed every ten years or so.

Amino sugar compounds are constantly being broken down, rebuilt and recycled as cells grow, divide, multiply and die, and the rate of re-building is limited by the speed with which the body can manufacture glucosamine. Rapidly renewing tissues like skin or the lining of the gut need supplies of amino sugars constantly. Other tissues need extra amino sugar whenever there is extensive damage and regrowth.

This implies that glucosamine supplements should not only help wound healing after injury or surgery, but also in the treatment of inflammation. Inflammation is a basic element in many diseases where the rate of tissue damage exceeds the rate of tissue regeneration, as in arthritis.

In these cases, a glucosamine supplement can boost the repair process, tipping the balance away from tissue destruction towards reconstruction and health – especially when combined with anti-inflammatory agents such as the flavonoids and Omega 3 oils.

Arthritis

Cartilage, tendon and bone are all living tissues. They grow and regenerate relatively slowly – very slowly in the elderly. But as long as the rate of tissue repair keeps up with the rate of tissue loss, the bones and joints will stay healthy.

In arthritis, however, the rate of tissue breakdown outstrips the rate of repair. As a result there is a progressive loss of cartilage, leading to pain and disability.

The standard medical response is to give pain-killers, and anti-inflammatory drugs. But the problem is that these drugs can **increase** the rate of cartilage loss, and although they may relieve the pain in the short term, in the long run they may make matters worse[44-46, 73-75].

There is evidence that it may be more effective, kinder, and more rational to increase the rate of tissue repair in the affected tissue[20-22, 50, 51, 59-61].

This is where glucosamine comes in. By giving glucosamine, the cells that build ligaments and joints get the material they need to carry out repairs and maintenance. In this way the body's capacity to heal itself is boosted.

Based on our current understanding of arthritis, a nutritional programme which combines glucosamine with natural anti-inflammatory flavonoids (see Chapter 6, Flavonoids & isoflavones) should greatly reduce the symptoms and the risk of the disease.

This is likely to produce the best results in the elderly, who are more depleted in glucosamine and anti-oxidants, such as flavonoids. It's a combination which has not yet been properly tested, but it seems logical that such a nutritional programme could halt, or even reverse the progress of arthritis.

Combating arthritis

Combine glucosamine with a natural anti-inflammatory such as ginger or turmeric.

This reduces the rate of tissue breakdown **and** increases the rate of fibre repair – a dual approach to cartilage regeneration.

Glucosamine should generally be combined with manganese. This trace element is an essential co-factor when glucosamine is built into joints and other tissues[68], and many people are depleted in manganese[69].

Chondroitin is a cheaper alternative to gluco-samine, but is probably less effective.

THE POWER OF AMINO SUGARS

In one double-blind study, subjects with arthritis of the knee were treated either with the amino sugar glucosamine, or a standard anti-inflammatory painkiller. The glucosamine group did significantly better[20].

In a second trial of subjects with chronic arthritis, 14 days of treatment with glucosamine sulphate resulted in a 71 per cent improvement in pain, swelling, tenderness and function[21]. Six more trials which were fundamentally similar in design obtained almost identical results[22, 50, 51, 59, 60, 61]. More recently, glucosamine treatment has been shown to lead to a normalisation of joint function in animal models of arthritis[62].

Bones too

Glucosamine is also essential for the growth of new bone – especially critical in the elderly.

How arthritis develops?

One way of getting osteoarthritis is via repetitive stress injury. Stress on a joint causes compression of that joint. Compression higher than the blood pressure stops blood flow in the capillary beds. This reduces the amount of oxygen reaching the tissues, which triggers free radical formation.

If compression on the joint is severe and frequent, the bursts of free radicals overwhelm local anti-oxidant defences. Oxidative damage follows, with breakdown of hyaluronic acid in the synovial fluid and phospholipids on the articular surfaces.

The resulting loss of lubrication and shock absorption in the joint leads to further tissue damage, more free radicals, inflammation, and an increasing rate of tissue destruction which eventually overtakes the body's regenerative capacity.

This is not the whole story. New research suggests that changes in local bone pre-date and contribute to the loss of cartilage. This underlines the importance of a total health approach, which incorporates bone support (see Chapter 15, Bones).

The other main type of arthritis, rheumatoid arthritis, is an auto-immune disease, where the joint is attacked by the body's own immune system.

This probably happens after infection with certain bacteria, such as the bacteria which cause urinary tract infection. These bugs carry molecules on their surface which resemble molecules in the joints. The body generates an immune response to the bacteria, which has the unfortunate side effect of attacking the similar molecules in the joints.

This produces inflammation in the joint, which leads to the release of free radicals – which once again triggers the breakdown of hyaluronic acid and phospholipids, the loss of lubrication, and further tissue destruction.

Whatever the original cause of the condition, pain and stiffness eventually indicate that the joint has been attacked by arthritis.

But does this means that it's too late to tip the balance towards repair and renewal? Glucosamine combined with high dose anti-inflammatory flavonoids (such as those in turmeric) and fish oil, can improve joint function dramatically within 1-2 months.

I would also recommend betaine, which encourages GAG and PG synthesis[53-57]; manganese[68], Vitamin K[11] and the bone health package described in Chapter 15, Bones.

Other applications

Defective amino sugar metabolism has been reported in rheumatoid arthritis and osteoarthritis[11]; diabetes[13]; nephrotic syndrome[14]; inflammatory bowel syndrome[15, 16, 17]; and cystic fibrosis[18].

Glucosamine may be helpful in all these conditions.

Irritable Bowel Syndrome (IBS)

The cells lining the gut have a very high turnover rate. In chronic inflammatory conditions, the rate is even faster.

In these conditions, the rate of cell growth may outstrip the rate of glucosamine and GAG (glycosaminoglycan) production. In fact, the inflammation itself may inhibit the making of GAGs, and increase the rate at which they are broken down[23-27].

Patients with active inflammatory bowel disease (including Crohn's Disease and Ulcerative Colitis) have very low levels of GAGs in their intestinal walls[17]. A depletion here would be expected to cause local vascular problems, increasing leakage of fluid into the surrounding tissues, and contribute to several distinct types of local tissue damage that are, in fact, all found in chronic inflammatory bowel disease[28-33].

Low levels of amino sugar compounds bring another set of problems. They would eventually affect the thin but vital glycolipid layer which protects the intestinal wall[16]. Since the gut, more than any other organ, is constantly challenged by bacteria, viruses, digestive juices and dietary antigens, losing this vital protection could lead to health problems[34], including food allergies, which are thought to occur in conditions where the gut wall is abnormally permeable.

All this suggests that a glucosamine supplement might be very helpful in treating IBS and food allergies, and there is a substantial body of anecdotal data that this is indeed the case. However, this is a new area, and much more work needs to be done; including, of course, properly designed clinical trials.

Coronary Artery Disease and Thrombosis

Amino sugar therapy suggests an entirely new approach to the huge health problem of coronary artery disease. This is because GAGs play a key role in determining the risk of blood clots forming inside the blood vessels.

GAGs in the blood vessel walls carry electrically charged sulphate groups which repel platelets and discourage them from sticking to the vessel walls[7]. GAGs also stimulate two important anti-clotting factors[5, 6]. **So if amino sugar levels in the blood vessel walls fall, the risk of clots would increase**[32, 33]**, and so would the risk of heart attacks and strokes.**

Does this ever happen? Interestingly, there are two conditions where this may be important.

In Irritable Bowel Syndrome, low GAG levels are thought to be the cause of an abnormally high rate of thrombosis, not just in the gut itself but elsewhere in the circulation too[35, 36]. Old age, when the rate of GAG formation slows, is also when the risk of thrombosis and related complications increase.

Glucosamine and skin complaints

Anecdotal reports suggest that amino sugar supplements may help in the treatment of eczema and psoriasis.

These skin conditions are characterised by an increased skin cell turnover and a possible amino sugar deficiency [23-25].

Reduced risk of thrombosis

Glucosamine supplements may help to maintain the integrity of the blood vessels; and thereby reduce the risk of thrombosis.

Skin Ageing

In the exposed skin of the face and hands, much of the ageing is caused by free radicals liberated by sunlight.

Free radicals damage collagen and elastin fibres in the skin, and the GAGs and PGs. This damage to the extra-cellular matrix leads to a loss of firmness, plumpness and elasticity, and is a large part of skin ageing.

The amino sugar compounds in the skin are constantly being broken down and replaced. As much as one fifth of the glucose in the blood is destined for connective tissue formation. But if the glucosamine-producing enzymes slow down, as they do with age, they cannot keep pace with the deterioration caused by exposure to ultra-violet light (UV), cigarette smoke, pollution and other sources of free radicals.

The connective tissue that gives the skin strength, elasticity and firmness deteriorates, with all-too-obvious results.

To protect the skin, you need amino sugars such as glucosamine, and Vitamin C and zinc for collagen and elastin synthesis. To maintain the exta-cellular matrix requires an anti-oxidant mix containing the procyanidin flavonoids (eg bilberry or grapeseed), which concentrate in the connective micro-fibres and protect them from free radical damage; plus mixed carotenoids, which have a similar effect[36].

You also need an anti-glycosylant. Glycosylation (the attachment of sugar molecules) of collagen and elastin increases with ageing. This disrupts the connective tissue in a process known as cross-linking. This has the unfortunate effect of leaving the skin less elastic, less permeable and more prone to wrinkles.

Half a tablet of aspirin helps prevent glycosylation[43], as does a tablespoon of turmeric[77]. Vitamin C has a similar effect[58], and is another essential part of the anti-ageing programme; especially as it is essential for the synthesis of the skin protein collagen[52].

A supplement of silicic acid may also be appropriate. High levels of aluminium damage the fibroblasts and other cells responsible for building and repairing the extra-cellular matrix, in

UV and ageing

To see clearly the ageing effects of UV, compare the texture of middle-aged facial skin to that of underarm skin, which is rarely exposed to UV and ages considerably less rapidly as a result.

Further benefits

Some nutritionists recommend GAG therapy, using such molecules as chondroitin (extracted from cartilage) for coronary artery disease and even certain cancers[39-41]. Further work is needed.

Cross-links

Glucose-induced cross-linking in the extra-cellular matrix is an important part of the ageing of skin and other tissues (and is accelerated in diabetes). Other cross-links (ie pyridine) are essential for all connective tissues.

the skin and elsewhere. Silicic acid is the most effective shield against ingested aluminium, and can enhance the regeneration of the extra-cellular matrix[12, 65-67].

For more information on skin ageing turn to Chapter 18, Skin.

Which silicon?

Silica (eg in horsetail extract) is inert, and ineffective. Silicic acid in colloidal form is recommended – and available in some countries as 'Silicol'.

SUMMARY

Amino sugar guide

▶ There are several different amino sugar supplements – n-acetyl glucosamine (NAG) and glucosamine (sulphate or hydrochloride).

NAG is more rapidly absorbed than glucosamine[37, 38], but is more expensive and no more effective[47-49].

▶ I prefer glucosamine hydrochloride. The sulphate products contain large amounts of salt (which can raise blood pressure); and the sulphate itself is tentatively linked to colon diseases.

▶ Take amino sugars with anti-oxidants. Amino sugars are very susceptible to oxidation, and anti-oxidants protect them.

▶ Vitamin C protects amino sugars while they are in circulation, but not necessarily once they have been taken up into the areas where they are required.

▶ Procyanidins, the flavonoids which target the connective and supportive tissues, protect amino sugars against attack by the destructive MMP enzymes (see Chapter 6, Flavonoids & isoflavones).

▶ Smoking, heavy drinking and diabetes increase the free radical load and the oxidative damage of the amino sugars, reducing their effectiveness.

▶ The glucosamine level needed to help alleviate arthritis symptoms may be 1-2g a day. Combine with ginger or turmeric.

▶ The glucosamine level needed to help slow the ageing of the skin may be about 1-2g a day.

Combine with a supplement that contains Vitamin C, flavonoids and mixed carotenoids (see Chapter 18, Skin).

Chapter 11

Betaine – a new 'vitamin'

Methyl groups, like vitamins, are essential in our diet. Foods that contain significant levels of the methyl groups are, in descending order, sugar beet, sugar cane, prawns, shrimps and eggs.

To give an idea of the importance of methyl groups, the nervous system, the immune system, the heart and blood vessels, the kidneys and the liver all depend on methyl groups to function normally[10, 25].

A diet low in methyl groups damages all the above systems. Stress becomes more destructive, toxins become more toxic, carcinogens more carcinogenic.

In fact, a lack of methyl groups in the diet is the only dietary deficiency known to be directly carcinogenic. If there are not enough methyl groups, DNA reproduction can go wrong, leading to the activation of oncogenes[29] (cancer-causing genes).

To appreciate why a deficiency of methyl groups in the diet is so dangerous, we need to understand a process called the methyl group cycle (see diagram on next page). It's also important to know that excessive levels of the amino acid homocysteine in the body are a major risk factor for heart disease and Alzheimer's (see Chapters 14, Heart disease and 17, A healthy brain).

Methyl groups are a simple combination of carbon and hydrogen atoms. You will see from the diagram that methyl groups from the diet combine with homocysteine in the body to form methionine. Methionine is then turned into S-adenosyl methionine (SAM).

TOP BETAINE FOODS

Sugar beet, eggs, and freshwater shrimps and prawns.

SAM passes on the methyl groups in the body to produce many essential compounds[12]. These include creatine and carnitine (important in energy production), phospholipids, (essential molecules involved in cell membrane and especially nerve health), RNA and DNA, the stress hormones epinephrine and nor-epinephrine, and the neurotransmitters involved in mood (see Chapter 17, A healthy brain). Methyl groups are also essential to the basic functioning of the immune system[1, 13, 14, 31, 34, 35].

If there are inadequate methyl groups in the diet, all these functions are impaired. But there is a further serious implication of insufficient methyl groups in the diet.

After SAM has donated its methyl group it becomes S-adenosyl homocysteine, which breaks down into the toxic amino acid homocysteine.

If there are too few methyl groups from the diet to transform this homocysteine back again into methionine, levels of homocysteine rise and so therefore does the risk of cardiovascular disease[24, 26, 37] **and Alzheimer's disease** (Optima Report '97).

> **How Betaine reduces heart disease risk**
>
> High levels of homocysteine are predictors of heart disease and are very prevalent. This is because an estimated 90% of us have an insufficient intake of methyl groups.
>
> Supplementation with betaine is the logical answer – and has been shown to reduce homocysteine levels (see Chapter 14, Heart disease).

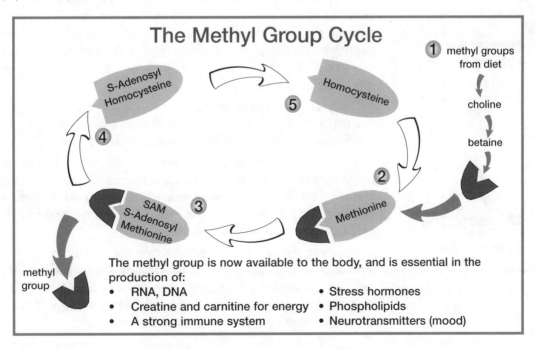

The Methyl Group Cycle

S-Adenosyl Homocysteine — 4

Homocysteine — 5

1 methyl groups from diet
↓
choline
↓
betaine

SAM S-Adenosyl Methionine — 3

Methionine — 2

methyl group

The methyl group is now available to the body, and is essential in the production of:
- RNA, DNA
- Creatine and carnitine for energy
- A strong immune system
- Stress hormones
- Phospholipids
- Neurotransmitters (mood)

THE DEFENCE BOOSTERS : Betaine

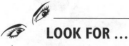
The body cannot synthesise methyl groups, and therefore a constant dietary intake of methyl groups is essential to maintain the cycle, in order to keep levels of SAM up and levels of homocysteine down.

The principal dietary sources of methyl groups are, in descending order, the nutrients betaine, choline and methionine; and to a lesser extent the Vitamins B6, B12 and folic acid. The vitamins are not the best donors; betaine is far more effective[1, 2, 7, 15, 18-21, 33, 36].

Under conditions of stress (such as disease), the need for methyl groups increases. This is because methyl groups are needed for the formation of stress hormones, for various defence mechanisms and for the synthesis of polyamines, RNA and DNA[34, 35], all of which are needed for tissue repair.

When stress increases the demands for methyl groups, the resulting shortfall in methyl groups inevitably leads to an increase in homocysteine – another reason why stress is bad for your health.

As an excellent methyl group donor, betaine is very effective at lowering levels of homocysteine. Most humans, however, do not consume much betaine; and in this situation, the B vitamins become the next line of defence. One recent study found that people who ate high levels of folic acid (a B vitamin) were 69% less at risk of a fatal heart attack than those whose diet contained low levels of folic acid[22].

Sadly, B vitamin deficiency is also all too common[24, 26, 37] – and this explains why excessive levels of homocysteine (and therefore heart disease and Alzheimer's disease) are so common[23, 27, 28].

A strong B complex preparation reduces levels of homocysteine[38, 39]. This is why supplements of folic acid and Vitamins B6 and B12 are increasingly being used to reduce homocysteine levels, and the risk of homocysteine-related cardiovascular and neurological diseases.

However, nearly 10% of the population cannot metabolise folic acid, and in these subjects its physiological benefits are greatly reduced[41]. Industry is now promoting the use of activated folic acid; but this is an expensive and inappropriate strategy. Betaine is the best donor of methyl groups to the cycle.

What is betaine good for?

Betaine's functions follow logically on from its role in the methyl group cycle. It reduces levels of homocysteine in the body, and thereby reduces risk factors for coronary artery disease and probably neo-natal neural tube defects and Alzheimer's disease also.

Betaine is also essential for the process by which dietary lipids (fats) are turned into phospholipids; and so it supports liver function, as methyl group deficiency leads to fatty infiltration of the liver.

Betaine offers considerable protection against fatty degeneration of the liver, even during extreme alcohol intake[3, 4]; and this protective effect, together with betaine's other physiological role as an osmoprotectant (it protects against dehydration, and hangovers!), makes it **the** supplement for drinkers.

By feeding methyl groups into the methyl group cycle, betaine has been shown to increase resistance to various stresses, including infection[5]. So it has an immuno-strengthening role.

Finally, methyl groups are needed by the body to make neurotransmitters involved in controlling mood – which explains why betaine is also a strong anti-depressant – see Chapter 17, A healthy brain.

Betaine is non-toxic and, although it occurs in low levels in many species of plants and animals[6], the only sources with significant levels are in plants belonging to the sugar beet (Chenopodiaceae) family, and freshwater invertebrates, which contain betaine at levels of up to 1.5g/kg[16, 17]. The only realistic way to get the 500mg a day that I believe to be optimal is supplementation.

Help for heavy drinkers

A betaine supplement is especially important for the heavy drinker.

Betaine helps protect the liver from damage linked to alcohol and reduces hangovers[3, 4, 40].

Anti-depressant

Betaine is the best source of the methyl groups, and is, therefore, the anti-depressant of choice where methyl group depletion is indicated – see Chapter 17.

Nutritionists – should prefer betaine to choline

Some nutritionists still recommend choline, without necessarily understanding why they are using it. But choline is not a methyl donor: it must be transformed in the mitochondria into betaine[21], and it is betaine which is the ultimate provider of essential methyl groups into the methyl group cycle.

Another argument against using choline as a methyl donor is that much of it is used in the body to form acetyl choline and phosphatidyl choline, rather than betaine[2, 33]. This is one reason why the rate of formation of betaine from choline is too slow to make enough betaine to supply the methyl group cycle[1, 18, 20].

This is why betaine is termed a quasi-vitamin. It is the only nutrient which can supply enough methyl groups to maintain optimal methyl group levels, even under conditions of stress[9].

S-adenosyl methionine is far more expensive and far less effective – see diagram on page 163.

SUMMARY

Betaine – 'Vitamin B10'?

▶ The heart, blood vessels, kidneys, liver and immune system all depend on methyl groups to function properly.

▶ Under stress the need for methyl groups increases.

▶ A shortfall of methyl groups leads to increased levels of homocysteine, which has been linked to an increased risk of cardiovascular and neurological diseases.

▶ Methyl groups are essential for phospholipid synthesis in the liver. Betaine increases phospholipid synthesis. This raises HDL cholesterol ('good cholesterol') levels, and supports cell membranes, which helps maintain a healthy heart and brain.

▶ Methyl groups must be sourced from the diet.

▶ Betaine is the most important source of methyl groups.

▶ Betaine offers protection against liver damage caused by high alcohol intake.

▶ Betaine is non-toxic and comes from sugar beet and freshwater seafood.

▶ Choline and Vitamins B6 and B12 and folic acid can also contribute methyl groups, but are less effective than betaine.

▶ S-adenosyl methionine is expensive and not very effective.

> Being unfit increases your risk of heart disease by 250%. It increases your risk of heart disease as much as smoking.

> Exercise lowers blood pressure and cholesterol, produces anti-oxidant enzymes and cuts heart attack risk by up to two thirds[7].

> Sex reduces stress and boosts the immune system.

> A whole range of vitamins and minerals are also needed to maintain the immune system and produce the hormones that increase the sex drive.

Chapter 12

Body weight, exercise, sex and cigarettes

Washing machines, cars and lifts all make our lives easier – and shorter.

The problem is that our bodies and our way of life are out of step. We were designed for a physical lifestyle, with high energy requirements and a high food and micro-nutrient intake.

Instead, modern technology means that most of us live a low energy lifestyle, with a low intake of calories and micro-nutrients. The main reason most of us in the developed countries are getting fatter is not so much that we are eating more, but rather because we are burning 500-800 fewer calories per day than our grandparents did.

The combination of exercising less, and consuming richer and more diverse foods explains why the number of overweight people shot up from 25 per cent of the adult population in 1986 to an astonishing 35 per cent today, a trend which shows no sign of slowing down[80, 81].

Where will it end? In the USA, nearly two-thirds of all adults are overweight. It's reached the point where obesity is considered by some to be as serious a health problem as Alzheimer's[82]. Are we all doomed to follow, waddling, in their footsteps?

Keeping warm

Central heating, double glazing and thermal clothing reduce our exposure to cold – and reduce the number of calories we would otherwise burn in keeping warm.

Overweight = unfit = unhealthy?

Being overweight is a major risk factor for disease. When overweight tips into obesity, the risk of coronary artery disease increases by two and a half times[1]. The risks of hypertension, diabetes and certain cancers are also raised ... but why is being overweight dangerous?

Overweight people tend not to take a lot of exercise. And there's a growing body of evidence that suggests that this is one of the reasons that being overweight causes ill health.

But lack of exercise doesn't just affect the overweight – it affects all of us, whatever build.

In fact, inactivity is as great a risk factor for heart disease as a 20-a-day cigarette habit, and is as bad as having hypertension or raised cholesterol[2, 3]. The unfit have two and a half times more risk of early cardiac death than the fit[5]; which is, interestingly, the same increase in risk associated with being overweight.

Taking exercise, on the other hand, has such a good effect that it overrides or neutralises any and all bad eating habits[2,3].

And if you have other risk factors such as smoking, hypertension or high cholesterol, a good exercise programme reduces the risk of early cardiac death an amazing five-fold![5]

Another way of looking at this is that you may have several risk factors, but if you are fit you are 1.7 times less at risk than your colleague who has no risk factors, but who is unfit[5].

Just to prove the point, one large and long-term study at Harvard showed that men who took up moderate physical activity reduced their death rates by 17 per cent. Those who took up vigorous activity cut their death rates by 41 per cent, from coronary artery disease and all other causes[6].

Lack of exercise may be the most important risk factor of all, because it is the most common risk factor, affecting 70% of all adults[4].

Get up – and lose weight!

Increase the amount of daily exercise you take – walk up stairs rather than take the lift, get off the bus one stop early, throw the TV remote control away. Just 100 calories extra of physical activity a day could mean up to 6kg of weight lost in a year.

Move!

Weight loss diets are more successful when combined with exercise. This prevents metabolic slowdown[20], which makes so many diets fail[23].

HOW TO CALCULATE YOUR BODY MASS INDEX

The Body Mass Index (BMI) is calculated by dividing your weight in kilos by your height in metres squared. For optimum health your BMI should be between 21 and 25. To save you having to use a calculator, we have worked out the figures for you.

Height	BMI = 21	BMI = 25	Height	BMI = 21	BMI = 25
5' 0"/1.52m	7st 5lbs/46.7kg	8st 11lbs/55.8kg	5' 9"/1.75m	10st lbs/64kg	12st 1lbs/76.6kg
5' 1"/1.55m	7st 12lbs/50kg	9st 6 lbs/59.9kg	5' 10"/1.78m	10st 5lbs/65.8kg	12st 6lbs/79kg
5' 2"/1.58m	8st 2lbs/51.7 kg	9st 10lbs/61.7kg	5' 11"/1.80m	10st 10lbs/68kg	12st 10lbs/80.7kg
5' 3"/1.60m	8st 7lbs/54kg	10st 1lbs/64kg	6' 0"/1.83m	11st 0lbs/69.8kg	13st 1lbs/83kg
5' 4"/1.63m	8st 10lbs/55.3kg	10st 5lbs/65.8kg	6' 1"/1.85m	11st 4lbs/71.7kg	13st 7lbs/85.7kg
5' 5"/1.65m	8st 13lbs/56.7kg	10st 10lbs/68kg	6' 2"/1.88m	11st 9lbs/74kg	13st 12lbs/88kg
5' 6"/1.68m	9st 4lbs/59kg	11st 0lbs/69.9kg	6' 3"/1.90m	11st 13lbs/76kg	14st 5lbs/91kg
5' 7"/1.70m	9st 8lbs/60.8kg	11st 4lbs/71.7kg	6' 4"/1.93m	12st 5lbs/78.4kg	14st 8lbs/93kg
5' 8"/1.73m	9st 13lbs/63kg	11st 11lbs/74.8kg			

Why exercise works

The Honolulu Heart Programme Study, published in 1994, showed that physical activity reduces the risk of heart attacks by lowering blood pressure, improving blood sugar control in diabetics, and improving plasma cholesterol profiles[9].

Specifically, exercise lowers levels of the 'bad' LDL cholesterol, and raises levels of the 'good' HDL cholesterol[10, 13]. Increased HDL levels help to remove cholesterol from the arterial walls, which is why exercise stops arteries furring up[11].

More, the increase in free radicals triggered by using extra oxygen to exercise causes the body to boost production of its own anti-oxidant enzymes. These remain active even when the exercise stops[78], which means you get better protection against oxidative stress, heart disease, and cancer as well[5, 25].

How fit and how much exercise?

Fitness is most easily and conveniently measured by taking the resting pulse. If this is high, you're unfit[14] and may be at risk[15] (see the chart below). Regular exercise will bring it down[16].

The crucial threshold appears to be 20 minutes of exercise, repeated three times per week[3]. This should be enough to raise

Health Warning

If you're unfit, you're over **twice** as likely to die from a heart attack.

Inactivity is more dangerous than simply being overweight. It's as unhealthy as smoking 20 a day, high blood pressure or high cholesterol.

Conversely, you can be overweight, have high blood pressure, high cholesterol, or smoke, but if you exercise you are less at risk than your unfit neighbour.

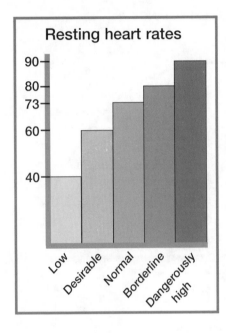

Resting heart rates

90 –	
80 –	
73 –	
60 –	
40 –	

Low Desirable Normal Borderline Dangerously high

a sweat, and your breathing and pulse rate by at least 30 per cent.

Try to take your exercise just before your main meal of the day. A brisk walk before a meal speeds the removal of fats from the blood after eating[12]. This almost certainly helps to reduce the risk of both heart disease and diabetes.

Good habits should start as early in life as possible. In children, low levels of physical inactivity correlate very strongly with a tendency to fatness, and set up a pattern of life-long overweight[17]. This could be partly genetic – but good training can reduce the impact of bad genes. It's never too late!

Exercise – moderation!

Very intensive exercise reduces blood glutamine levels, which suppresses the immune system and leads to a fall in IgA immuno-globulins in the saliva[18]. These immuno-globulins are designed to protect the mucous membranes of the mouth and throat from infection.

This fall in IgA explains why athletes are prone to infections of the upper respiratory tract. The run-down in immuno-globulins is probably caused by the excessive free radicals produced by intensive exercise, together with substantial reductions of plasma glutamine. (The amino acid glutamine is the basic fuel of the immune system.) The incidence of infection in athletes can be considerably reduced with combinations of anti-oxidants[19, 79] (see Chapter 5, Anti-oxidants), and glutamine at 2-4g immediately before and after strenuous exercise[86].

Doctors recommend ...

The American College of Sports Medicine recommends:

- Walk two miles in under 27 minutes at least three days a week, OR

- Two miles in under 40 minutes six days a week, OR

- Two miles a day in three periods of 10 minutes.

How fit are you?

After exercise, how long is it before your pulse returns to the pre-exercise rate? If more than 10 minutes, you're unfit.

One third of the risk

One study in Finland, where heart attack rates were until recently the highest in the world, found that those who took a lot of exercise had only a third of the risk of the unfit, regardless of diet[7].

Another trial showed that physical activity protects against strokes[8].

THE DEFENCE BOOSTERS : Body weight, exercise

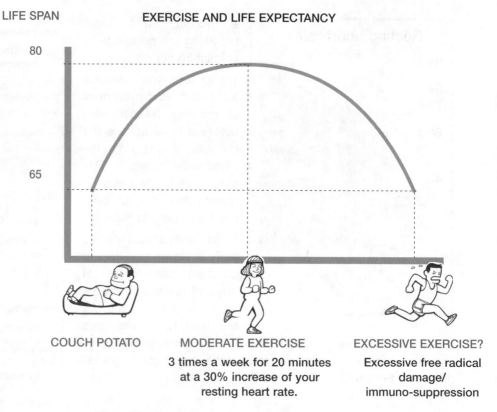

LIFE SPAN   EXERCISE AND LIFE EXPECTANCY

80

65

COUCH POTATO	MODERATE EXERCISE	EXCESSIVE EXERCISE?
	3 times a week for 20 minutes at a 30% increase of your resting heart rate.	Excessive free radical damage/ immuno-suppression

The stiffness and pain the next day, which puts many would-be exercisers off is due to free radical damage in the muscles, and can be minimised, or avoided, with a well-designed, high-dose anti-oxidant programme[21-24, 27, 28].

At risk from heart attacks:

- **The 25% who have cholesterol over the recommended 6.5 mmol**

- **The 30% who smoke**

- **The 70% who don't take enough exercise[4]**

A weight loss combination

The problem with weight loss programmes is that, in the long run, they generally fail. Psycho-social pressures and other factors such as metabolic slowdown[20] undo the initial progress. Exercise helps[20]; but there may be more you can do. Thermogenics are substances which increase the rate at which you burn calories. Combined with appetite suppressants, they should theoretically enhance early weight loss, reduce metabolic slowdown, and ease the psycho-social pressures which can break the diet routine.

The 'best' thermogens, in the sense that they are safe and there is some data to support their use, are capsaicins, the 'hot stuff' extracted from chilli peppers; and guarana and/or coffee.

Capsaicin may work by inducing a rise in body temperature after eating (Dietary Induced Thermogenesis or DIT)[49]. It's also a powerful anti-oxidant and can protect against oxidative damage to lipids and DNA[30].

Guarana acts rather like ephedrine (shown in Danish and British research to achieve weight loss when combined with caffeine). The net effect is that you burn a few more calories.

You could add Vitamin C to counter the increase in free radicals produced by an increased metabolic rate.

One interesting appetite suppressant is alpha hydroxy citrate (HCA). This is extracted from Garcinia cambogia – the Malabar tamarind[31, 32]. HCA stops the body storing calories from carbohydrate foods as fat, and stores them as glycogen in the liver instead[33-45]. The brain interprets this as meaning it has just had a large meal[69-73], so appetite is reduced[46-48], **providing you are eating a high carbohydrate diet**.

Consider also organic chromium, usually derived from chromium enriched yeast, which can help to stabilise blood sugar levels. Chromium is an essential part of the Glucose Tolerance Factor, which is needed for the body to metabolise sugar and other carbohydrates[51,52]. Chromium depletion is surprisingly common[53-55, 63, 65-68] and causes hypoglycaemia, a condition characterised by erratic glucose tolerance, mood swings, sugar craving and overweight, and which may be a form of latent or incipient diabetes.

Hypoglycaemia responds well to chromium supplements[50, 56-61]. If sugar craving is your thing, a chromium supplement may help.

Finally, fibre-rich foods containing inulin or non-digestible oligosaccharides (such as artichokes or oats) are bulking agents which produce a feeling of fullness in the stomach **and** form metabolites which may affect appetite (See Chapter 7, Pre-biotic fibre). Combined with the other ingredients, this may contribute to an overall lessening of appetite.

This combination approach has not to my knowledge been tested – but seems worth trying.

A natural diet cocktail?

A combination of five natural extracts – tamarind, chilli, guarana, organic chromium and inulin – may help weight loss.

Chromium

If you have adult onset diabetes, chromium supplements reduce serum triglyceride levels[50], and probably reduce the risk of coronary artery disease.

Work with diabetic models shows that chromium supplements have additional benefits, and can help to reduce blood sugar levels, excessive water drinking and polyuria[50, 62, 64].

Chromium/yeast supplements

Glucose tolerance, which often deteriorates with old age, can be normalised by non-toxic[74, 75] chromium-containing yeast supplements[56-60].

Avoid inorganic chromium supplements[76].

It should have additional benefits including a reduction in cholesterol and homocysteine levels and, in some cases, a normalisation of blood glucose.

Conjugated linoleic acid (CLA) is currently fashionable but, in my view, there is not yet sufficient data to support its use in weight loss regimes.

Lose weight now?

Our genes and lifestyles may give us more or less risk of becoming overweight, but we can (if we wish) overcome them.

Be sceptical of ...

Combination Diets: These have had a lot of publicity but most nutritionists say the theory is rubbish, and they only work because they are camouflaged low calorie diets.

Crash diets: Cycles of weight loss and gain may increase the risk of heart disease. During every period of weight loss, fat metabolism is altered in a way which could theoretically put your arteries at risk[83, 84].

Furthermore ...

Your metabolism plays a nasty trick on you when you diet. After a couple of attempts at dieting, the body learns to store fat more efficiently.

Not only do you find it harder to lose weight with every subsequent diet, but it also comes back more quickly when the diet is replaced by a binge!

Try less ...

Clothes: Wear fewer layers of clothing, and turn down the thermostat a little, you'll use up more calories just staying warm.

Workers in the Arctic Circle need up to 7,000 calories a day just to maintain their weight. (Not for the inactive elderly, who must be careful of hypothermia!)

Fats: Watch your balance of fats (no more than 30 per cent of your calories should come from fat), and reduce that if you can to 25%.

Starches and proteins are less liable to be turned into body fat, while fibre helps you feel full.

Try more ...

Meals: rather than snacks.

Food eaten as a meal gives you less calories than the same amount of food nibbled throughout the day, as more of its energy is burnt off as DIT (see page 173).

Coffee: Drunk with a meal, coffee will help you burn off some of those excess calories.

Activity: A recent study of Cambridge housewives found they used 100 calories per day less than in 1980, because they used so many labour-saving devices.

Exercise three times a week for 20 minutes. Don't drive to the shops when they're only 200 yards away!

Find a form of exercise you enjoy. And on that note ...

Sex is good for you

The hazards of unprotected sex in non-monogamous relationships are well known. Less well known is the fact that anti-ageing researchers have commented that people showing the slowest ageing rates have, in general, a particularly well-developed libido and sex-life[85].

This may be because good sex is profoundly de-stressing – and stress certainly accelerates the ageing process.

Not tonight, darling

But when the lights are low, is your libido too? Look in the back of most newspapers and you'll find small ads offering help to men suffering from low sex drive.

You won't find offers of similar help for women – which seems unfair, as women can also experience periods of low libido. Society puts much more pressure on the male to be virile, so he's far more likely to think of his symptom as a problem, and run for help, than the female. But sometimes she needs help too.

Sexuality is a complex and sensitive thing, and the lack of desire can have many different causes. Partnership difficulties often manifest themselves in bed, or there could be psychosexual problems; but, where a relationship is otherwise healthy, the problem may be rooted in the body rather than the mind.

> **Sex and the immune system**
>
> IGA is an antibody found in saliva which defends against colds and flu.
>
> Stress reduces IGA levels; but regular sex can increase levels of IGA in the blood by up to 30%.

It could be your hormones

Some cases of decreased sex drive have medical causes. Thyroid insufficiency, for example, can squash the libido to almost zero. Treat the underlying medical malfunction, and a whole range of symptoms, including the sexual ones, disappear.

Hormonal changes associated with the menopause are a more common cause of low libido, and can be reversed by HRT or the phytoestrogens in soy. But it's not just a question of oestrogen: the main libido-determining hormone, in women as well as men, is testosterone.

In some women, a fall in sex drive is caused by low levels of testosterone, and testosterone replacement therapy, available from some private clinics and hospitals, can help.

Sexy sauna ...

The sauna could not have been better designed to raise the sexual temperature.

The heat, cold and birch twigs all combine to raise noradrenaline levels – and what do we associate with saunas, if not sex?

TESTOSTERONE – HANDLE WITH CARE!

Testosterone replacement therapy should **only** be administered by a professional.

One couple turned up at a Harley Street clinic with the husband complaining of his wife's lack of interest in sex. Her testosterone levels were indeed on the low side – but not low enough, in the consultant's opinion, to merit replacement therapy.

Two months later the husband returned. He had obtained testosterone tablets, illegally, and had been putting very large doses in his wife's food. Her sexual appetite had risen dramatically, to the point where he was finding it difficult keeping up with her.

She had begun to grow a moustache and had become so assertive that he was no longer able to cope. He felt sexually inadequate and was convinced she was having affairs with at least two other men.

At this point he decided to confess his sins. Unfortunately his wife was still under the influence of the unofficial testosterone therapy. In the ensuing argument she beat her husband severely, wrecked the family home and trashed the car. No charges were filed!!

... and sexy swimmers

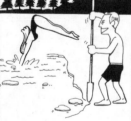

Swimming in cold water gives your levels of the 'sexy' hormone noradrenaline a boost. So do rows, mild pain, exposure to cold and danger!

More hormones

Lack of exercise lessens desire. Don't start running marathons, however, as the hormonal changes caused by serious athletic training kill sexual appetite. Moderate exercise, however, has quite the opposite effect.

Swimming, in particular, has put a sparkle in many a woman's eye. Why swimming? Dr John Moran, a well-known psycho-sexual consultant based in London's Harley Street, explains: "Swimming twice a week definitely gives the libido a boost. The loss of body heat during swimming triggers a surge of noradrenaline into the bloodstream, which tickles the pleasure centres in the brain and makes you feel sexy."

This might explain the otherwise incomprehensible behaviour of those dedicated men and women who break the ice on frozen rivers and lakes to go bathing on New Year's Eve.

There are some, however, who become addicted to the noradrenaline rush. These are the compulsive thrill seekers, the bungee jumpers and the devotees of sado-masochism. "Mild to moderate pain," says Dr Moran, "produces the same surge of noradrenaline as cold does, and this is one of the aspects that gets some people involved in the S & M scene. But it goes farther than that, because any sort of aggression can produce noradrenaline.

"A row has the same effect, and you know how many rows are followed by sex. Some people learn this subconsciously, and use rows as a kind of foreplay."

Seasonal sex

If cold was critical you'd expect people to feel sexier in the winter, but it's more complicated than that. For one thing there's central heating; for another, the dim days and long winter nights bring on melatonin, the 'dark hormone'.

Bright light brings melatonin production grinding to a halt, but switch the lights off and levels of the hormone shoot up. Melatonin is a calming hormone, which is one reason we prefer to sleep in the dark, and one reason why many couples prefer making love with the lights on.

Melatonin is also involved in Winter Depression, or Seasonal Affective Disorder. SAD sufferers have little interest in sex; all they want to do is binge on carbohydrates and sleep, almost as if they were trying to hibernate. Intense light lifts their depression and boosts their sex drive. (Sparrows are surprisingly similar. City lighting allows metropolitan birds to enjoy sex all year round while their rural counterparts only do it in the summer months.)

The sexiest weather conditions combine cold to boost noradrenaline, and bright light to reduce melatonin. This is an uncommon combination in many cities but not in the ski resorts, which could explain both après-ski and the legendary reputation of the ski instructor!

Paris in the Spring

If you're no good on skis, take a spring break in Paris. For centuries the town gallants have been in the habit of walking their fiancées in parks where the horse chestnut trees grow.

The animal and plant kingdoms use the same sexual attractant pheromones, and horse chestnut blossom reproduces the steamy atmosphere of a bedroom where tumultuous sex has just taken place. The effects are claimed to be rapid, and sustained.

Dark days – dark nights

The calming hormone melatonin is produced in the dark. Too little light can trigger SAD in the winter and switches off your sex drive.

In-built aphrodisiacs

Various hormones are involved in regulating sex drive, including oestrogen, progesterone and testosterone. Their synthesis requires niacin (B3), Vitamin B5, Vitamin A or beta carotene, zinc, and manganese.

The vitamins and minerals cited above should be taken regularly for at least 20 days before any effects can be expected. In addition, in cases where it may be necessary to address significantly low levels of sexual desire, you might try the amino supplements tyrosine and arginine, which are involved in the production of neurotransmitters that stimulate alertness, excitement, desire and physiological arousal.

If pure amino acids are unavailable, two or three tablespoonfuls of a high-grade micro-algal product such as spirulina or chlorella will provide most of them. Unfortunately, they also stain your lips and tongue green (temporarily!).

Male impotence

Most cases of male impotence have a physical cause. Various anti-hypertensive, anti-ulcer and other drugs have been implicated and a simple change of prescription can often help.

Where severe, chronic impotence has been caused by damage to blood vessels or nerves supplying the penis, a different approach is called for.

Blockage of the penile arteries is generally caused by the same process that blocks the arteries supplying the heart. Damage to the nerves is often caused by the oxidative stress that is also associated with diabetes.

In both cases, a high-dose anti-oxidant and PUFA replacement programme (see Chapters 14, Heart disease, and 16, Diabetes), maintained over a period of at least 12 months, may help to regenerate the damaged tissues.

The programme should include Vitamins C, E and the B group; mixed carotenoids; grapeseed extract; and a balanced Omega 3 and 6 oil mix (eg flax oil or hemp oil). And stop smoking!

BONUS!

The preventative health-care formula I recommend on page 338 contains most of the nutrients needed for a good sex life.

DHEA

The steroid DHEA may be another key element in male and female sexuality. It is associated with increased libido in both sexes.

No sex please – we're cyclists

Male cyclists beware! Badly designed bicycle saddles put pressure on the penile nerves and arteries, resulting eventually in tissue damage.

Too many hours in the saddle lead to down-time in bed.

17 ways to kill yourself with cigarettes

You already know that smoking is seriously bad for you. The decision not to smoke is the biggest single contribution you can make to your own health and long life. If you – or anyone near you needs convincing – read on.

Thanks to the tobacco multinationals, lung cancer has overtaken breast cancer to become the leading cancer death in most developed countries[69, 113] and is rapidly moving towards the number one slot in the developing countries too.

Cigarette smoke hits the immune system hard. In the airways, it harms the immune cells which normally protect us against the inhaled micro-organisms that cause coughs, colds, sore throats and bronchitis.

This is why smokers are more prone to all these illnesses; but, more worryingly, tobacco smoke damages immune cells elsewhere in the body too. This is why smoking is associated with an increased risk of cancer not just of the lungs, but also the mouth, larynx, oesophagus, bladder, pancreas and cervix![95]

Smoking is linked to increased levels of rheumatoid factor and other auto-antibodies in the blood[103], and almost certainly increases the risk and the severity of arthritis[104]. Arthritis is more common in women, and there is mounting evidence that women are especially at risk of tobacco-related disease.

Smoking advances the menopause by two to three years, erodes the bones[129], and increases the risk of osteoporosis and osteoporotic bone fractures[97], a major cause of pain and disability in later life.

In younger women who smoke during pregnancy, cigarettes increase the risk of miscarriage by over 25 per cent[98]. In surviving babies, the risk from disease and death in childhood is also increased[98].

In another blow against equal opportunities, recent evidence indicates that women smokers may be up to twice as likely to get lung cancer than men, even if they smoke less[109].

However, although the 35-year-old woman smoker can expect to live five years less than her non-smoking sister, men fare even worse.

How cigarettes damage your health

Each puff of smoke you inhale from a cigarette or joint contains over 10^{14} (100,000,000,000,000) free radicals[115].

This huge intake of free radicals uses up the body's natural anti-oxidant defences[143], which is why smokers have lower levels of Vitamins C, E, glutathione, selenium, the carotenoids and other anti-oxidant micro-nutrients[126-128, 130,131].

Vitamin C is one of the first anti-oxidants to be used up: even passive smoking reduces your Vitamin C levels[119]. Stopping smoking has the opposite effect: within days, levels of Vitamin C and other anti-oxidants in the blood rise towards normal[144].

Reduced levels of anti-oxidants damage lung tissue, leading to bronchitis and emphysema[114]. They also damage vessel walls and cause cholesterol oxidation, and increased platelet stickiness. Nicotine narrows the blood vessels and raises blood pressure – a perfect recipe for heart attacks.

Free radicals cause DNA damage, leading to cancer.

A male smoker at age 35 can expect to die seven years before his non-smoking brother, because of the higher rates of heart attacks in middle-aged and elderly men[95]. As if that weren't enough, male smokers are more likely to become impotent, due to degenerative changes in the blood vessels supplying the penis[142].

You may think that none of the above applies to you, because you don't smoke that many cigarettes, and the ones you do smoke are low tar. But one in two smokers will die of their addiction, and the majority of those who die are not the heavy smokers, who are fewer in number to start with[107, 108], but the light to moderate smokers. And if all that isn't enough to persuade you to stub out your last cigarette, consider the following summary[95, 106]:

Cigarettes cause:

- 4 out of 5 cases of lung cancer
- 3 out of 4 cases of bronchitis and emphysema
- 1 in 5 heart attack deaths
- Low immune system – leading to illnesses and cancer
- Worsening arthritis
- Earlier menopause
- More osteoporosis
- Male impotence
- Greater risk of miscarriage and childhood death
- A shortened lifespan – smokers on average lose one day of life for every week they smoke
- One death in every six

The only good news I can possibly offer is that, **while** you are giving up smoking the combination of anti-oxidants, flavonoids, isoflavones and PUFA (Omega 3) supplements that I recommend on pages 338-339 will provide some measure of protection.

The good news ...

- People do quit. Nearly 25 per cent of the British population are ex-smokers and the health benefits of stopping are vast.

- Within weeks of quitting, the sense of taste and smell improve. The lungs are already cleaner, and you'll feel less wheezy and short of breath. General health improves, and you'll need less time off work due to sickness.

- Within one or two years, your risk of heart attack is reduced to half of the smoker's risk.

- At three years, your risk of heart attack has fallen to that of a non-smoker.

- At 10 years, the risk of lung cancer has fallen by half[172].

A safer smoke?

The human body is extremely resourceful and adaptive. As part of the body's response to the insult of smoking, it boosts its levels of anti-oxidant enzymes – but not by enough.

Even though anti-oxidant enzymes are raised in the red blood cells of smokers, the cells' much reduced content of anti-oxidant vitamins means that they are still more vulnerable to oxidation than the cells of non-smokers[111,135].

Much of the damage caused by cigarettes is due to free radicals. So could taking anti-oxidant supplements make tobacco safer? We know that lifestyle habits can modify the risk of tobacco-induced illness. For example, the French and the Japanese smoke as much or more than British and Americans do, yet suffer from less heart disease and less lung cancer.

Many scientists believe that this relative immunity is due to their increased anti-oxidant intake. Many also believe that anti-oxidant supplements offer a degree of protection against some of the dangers of cigarette smoking[132-134].

The case for anti-oxidants

- Anti-oxidant depletion in smokers contributes to their reduced sperm counts and low fertility. Vitamin C supplements, at over 200 mg/day, improve sperm quality in smokers[117]. Vitamin E reduces platelet damage in female smokers[142].

- Vitamins C and E protect against lipid oxidation[135, 138-140] which should help to protect against heart disease. To protect proteins from oxidation, glutathione is needed, although Vitamin C has some protective effect[110].

- A genetic error in one of the major anti-oxidant enzymes, glutathione-S-transferase, has been linked to an increased risk of lung cancer in smokers[112].

A 50% risk

One in two smokers dies from his addiction.

Light to moderate smokers, even those smoking low tar, still run a substantial risk.

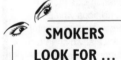

SMOKERS LOOK FOR ...

a supplement with
at least
Vitamin C 600mg
Vitamin E 400IU
Mixed carotenoids
50-100mg
Mixed flavonoids 500mg
plus copper, zinc,
magnesium and
selenium

The case against beta carotene for smokers

Two studies[147, 148] found a significant **increase** in lung cancers in smokers who were given beta carotene supplements. In these men, many of whom already had cancer when the trial started, the supplements encouraged tumour growth.

When beta carotene (or any carotenoid) is oxidised, it becomes a pro-oxidant, unless it is recycled by Vitamin C. A smoker's lungs are full of oxygen and free radicals, and low in Vitamin C; exactly the conditions which produce beta carotene radicals, which in turn cause increased DNA and other tissue damage.

Carotenoids should, therefore, always be combined with Vitamin C, and a compre-hensive package of the other anti-oxidants.

That's why I recommend that good nutritional supplements should contain a full spectrum of the protective nutrients; and why you should eat a variety of fruits and vegetables.

• Combination anti-oxidant supplements decrease the amount of oxidative damage in smokers' white blood cells[116]. The supplements also reduce the amount of DNA damage[118, 137], which should mean a reduced risk of cancer.

There is general agreement among scientists and clinicians that eating more fruit and vegetables is a good thing. The health hazards of smoking are probably exacerbated by the fact that smokers eat, on average, less fruit and vegetables than non-smokers. As a result, they have a lower intake of anti-oxidant vitamins[141, 145, 146] and other protective phyto-nutrients.

In addition, the fact that they take less exercise means that they tend to have lower levels of the 'good' cholesterol, HDL. All the above factors would increase the risk of coronary artery disease and cancer[105, 145].

Smokers who cannot cure their addiction but who wish to protect themselves as far as possible from its ill effects, should do so by increasing their intake of fresh fruit and vegetables. The vegetables should include plenty of cabbage, broccoli, Brussels sprouts and beans. In addition, supplements containing Vitamins C, E and the B group, mixed carotenoids and flavonoids; and the minerals selenium, copper, manganese and zinc, are well worth taking.

Finally, eating more oily fish (mackerel, sardines, trout, etc) would seem to be a good thing. This has been shown to improve lung function, even in smokers[122, 123], and to significantly reduce the risk of chronic bronchitis and emphysema[124]. This should be combined with anti-oxidant and other supplements.

WHAT CIGARETTE COMPANIES REALLY THINK

"It's the perfect product – costs a dime to make, a dollar to sell, and it's addictive."

"We don't smoke the stuff, we just sell it. We reserve the right to smoke for the young, the poor and the stupid."

(Quotes from known senior tobacco company executives, but non-attributable due to the libel laws)

SUMMARY

Slim and fit:

▶ Eat more carbohydrate-rich vegetables and cereals – they are less calorie-dense and take more energy to digest.

▶ Exercise for 20 minutes, three times a week – that's walking two miles in under 30 minutes, or walking two miles a day, in three 10 minute periods.

▶ Exercise before a main meal.

▶ Make your body work to keep you warm – fewer clothes, turn the heating down, and sleep cooler.

▶ Drink a cup of strong coffee with each meal to burn up calories, or try caffeine tablets.

▶ Sugar cravers and adult-onset diabetics should try organic (trivalent) chromium supplements and a pre-biotic.

Sex and health:

▶ Sex reduces stress and increases immune levels.

▶ Moderate exercise boosts interest in sex – swimming twice a week is recommended.

▶ Forget mood lighting – try turning up the house lights.

▶ Learn a de-stressing technique. Stress reduces testosterone levels, and relaxing brings them back up again.

▶ Take Vitamins C, B complex, E, the carotenoids, zinc, manganese. These enable the body to produce the hormones and other compounds needed for arousal.

▶ If all else fails, try a good bed-time row!

Smokers should:

▶ Stop!

▶ Eat more vegetables, particularly cabbage, broccoli, Brussels sprouts and beans; and fruit, especially red, orange and blue fruits.

▶ Eat more oily fish such as mackerel, sardines, trout, etc.

▶ Supplement with Vitamins C, E and B, alpha lipoic acid, a full spectrum of carotenoids and mineral supplements containing selenium, copper, manganese and zinc.

▶ Try an anti-inflammatory flavonoid such as green tea or turmeric extract.

Part 3

DIETS WHICH FIGHT DISEASE

Cancer, heart disease, osteoporosis, diabetes and Alzheimer's – the biggest killers, the most dreaded diseases.

We associate each with age and deterioration. It seems almost inevitable that each of us will succumb to at least one. With all the advances of medical science, there seems to be little we can do to prevent them. And once they strike, medicine has treatments, but rarely cures.

Nutritional science, however, offers:

- *Answers – and treatments, even for the 'untreatable' Alzheimer's.*

- *Prevention, even for hidden killers like osteoporosis and hypertension.*

- *And cure, even for heart disease.*

For each there are identified patterns of cause and effect. For each, nutrition offers a long-term way to stave off, treat, even reverse disease.

It's safe, effective and in your own hands.

- Four in every ten of us will develop cancer

- Your diet can greatly increase or reduce your risk of cancer

- Anti-oxidant supplements alone are not enough to stop a poor diet leading to cancer – food offers at least eight distinct anti-cancer families of nutrients

- Eating the right foods leaves your cells swimming in a sea of anti-cancer compounds, backed by a strong immune system

- Upping the amount of fruit and veg you eat can cut your cancer risk in half

- Four servings of tomato a week may cut prostate cancer by a fifth; eating cabbage once a week could cut bowel cancer by two-fifths

- Soy beans, shark cartilage and bilberries contain substances that can slow or stop cancer spreading

- Poly-unsaturated fatty acids in grains, nuts and fish oils have been shown to destroy cancer cells, and may obliterate many before they become tumours

- The anti-cancer diet is almost identical to the anti-heart disease and anti-diabetes diet

Chapter 13

Fighting cancer with food

A s a potential cancer victim (along with everyone else), I'm almost as afraid of the treatment I'd receive as I am of the disease itself.

Chemotherapy, radiotherapy and surgery are not kind to patients, even though cure rates for certain cancers are creeping up. We're still waiting for that elusive breakthrough – like the antibiotics that turned the tables against bacterial diseases.

The health philosophy that prevention is better than cure holds true for all disease – but none more so than cancer.

Causes and effects

The four main causes of cancer are radiation, toxins, infections and food.

Radiation includes solar, nuclear and geological, such as the radioactive gas radon released by granite.

Toxins include tobacco, lead, diesel exhausts, dioxins and asbestos.

Infection includes certain viruses (linked to cervical cancer, liver cancer and leukaemias); bacteria (associated with stomach, colon and other cancers); and fungi, a significant cause of cancer in tropical and sub-tropical regions[1].

Smoking causes 35 per cent of all cancers[245]; another 30 per cent are related to dietary factors[2-4]. Certain foods contain carcinogens; but on the other hand foods also contain a rich mix of anti-cancer compounds. The anti-oxidants have received an enormous amount of publicity, but they are only one element in the protective mix.

It's fine to take anti-oxidants, and there's plenty of evidence that this will improve your long-term health – but there's more to it than that. This chapter spells out just what else you can do to reduce your risk of cancer or, if you already have cancer, how to improve your prospects with nutritional means alone.

THE CHINESE EVIDENCE

One of the best-known trials which showed the protective effects of anti-oxidants was the massive Linxian trial, held in China. Thirty thousand men and women were given Vitamin A and zinc; or riboflavin and niacin; or Vitamin C and molybdenum; or Vitamin E, beta carotene and selenium.

These are sub-optimal combinations of nutrients, and the doses used were relatively small, but there was a 13 per cent decline in total cancer deaths[15]. The problem with the Linxian trial, as far as we are concerned, is that it may not be relevant in the developed countries. Linxian is an area with very poor nutrition and a very high cancer rate, especially of the stomach and oesophagus; would anti-oxidants be as effective in populations who are better nourished?

Various smaller trials suggest that anti-oxidant supplements benefit us too. For example, a high Vitamin C intake has been shown to reduce the risk of cancers of the digestive tract[143], probably by inhibiting nitrosamine formation.

In another trial, supplements of Vitamin E reduced the risk of oral cancer[16]. Conversely a low intake of carotenoids, Vitamin E and other anti-oxidants is associated with high cancer risk[140].

Anti-cancer clues

Some recent techniques, one such is cancer 'immunisation', are very promising and will undoubtedly help to make cancer therapy more effective, and less painful. But they are high tech, and not available just yet. They will be expensive, requiring medical professionals and services.

Factors in the diet which can cause cancer include

- aflatoxins (eg in stale peanuts) and nitrosamines (eg in hot dogs)
- probably sulphate and sulphite preservatives
- charred meats

Dietary factors which help protect against cancer include

- anti-oxidants, enzyme inducers, immuno-supportive nutrients

Food factors which can help suppress a cancer include

- re-differentiators such as genistein, butyric acid, lycopene and alpha carotene
- angiostats such as genistein and various flavonoids
- apoptosis (cell 'suicide') inducers such as genistein, various flavonoids, and carotenoids such as lycopene and alpha carotene

In the meantime, there are a series of safe, inexpensive, nutritional steps you can take which will reduce your own risk of cancer dramatically.

A predominantly vegetarian diet helps, but this is just the beginning. If we knew which fruits and vegetables had the strongest anti-cancer effects, we could select our diet accordingly, and cut the cancer risk still further.

Many important cancers (including cancer of the prostate, breast, stomach, liver, colon, oral cavity, oesophagus and ovaries) are significantly reduced by a fruit and vegetable diet, and are up to 20 times less common in some countries than in others[14].

If we knew just what it was in the fruit and vegetables which protected us against cancer, we could try to breed new strains of those crops which contained higher levels of the crucial ingredients. Alternatively, we could take concentrated extracts of fruits and vegetables in pills and capsules, to gain a similar advantage.

The pharmaceutical industry isn't very interested in marketing such things, as they can't be patented; but they are busy making their own versions of some of the key compounds, and these will start to enter the market in the next few years.

And that gives the game away. Many important anti-cancer compounds in plants have been identified. What's more, they have been grouped into several distinct categories, on the basis of the type of risk reducing effect each one offers.

Different scientists have proposed different sorts of categories, so the one which follows is a compromise, but it will give you a reasonably comprehensive guide as to what food has to offer.

Eight vital elements in the fight against cancer

Cancer avoidance

1 First there are the **classical anti-oxidants**, which neutralise the dangerous free radicals produced inside the body by radiation and by some toxins.

These include:

- Vitamins A, C, E, D, K and some of the B group
- Co-enzyme Q10
- alpha-lipoic acid
- the plant compounds called the flavonoids
- the carotenoids, such as lycopene
- melatonin.

2 The second group of cancer-protective substances in food are the **enzyme inducers**. These are compounds which stimulate the body into producing higher than normal amounts of 'de-toxifying' enzymes.

Some of these enzymes can neutralise free radicals. Another group (Phase 2 enzymes) speed the removal of carcinogens from the body.

In this category are compounds like quercitin and sulphorophane – found in onions, cabbage and broccoli.

3 A group of compounds which have the ability to wrap themselves round the fragile DNA inside our cells, providing a **shield** against harmful influences. Most of these appear to be flavonoids.

4 A group which **binds directly to potential carcinogens** and speeds their excretion from the body. Chlorogenic acid, a flavonoid found in tomatoes, is one example.

5 **Immuno-enhancers** are substances which improve the immune system's ability to mount a defence against foreign organisms such as cancer cells.

- Various herbs like echinacea have been shown to increase the number of natural killer cells (which can kill cancer cells). They also boost production of interferon, a natural anti-cancer 'hormone'.

- Some ingredients in plant fibre, such as the pectic polysaccharides, have a similar effect; as do related polysaccharides found in certain mushrooms, fungi, the cell walls of some bacteria and the gritty particles in pear skin.

50% potential risk reduction

By increasing your intake of fruits and vegetables, evidence is accumulating that you can potentially cut your risk of cancer almost in half, and the risk of certain cancers by 75 per cent[3, 12, 13, 120, 181, 211].

People who eat fruits and vegetables rich in anti-oxidants have less genetic damage[81] – one of the precursors to cancer.

Cut skin cancer by 70%

One recent study indicated that taking Vitamin A could reduce the chance of basal cell carcinoma – the most common form of skin cancer – by 70 per cent[133].

- Some bacteria which live in the gut have been reported to improve immune performance: these are the lactobacilli and bifidobacteria, the organisms in live yoghurt. These can be increased in the gut by eating non-digestible oligosaccharides found in foods like oats, onions and Jerusalem artichokes (see Chapter 7, Pre-biotic fibre).

- Co-enzyme Q10 is not strictly speaking an immuno-enhancer, but should be used in conjunction with all the above agents, as it increases the energy with which the immune system can go to work. Interestingly, there are reports that indicate that high doses of Q10 alone (around 400mg/day) can induce remission in some cases of breast cancer[182-184] (see Chapter 9, Co-enzyme Q10).

- Glutamine – this amino acid prevents the immuno-suppression caused by excessive physical exercise.

- Adaptogens – such as Siberian ginseng – can prevent the immuno-suppression caused by excessive stress.

Cancer containment

6 **Anti-cancer nutrients** improve connections between cells, and help to bring cancer cells back under normal control. The carotenoids are important members of this group, and are found in orange and red plant foods such as peppers, carrots and tomatoes, and in dark green leaf vegetables. Genistein, an isoflavone from soy, is another, as is selenium.

7 **Anti-growth factors**. These work in different ways, but all have the ability to inhibit the growth of tumours, to slow the growth of new blood vessels to supply those tumours, and to impede the tumour's ability to spread (metastasis).

Into this category fall:

- protease inhibitors, such as lectins (found in beans like soy beans).

Could we eliminate most cancers?

By identifying the anti-cancer elements in the diets of the low risk countries, we too may be able to achieve the same low risk status.

This chapter will look at those elements.

- matrix stabilisers such as flavonoids (in grapeseed, the bark of maritime pine, quince, etc), flavolignans (flaxseed) and flavonoid-like compounds found in herbs such as echinacea: and the closely related …

- angiostats, such as genistein (in soy), or the glycoproteins found in shark cartilage (see page 197, and Chapter 6, Flavonoids & isoflavones).

8 **Redifferentiators**. These compounds can force cancer cells back to normal or in some cases to commit suicide ('apoptosis'). They include butyrate, a fatty acid produced in the large bowel by (friendly) bifido-bacteria (see Chapter 7, Pre-biotic fibre); flavonoids including genistein and resveratrol, carotenoids including lycopene, and lectins including chokeberry and elderberry lectins.

THE ANTI-CANCER STORY SO FAR

Increase your intake of cruciferous vegetables like cabbage and broccoli, tomatoes, mushrooms, live yoghurt and soy-based foods. Your supplement regime should include a broad spectrum vitamin/mineral anti-oxidant supplement (at levels shown on page 338), a flavonoid complex (eg grapeseed, bilberry, etc.), Co-enzyme Q10, betaine and occasionally echinacea, plus a pre-biotic supplement.

When cancer begins

You can see that, although I placed anti-oxidants first in the list, they are merely one of a large number of categories of anti-cancer compounds.

This is why you cannot make up for a bad diet with anti-oxidant supplements alone. And when you consider that there are hundreds of carotenoids, thousands of flavonoids, and an unknown number of examples in most of the other categories, it all begins to seem rather confusing. But here's another way of looking at it, which should help to put it into some sort of perspective.

A summary of the anti-cancer shield

- **Anti-oxidants**

- **Enzyme boosters – especially found in cruciferous vegetables like cabbage, broccoli, kale and onions**

- **Flavonoids**

- **Carcinogen neutralisers, eg chlorogenic acid found in tomatoes**

- **Immuno-boosters – found in certain mushrooms, lactobacilli and increased when you eat oats, onions, inulin, soluble fibre and butyrate**

- **Redifferentiators such as carotenoids and genistein**

- **Compounds that inhibit the flow of blood to tumours, eg the soy derivative genistein, and other flavonoids**

DIETS WHICH FIGHT DISEASE : **Cancer**

Throughout our lives, cells in our bodies are dying, multiplying, and being replaced. Each time our cells divide, they have to copy the DNA they contain as accurately as possible; but they're only human. Mistakes creep in – mistakes that can lead to cell death or the uncontrolled growth of cancer.

To make matters worse, there is a constant background of low level radiation (unless you are a frequent flyer – one trans-Atlantic flight = four whole body x-rays!). Even at the best of times, our cells are constantly being irradiated. It's been calculated that the DNA in each cell receives around 1,000 hits per day, although a diet rich in anti-oxidants reduces the rate of DNA damage[204, 222].

The repair systems are very good indeed at spotting damage and repairing it, but they're not perfect and there is a steady accumulation of DNA errors with age. There is a constant risk of a cell somewhere in the body taking a wrong turn and becoming cancerous, a risk which increases with age as genetic errors accumulate and repair mechanisms slow down.

If our immune system is working properly it may spot the cancers early on, and kill them. But when the immune system is damaged (by immuno-suppressant drugs, malnutrition, stress or HIV), the incidence of cancers increases very significantly.

This is where our diet comes in. As you can see from the long list of protective food substances, our cells are swimming in a sea of anti-cancer compounds derived from the food we eat, and these act as a second safety net.

When you remember that almost all of these anti-cancer compounds come from the fruits and vegetables in our diet, it's easy to see why a vegetarian diet reduces the risk of cancer.

So what are the key anti-cancer compounds, where do you find them, and how should you put them together?

Anti-cancer strategy – Level 1 – Avoidance

The following are suspect, potential or actual carcinogens (cancer causing elements). Reduce your exposure whenever you can.

- Tobacco smoke
- Petrochemical compounds
- Preservative nitrates in bacon, hot dogs
- Smoked fish or meat
- Fats heated to high temperatures – 200°C or over
- Saturated fat in excess amounts
- Pesticide and insecticide residues
- Charred meat
- Mould on nuts and grains
- X-rays
- Solar radiation

However, you don't get cancer by simply being exposed to carcinogens. You get cancer when the carcinogen load your body suffers overwhelms your body's natural repair ability.

That's why it makes sense to continually support your natural defence mechanisms with anti-oxidants, immuno-strengthening nutrients and other protective dietary factors.

Plants and protective enzymes

Fruits and vegetables contain anti-oxidant vitamins and other compounds, which shield us from free radicals which can otherwise cause cancer. But, although the anti-oxidant nutrients are important, they are the body's second line of defence against free radicals. The first line of defence is the anti-oxidant enzymes that our cells make themselves.

And we now know how to boost enzyme levels quickly and cheaply – by eating more fruit and vegetables.

Many fruits and vegetables contain substances which stimulate the body to speed up production of the major anti-oxidant enzymes. At the world-famous Food Research Station at Norwich, Dr Gary Williamson's team have carried out a survey of hundreds of different foods, looking for their ability to boost levels of the anti-oxidant enzyme quinone reductase.

Your anti-cancer strategy can be visualised in three levels:

Level 1 – Avoid it

Level 2 – Contain it

Level 3 – Kill it

Enzyme production needs minerals

The body will try to boost its own levels of anti-oxidant enzymes whenever levels of free radicals increase, whether this is caused by smoking, exercise or infection[153-154].

But these anti-oxidant enzymes need the trace metals selenium, zinc, manganese and copper to work properly.

As so many of us are depleted in these trace metals, we cannot always protect ourselves adequately.

Natural phase 2 enzyme boosters:

- **Cabbage – particularly Savoy**

- **Brussels sprouts**

- **Broccoli**

- **Red peppers**

- **Garden peas**

- **Fresh rosemary**

- **Onions, leeks, etc**

- **Citrus fruits**

Eat your greens!

Eating cabbage at least once a week is reported to reduce the incidence of cancer of the colon and rectum by as much as two thirds[80] (although this has been disputed).

Brussels sprouts, broccoli and kale are probably better anti-cancer foods.

The new 'super-broccoli' will be better still.

Their theory is that eating those foods which increase levels of quinone reductase will improve our defences against free radicals and offer protection against cancer[77].

Various foods also stimulate the formation of two other groups of detoxifying enzymes – called the Phase 1 and Phase 2 enzymes. These enzyme groups are important in breaking down dietary carcinogens and toxins and removing them from the body.

Phase 1 enzymes are oxidative enzymes; Phase 2 enzymes make potentially dangerous compounds more soluble, so that they can be more easily excreted in the bile or in the urine.

Specific foods improve the performance of these enzymes, and improve the body's ability to deal with carcinogens.

Most scientists are concentrating on Phase 2 enzymes. The cabbage and onion families score highly here[78]. One interesting study found that the amount of genetic damage in smokers was reduced when they ate large amounts of Brussels sprouts[81].

Other vegetables which are good at inducing Phase 2 enzymes include red peppers (raw), and garden peas (raw or cooked).

Different kinds of cabbage had different effects: Savoy Rhapsody was very effective, other strains of cabbage less so. Raw basil is very effective at stimulating the body to make its own anti-oxidant enzymes, as is rosemary, which should be given pride of place in the spice rack because it is also a very potent anti-oxidant.

The best inducers of Phase 2 enzymes, however, were Brussels sprouts and broccoli, especially when eaten raw[77]. As no-one in their right mind wants to eat raw Brussels sprouts, I would personally choose broccoli, in a salad or served with a dip, as the most painless and effective way of getting the body's enzyme defences up and running.

I would also put onions or leeks on the menu because quercitin, a flavonoid found in high concentrations in the outer layers of leeks, onions and shallots, is a powerful enzyme inducer and anti-oxidant[82], and also is linked to a reduction in cancer risk[202].

To summarise this section – the first level in the anti-cancer strategy is to minimise exposure to carcinogens, and to strengthen the body's anti-cancer defences.

This will undoubtedly reduce the risk of many cancers – but not to zero. Some cancers will still emerge. What can enhanced nutrition do for the cancer sufferer? For one thing, it offers the prospect of cancer containment.

FOOD PREPARATION, COOKING AND STORING AFFECT NUTRITION

Dr Williamson's work showed that the breed of plant and the method of preparing the food make a big difference; and the length of storage may also be a factor. These variables are being studied, and it may soon be possible to make more detailed recommendations regarding dietary intake. It is already clear that cooked cabbage, sprouts, kale, and broccoli; mustard, radish and horseradish; citrus fruits; raw peas and red peppers are all good at upregulating the Phase 2 enzymes[77].

Anti-cancer strategy – Level 2 – Containment

Many cancer specialists no longer talk about cancer killing, but cancer management, or containment. Killing cancers with radiotherapy or drugs is still very toxic, although some clever targeting systems will make the killing strategy safer. Cancer containment is intrinsically less aggressive, and easier on the patient. The basic idea is that, if we could stop cancers growing and spreading, we could live with them.

Co-habitation with a cancer may seem scary, but if held in check, a tumour could remain in situ for years or decades – and perhaps eventually be down-graded to a minor inconvenience.

The extra-cellular matrix

All our cells are normally held in place by the three-dimensional mesh of micro-fibres known as the extra-cellular matrix (See Chapter 10, Amino sugars). If a cancer is to grow, or spread ('metastasise') from its site of origin, it must break through the matrix; and aggressive cancers do this by secreting a group of very destructive enzymes called the Matrix Metallo-Proteinases (MMPs). There are over twenty of these, and between them they break down the micro-fibres, eating holes in the matrix which

Hey Pesto!

Pesto sauce has a high basil content. And it's made with olive oil.

Blocking cancer by limiting its growth

- **Genistein, a compound found in soy beans (see Chapter 6)**

- **Sulphated glycosaminoglycans**

- **Tetrahydrocortisone, a hormone formed in the adrenals, is regarded as one of the body's natural anti-tumour agents (angiostats)**

- **Shark cartilage (see following pages)**

- **Flavolignans found in flaxseed and linseed**

- **Many flavonoids (green tea, tumeric, red wine)**

- **Lectins (soy beans)**

permit the ingrowth of new blood vessels (essential for tumour growth), and the outgrowth of cancer cells (metastasis).

Blocking the matrix metallo-proteinases is the key to cancer containment, as this strategy inhibits both cancer growth and metastasis.

Cancer growth

When a cancer first starts to grow, it can only reach the size of a pinhead before it runs out of oxygen, and starts to choke on its own waste products. To grow any further it needs its own blood supply, new capillaries to bring in oxygen and nutrients and take away the waste products.

At this point the low nutrient/high waste levels attract new blood vessels towards the cancer. Now it can start to grow very much larger[159-161].

Certain compounds are able to prevent the formation of new blood vessels, thereby starving the cancer and preventing it from expanding.

These anti-growth compounds are known as angiostats. They are an enormously promising new class of natural and non-toxic anti-cancer agents[61]. One is genistein found in soy beans; another occurs in shark cartilage.

Drugs

Some drugs inhibit the growth of new blood vessels. One is thalidomide; another is captopril, which blocks many MMPs. These may become useful cancer management tools.

How genistein can block the spread of cancer

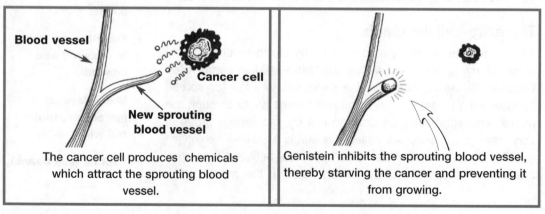

Blood vessel

Cancer cell

New sprouting blood vessel

The cancer cell produces chemicals which attract the sprouting blood vessel.

Genistein inhibits the sprouting blood vessel, thereby starving the cancer and preventing it from growing.

Natural angiostats

All the angiostats now being studied in the cancer research centres stem from a natural product breakthrough made by Dr Judah Folkman at Bethesda, who did the first work with bovine cartilage extracts[159-160].

It became public knowledge in the early '90s, when marine biologist Dr Bill Lane published a book on the anti-cancer effects of shark cartilage[251]. Here's how angiostats work.

Active cells anywhere in the body use up oxygen. This reduces oxygen levels in the local tissues and causes a build-up of potentially toxic waste products. This triggers new blood vessels to grow into the area and bring in more oxygen. So as the body grows, the blood supply automatically grows in step with it.

This is why the network of arteries and veins is so beautifully and efficiently laid out. It grows exactly to where it is needed, and in the right amounts. So there are blood vessels in skin, muscle, brain, bone, lungs – every tissue in the body – with one sole exception: cartilage.

Although cartilage (the medical term for gristle) is alive, it contains no blood vessels. This is because there are chemicals in cartilage that prevent the ingrowth of new blood vessels. These inhibitory chemicals are probably there because if arteries and veins were to grow into the cartilage they would weaken it.

This offers a completely new approach to the treatment of cancer.

While you are growing, the blood system grows with you. But when you stop growing you stop forming new blood vessels – except in a very limited number of situations.

Firstly, in women, blood vessels re-grow inside the uterus once a month, after every period, as part of the menstrual cycle.

Secondly, the tissue regrowth which occurs in the healing process after major surgery also needs new blood vessels.

Thirdly, there is some regrowth of blood vessels after a heart attack. And finally, there is cancer.

In adults, cancer cells represent a new localised area of tissue growth. As the cancer cells grow and multiply, their metabolic activity reduces local oxygen levels, and increases local levels of waste products.

Cartilage has no blood vessels

As a cancer grows it needs new blood vessels.

All body tissue has blood vessels supplying it – except cartilage, which contains compounds that inhibit blood vessel growth.

That's why cartilage extract is being used to slow tumour growth.

The lens of the eye is the only other tissue without blood vessels – and may contain similar compounds.

Sharks have 10 times more cartilage than mammals

Cartilage makes up six per cent of a shark's body weight, compared with less than 0.6 per cent in cows and other mammals. Compared to fish, they are relatively immune to cancer.

This stimulates the ingrowth of new blood vessels. With its own blood supply established, the cancer can really take off[159-161]. (If you film a tumour using time-lapse photography, you see all the nearby blood vessels sending offshoots towards the tumour, as if they were drawn in by a magnetic field. When they arrive, tumour growth accelerates.)

This was why, back in the '70s, researchers wanted to test substances that might stop the growth of new blood vessels. They thought that bovine cartilage might be a good place to look. Their hope was that cartilage extracts could stop the formation of new blood vessels, and starve cancers to death.

The first results were positive[252-254]. When cartilage extract was given to mice and rabbits, the growth of new blood vessels towards tumours stopped, and tumour growth was halted, with no toxicity. But although bovine cartilage clearly contained angiostat compounds, they were only present in very small amounts. It took a half kilo of cartilage to make 1 milligram of active compound. Because cancer patients would require about 10 grams of the active compound per day, a drug company would need to process 5,000 kilos of cow cartilage per patient, per day.

It was at this point that the shark made its contribution. Although most fish suffer from cancer just like any other higher life-form, sharks are nearly immune to cancer. It is perhaps no coincidence that sharks have skeletons composed entirely of cartilage.

The research group started with cartilage from the 20-foot long basking shark, and obtained positive results. The first assays revealed that shark cartilage was an extremely rich source of the angiostat factor, containing over a thousand times more of the compound than cow cartilage[255]. The researchers realised the importance of their findings. Other labs duplicated the results[62-66,127,128,256], and the rest of the medical profession began to take an interest.

A few doctors started to give shark cartilage extract to some of their 'hopeless cases'. In a few of these patients, the tumours shrank and disappeared. Patients who had been given up for dead, recovered. Sceptical clinicians became converts. As a result, further research into angiostats is now under way.

No side effects

The beauty of angiostats is that they don't affect any other part of the body, except in those few situations where new blood vessels are forming.

Compared to orthodox chemotherapy, angiostats are remarkably free from side effects.

Angiostats are not panaceas

Angiostats, whether natural or synthetic, work best to help suppress breast, cervical, prostate and other solid tumours, rather than leukaemias and lymphomas.

Shark cartilage and the soy compound genistein appear to attack cancers in a highly specific manner, and at one of their weakest points. The blood supply to a tumour is much more fragile than a normal blood network. The vessels are thin and incomplete, constantly breaking down and constantly needing to be replaced. Anything which inhibits the formation of new blood vessels is going to hit the tumour very hard.

But this approach won't treat every cancer. Breast, cervical, prostate, brain, and other solid tumours are likely to be the best targets. Lung cancer is unlikely to respond well, because lung tissue is so rich in blood vessels that a tumour could simply cannibalise the vessels already in the vicinity. Leukaemias and lymphomas are also unlikely to respond to this type of treatment, as they are less dependent on new blood vessels in their development.

HOW EFFECTIVE IS SHARK CARTILAGE?

Some scientists dismiss oral shark cartilage supplements because the proteins in shark cartilage are too large to be absorbed in the gut.

However, certain cancers and many anti-cancer treatments make the gut more 'leaky' and it may be in these subjects (about one in five) that shark cartilage has an effect – although only in large (100g/day) doses.

Shark cartilage would be more effective, and work at lower doses, if it could be given intravenously. The problem with even the best oral commercial shark cartilage is that it is too dilute.

Other roles for angiostats?

Angiostats also play an important role in one other group of diseases, namely the inflammatory diseases.

Although I am not yet aware of any major trials, there are many anecdotal stories of arthritis sufferers (and arthritic pets) who have responded well to shark cartilage treatment.

Inhibition of blood vessel growth pobably pays a role here; but trials have also found that shark cartilage contains substances which can modulate the activity of the immune system.

There is one more fishy story before we leave the shark, and that is to do with shark liver oil; which may turn out to be as therapeutically important as the cartilage.

Arthritis too?

In conditions such as rheumatoid arthritis, the continuing inflammation in the affected joints depends on the growth of new blood vessels into the damaged and inflamed tissues.

It seems quite logical, considering the way in which shark cartilage works, that it should also have some anti-arthritic activity.

Cartilage and auto-immune diseases

Some studies have shown that cartilage can boost the production of anti-bodies, and increase the activity of immune cells[257-261].

If shark cartilage were proven to enhance the body's natural immunity, it might eventually find a role in improving the effective-ness of vaccines.

Shark liver oil is a rich source of a peculiar group of compounds called alkoxyglycerols. These compounds occur in small quantities in many natural sources, including bone marrow, and human breast milk.

Alkoxyglycerols have a number of interesting properties. A Swedish team have shown that they stimulate the formation of antibodies after immunisation[262, 263]. They also help to minimise the suppression of bone marrow which occurs after radiation therapy[262, 264, 265]. They have been shown to protect against radiation injury caused by radiotherapy for cancer, especially when given prophylactically, ie in advance[266, 267]; when shark liver oil is given to cancer patients before radiation treatment, tumours are harder hit and mortality is reduced[267].

The shark has long been feared as the most ruthless and efficient of predators. But it looks as if the shark and its cousins, the skates and rays, may make an important contribution to the nutritionally based medicine of the future.

> **Matrix breakdown**
>
> There are three main elements in the extra-cellular matrix: collagen, elastin, and hyaluronic acid polymers.
>
> The matrix metallo-proteinase enzymes (MMPs) include enzymes which break down collagen (collagenase), elastin (elastase), hyaluronic acid (hyaluronidase) and gelatin (gelatinase).
>
> There are over 20 MMP enzymes known.

Cancer spread

The process of new vessel growth is complex, and can be blocked at several points. The matrix metallo-proteinases (MMPs) are an obvious target, as if there are no holes in the extra-cellular matrix there is nowhere the new blood vessels can grow. The other reason for targeting the MMPs is that they are equally involved in metastatic spread.

If a cancer is to metastasise, it must first attach to and then break through the extra-cellular matrix that would otherwise hold it in place. In order to do this, cancer cells secrete MMPs; the more MMPs a cancer secretes, the more invasive it becomes[126, 155].

These enzymes are so destructive that if a cancer cell tried to secrete them in active form, it would blow itself apart.

Instead, it secretes a form of the enzyme which is blocked with a sort of safety catch.

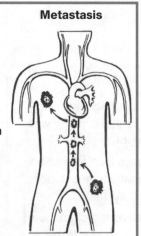

Metastasis

Cancer cells can break away from a cancerous site and travel via the blood stream to other parts of the body.

There they can attach themselves and start a new cancer or metastasis.

It's rather like the dispersal of seeds.

Once the inactive enzyme has been safely pushed out of the cancer cell, a second group of enzymes, called proteases, strip off the safety catch, and activate the matrix metallo-proteinase enzymes.

Cancer containment – a nutraceutical approach

The process whereby a cancer spreads can be blocked at a number of stages, using different food extracts.

Firstly, the rate of MMP production in cancer cells can be reduced by extracts (technically lectins) derived from the elderberry plant[236]; and by flavonoids such as the citrus flavonoids[237].

Secondly, the proteases responsible for activating the MMPs can be blocked by protease inhibitors such as the Bowman Birk compound (another lectin), which occurs in high levels in soy beans (see pages 202-203). These first two steps reduce both the amount of MMPs, and the degree of MMP activation.

Thirdly, those MMPs which have been activated can be blocked by various flavonoids. Some have the ability to bind the zinc atom at the heart of the MMP enzymes, others may block the enzymes' active site by bonding to specific amino acids on the site.

Fourthly, those activated MMPs which remain active can be prevented from attacking the matrix with flavonoids, which bind to elements in the matrix and shield them from enzyme attack.

Breast cancer risk

The protease/metallo proteinase story is very complex. Some MMPs, once activated by a protease enzyme, go on to activate other MMPs, so that the initial release of inactive precursors becomes a self-activating cascade of destructive enzymes.

The actions of lectins and flavonoids, therefore, overlap somewhat; but this does not invalidate the general scheme shown in the box below.

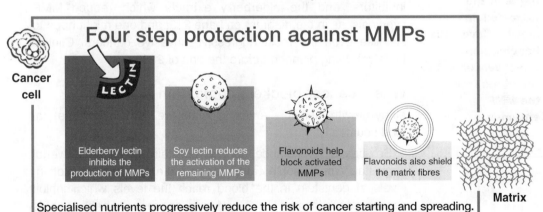

Four step protection against MMPs

Cancer cell

LECTIN

| Elderberry lectin inhibits the production of MMPs | Soy lectin reduces the activation of the remaining MMPs | Flavonoids help block activated MMPs | Flavonoids also shield the matrix fibres |

Matrix

Specialised nutrients progressively reduce the risk of cancer starting and spreading.

How flavonoids block MMPs

1 **MMPs require an atom of zinc to function – and many flavonoids can chelate (bind) this metal.**

2 **Flavonoids also bond to the amino acids proline and hydroxyproline. If these amino acids are in or near to the MMPs' active site, this will impair the enzyme's function.**

3 **Proline and hydroxyproline are also present in the micro-fibres of the extra-cellular matrix. Flavonoids bonding here effectively shield the fibres from the MMP enzymes.**

How effective is this nutraceutical approach to cancer management? The evidence is persuasive: for example, one group of flavonoids (termed proanthocyanidins) cause 100 per cent inhibition of key MMPs[74] at levels which are achieved in the body by taking grapeseed extract supplements, or by drinking 1/2 to 3/4 litres of red wine per day. This could explain the recent findings that red wine drinking is associated, not only with a reduced risk of cardiac deaths, but also of deaths from all causes[186-191].

Red wine contains the particular flavonoids resveratrol, which has a wide range of anti-cancer properties[241]; and catechin. In one particularly exciting experiment, when high dose red wine extract was given to cancer-prone mice, their life-span increased by 50 per cent or more[242].

In my experience, this group of flavonoids has the ability to stop even the most aggressive cancer cells in their tracks, at least in laboratory experiments[238]. What is more, these compounds achieve significant levels in the tissues, including the brain[239] – and they are non-toxic.

Other flavonoids which are almost as effective as the proanthocyanidins at blocking MMPs include luteolin, apigenin, kaempferol and silybin; and some of these have been shown to reduce cancer cell invasiveness also[185]. Olive oil, too, can inhibit MMP activity[240], and this is an important element in the health-promoting Mediterranean diet.

Add to the anti-cancer regime the soy-derived protease inhibitors, and the elderberry extracts which reduce MMP synthesis, as in the diagram on page 213; and one might hope to stabilise even the most aggressive, invasive cancers. Clinical trials are being planned before the end of 2000.

Where cancer blockers come from

Many growth inhibitors and angiostats are derived from natural food sources.

Soy beans, for instance, contain genistein, which is a powerful angiostat. When people eat a reasonable amount of soy protein, levels of genistein in the blood reach the levels which inhibit cancer growth in vitro[67, 68, 129], and force cancer cells back towards more normal behaviour[134] (known as redifferentiation).

Various experimenters have shown that genistein and other soy compounds are effective in suppressing the growth of breast cancer[131, 132, 139]; prostate cancer[137, 138]; colon cancer cells[133]; and leukaemias[130, 135, 136].

Soy is so much more widely consumed in Japan than in the West that levels of genistein in the urine of Japanese men and women are 30 times higher than in Westerners. This means that their blood and tissue levels are also much higher – probably high enough to keep many cancers in check. This would explain the four to fivefold increase in prostate and breast cancers in Japanese who relocate to the USA. They are no longer eating soy as a staple, and any cancer lurking in the body but being kept in check by the genistein, is suddenly free to grow[76].

Soy also contains at least five protease inhibitors, which prevent the activation of the matrix metallo-proteinase enzymes[76].

One of these is the Bowman Birk protease inhibitor. Recent work shows that this interesting and potentially therapeutic compound is rapidly absorbed from the gut, and spreads widely in the body, reaching the lungs, liver, kidneys, blood and the bladder[70].

Consider also blackcurrants, and the perennial herb Lady's Mantle. These plants contain flavonoids which are potent inhibitors of the metallo-proteinase enzymes, including the elastases, hyaluronidases, gelatinases and collagenases[71, 72, 74].

Don't forget ginkgo and pycnogenol. These contain flavonoids which are very good at stabilising collagen and elastin fibres and protecting them from enzymic attack – an equally important anti-cancer property[73, 75, 123-125, 185-191]. But for optimal cancer control, flavonoids should be combined with appropriate lectins and carotenoids.

Cancer-controlling carotenoids

The carotenoids – beta carotene is the best-known example – are a family of plant compounds which produce the yellow, orange, pink and red colouration in foods such as carrots, apricots and squashes.

Cancer blockers:

- **Soy beans and soy products**

- **Blackcurrants, elderberries**

- **Ginkgo**

- **Alpha-carotene**

- **Lycopene**

- **Flaxseed**

- **Green tea**

- **Grapeseed extract, raspberries**

LOOK FOR ...

a supplement that includes an angiostat (eg 40-100mg of soy isoflavones) that will help restrict blood supply to incipient cancers;

Plus flavonoids (especially from berries) which help block MMP enzymes and protect the extra-cellular matrix.

They are anti-oxidants, which explains their ability to protect against macular (eyesight) degeneration and coronary artery disease[193-195, 220] – a high lycopene intake appeared to reduce heart attacks by 40 per cent in the recent Euramic Study[295]. They are immuno-enhancing agents. They also have the special property of improving communications between cancer cells and normal cells, which is thought to force cancer cells to revert to normal behaviour[50, 83-86, 89].

Beta carotene and lung cancer

The relationship between beta carotene and lung cancer is particularly complex. A high beta carotene intake **reduces** the risk of lung cancer in non-smokers, but **increases** the incidence of lung cancer in smokers (shown by the ATBC[156] and CARET[213] studies).

The most persuasive explanation for this unexpected finding is that, under certain circumstances, beta carotene (in common with all carotenoids) becomes pro-oxidant and harmful.

This is most likely to occur when there are high concentrations of beta carotene, oxygen and free radicals, local tissue damage and, critically, low levels of Vitamin C. This is a precise description of the lungs of a smoker taking beta carotene supplements.

Carotenoids, as with Vitamin E, must not be taken without a Vitamin C foundation. When safely combined with Vitamin C, carotenoids should give pronounced health benefits to smokers and non-smokers alike. However, until further research clarifies the situation, it is wise for smokers **not** to supplement with beta carotene.

A novel anti-cancer effect

Many carotenoids have the ability to inhibit cancer development at low, non-toxic doses. The inhibition is generally reversible, so that, when the carotenoids are withdrawn, the cancer begins to grow once more. (Translated into dietary terms, this emphasises the importance of long-term nutritional prevention/maintenance regimes, rather than short-term treatment.)

Technically, the strength of this anti-cancer effect is related to the ability of carotenoids to improve inter-cellular communication; and to increase synthesis of connexin 43 (C43) protein, which forms part of the gap junction between cells[51, 52, 321, 322]. Increased C43 synthesis is strongly linked to growth control, and the suppression of neoplastic growth[83-86]. Cancer cells are deficient in terms of intra-cellular communication, C43 protein and contact inhibition. Carotenoids can return these parameters to near-

---

Mixed is best

Mixed natural carotenoids (ie not just beta carotene, but alpha carotene, lutein, lycopene[261], crypto-xanthin, etc.) can persuade cancer cells to revert to normal. Always combine with Vitamin C and selenium.

normal, and work best when combined with selenium, which is an essential element in C43 protein.

This is probably why the carotenoids can induce cultured cancer cells to revert to normal behaviour patterns[50, 89]. This finding is reflected in animal and clinical studies, where carotenoids have been used to prevent the development of pre-cancerous conditions in the upper respiratory tract, mouth, gut and cervix, with some success[16, 26, 34, 83, 88, 92, 93, 283, 286, 296, 304].

This potentially vital anti-cancer action is probably not a retinoid effect; the evidence suggests that carotenoids possess an intrinsic ability to regulate the key growth controlling genes[91, 173, 203, 276, 277, 294].

This would explain why high carotenoid levels in the diet are linked to a reduced risk of cancer in the stomach, oesophagus, cervix, throat and lung[8, 11, 17, 33, 87, 90, 176, 209, 278, 281, 287, 303]. But which carotenoid?

Many studies which found a lower cancer risk with a beta carotene rich diet were actually measuring the effect of a diet rich in fruits and vegetables, which contain a range of carotenoids and other potentially therapeutic compounds. In the last few years it has become apparent that beta carotene, *by itself*, appears to offer relatively little protection against cancer[156, 213, 218, 219, 221, 271, 272, 291, 292, 302, 312].

> ### Limits to growth
>
> Normal cells have C43 proteins on their surfaces. As they multiply the C43 proteins come into contact with C43s on other cells and this stops further growth. This is called cell contact inhibition.
>
> Cancer cells have few or no C43s, so their growth is uncontrolled.
>
> Selenium depletion impairs C43 function, which may be why it is linked to an increased risk of cancer.

Why organic foods are better cancer protectors

Protease inhibitors and flavonoids in soy beans and other plants (including tomatoes and potatoes) are part of the plant's defence system against insect predators.

For example, protease inhibitors stunt the growth of the insects and reduce the amount of plant consumed.

It's a generalised response. Even if only one leaf has been attacked by an insect, the plant begins to build up levels of its defence compounds throughout its leaves, shoots and other parts.

If the protease inhibitors and flavonoids are important in reducing our risk of cancer, it may therefore be healthier for us to eat organic food, which is exposed to more insect attack; because the plant will have developed higher levels of these defence compounds.

Immaculate fruits and vegetables, unblemished by insect attack, which are produced by intensively sprayed crops and designed for the supermarket shelves, are likely to contain less of the compounds which may be critical to lowering our cancer risk.

Genistein, the isoflavone in soy, also has anti-cancer properties. Genetically modified soy appears to contain less genistein – another argument for organic foods?

Lycopene – a strong anti-cancer carotenoid

The fact is that when researchers tested beta carotene, they probably picked the wrong carotenoid. Beta carotene is not as potent an anti-cancer agent as alpha carotene[199, 200], lutein or lycopene[314]. These carotenoids occur in some of the same foods as beta carotene, so the surveys which showed that a diet rich in beta carotene reduced the risk of cancer, were probably measuring the protective effects of other carotenoids, such as alpha carotene, found in carrots; and lycopene, found almost exclusively in tomatoes[318].

Of all the carotenoids found in human tissues, lycopene tends to have the most potent anti-cancer properties on a variety of human and other cancer cell lines in vitro[300, 315, 320].

In clinical studies, lycopene has been linked to a significant degree of protection against cancers of the gastrointestinal tract[282], breast[274, 323], the cervix[311, 319] and especially of the prostate[290]. In this context, it is probably relevant that lycopene is stored in the body in the testes, adrenal and prostate[279, 280, 317].

In sum, the balance of the evidence now available indicates that lycopene is an important micro-nutrient, and among the most potent anti-cancer dietary factors yet discovered[95-98, 288, 289, 309, 325-329].

Pasteurised tomato juice and tomato paste are good sources of lycopene, and have been shown to boost lycopene levels in the blood. Uncooked tomatoes do not have much effect, as the lycopene they contain is locked up inside the plant cell walls, and is unavailable for absorption[316].

Anti-cancer strategy – Level 3 – Killing

Cancer management as described in the preceding section may be able to hold many cancers in check for years, perhaps indefinitely. And it is very likely that some cancers managed in this way, starved of nutrition, unable to spread and forced to re-differentiate, will eventually die off. Other cancers however may persist, or become resistant. If this happens, cancer killing may become the only option – and nutrients have a role to play here too. Fish oil may be among the most important of these.

PUFAs are found in high concentrations in the membranes of all our body cells, in the form of phospholipids. They are very prone to being oxidised by free radicals[17].

When a PUFA molecule is oxidised it becomes a PUFA radical. This starts a chain reaction, oxidising other PUFAs into PUFA radicals. A chain reaction quickly becomes a cascade and, if not stopped, it kills the cell[20].

This doesn't usually happen, because anti-oxidants such as Vitamin E block the chain reaction. Another 'fire break' is that PUFAs in the membranes are kept apart from each other in separate compartments. But if the compartment bulkheads are damaged, and the PUFAs come into contact with one another, the chain reaction takes off and they all oxidise very rapidly indeed[17].

Cancer cells are different from normal cells in many respects, but one of the crucial differences is that they have sub-normal levels of PUFAs in their cell membranes[50-52].

They don't seem to be able to handle PUFAs well. If they are 'fed' on PUFAs, they produce more than normal amounts of PUFA radicals[19], because they are unable to protect them from oxidation in the way that normal cells do.

This isn't because they have less anti-oxidants. In fact, cancer cells tend to have above normal levels of Vitamin E and/or beta carotene[23-25, 180], and increased levels of the main anti-oxidant enzymes too[57, 58].

The reason why they cannot prevent the PUFAs in their membranes from being oxidised may be because the bulkheads that keep PUFAs apart in normal cells are not doing their job in cancer cells[26].

When levels of free radicals begin to increase inside a cell, they stop cell division. When they increase further, they trigger a cascade of radical formation that either makes the cell commit slow suicide, or kills it outright. And because cancer cells cannot store their PUFAs safely, so that they form PUFA radicals, they are uniquely vulnerable to PUFAs in their environment, or in your diet.

This may mean that many cancer cells self-destruct in a blaze of PUFA free radicals long before they can become a health problem.

Fried tomatoes

To obtain maximum benefit from tomatoes, use deep red tomatoes, which have the highest lycopene content. Then fry them in olive oil.

This makes their lycopene content more bio-available.

Cancer killing

Many flavonoids and carotenoids are capable of killing cancer cells, if used in large doses.

PUFAs trigger self-destruction in cancer cells

Cancer cells can be made to self-destruct if given high-dose poly-unsaturated fatty acids.

Most studies have used fish oil, rich in Omega 3 PUFAs. There is some rationale also for using an Omega 3: Omega 6 combination; a ratio of 2:1 – 3:1 may be best, which is the ratio in hemp or flaxseed oil.

It also means that, by definition, any cancer cells that survive and multiply for long enough to become a tumour must have learned, somehow, to protect themselves against PUFA oxidation.

<table>
<tr><td>

Conclusion

A daily Omega 3 supplement should form part of your anti-cancer strategy. Most people already eat enough Omega 6.

</td><td>

PUFA RADICALS

PUFA radicals may be more than mere agents of destruction. There is good evidence that the level of PUFA radicals is a critical signalling factor. Levels of PUFA radicals inside the cell go down just before the cell begins to divide, and may even be responsible for triggering the beginning of cell division[20-22].

This is completely logical because, when the cell divides, its DNA becomes extended, unshielded and very vulnerable to free radical damage. So a cell naturally wants to increase its anti-oxidant defences before the division process starts. This is probably why rapidly dividing tissues (like cancer cells) tend to have higher than normal levels of anti-oxidants[41].

</td></tr>
</table>

Removing cancer cells' defences

In fact, the potentially explosive PUFA chain reaction is so dangerous to cancer cells that they appear to have developed at least four different defences against them.

Firstly, they increase their levels of anti-oxidants such as Vitamin E[23-25]. Secondly, they have higher than normal levels of anti-oxidant enzymes[57, 58]. Thirdly, they tend to take up fewer PUFAs than normal cells[26]. And fourthly, the majority of cancer cells have reduced levels of PUFA synthesis[27-30].

These four steps all combine to reduce the levels of PUFAs and PUFA radicals in successful cancer cells. The better they are at keeping their PUFA levels down, the more malignant and metastatic they tend to be[31-35, 60].

If, on the other hand, you load cancer cells with PUFAs, their anti-oxidant defences are overwhelmed[142] and they self-destruct[42].

This theory predicts that pro-oxidants like iron and copper should increase the ability of PUFAs to kill cancer cells – and this does appear to be the case[43-48].

Cancer specialists will recognise this pattern, because many anti-cancer therapies work by generating free radicals inside the

<table>
<tr><td>

Limiting radio-therapy damage

To prepare for a course of radiotherapy or chemotherapy, stock up on high quality fish oil and evening primrose oil, with Vitamins C and E and red wine or red wine extract to minimise collateral damage[231].

A combination very like this is already being used in Europe to increase the effectiveness and safety of radiotherapy.

</td></tr>
</table>

cancer cells. As you might expect, cancer cells 'force-fed' on PUFAs become much more vulnerable to the free radical damage caused by orthdox anti-cancer drugs[18].

WARNING

Short courses of high-dose PUFAs may have significant anti-cancer effects. But long-term self-dosing with large amounts of PUFAs is not recommended, unless combined with high-dose anti-oxidants.

PUFAs are very susceptible to oxidation, which is why they are always, in nature, found combined with anti-oxidants. Plant sources of PUFAs, for example, are also good sources of anti-oxidants such as Vitamin E, which the plant uses to stop its PUFAs from going rancid.

If you take supplements of fish or plant oils without taking high-dose anti-oxidants, you are exposing yourself to increased free radicals, as well as potentially dangerous lipid oxidation products[53], which are toxic to the heart and blood vessels (see Chapter 8, Essential oils).

3:1

Human cell membranes contain Omega 6 and 3 fatty acids in an approximately 3:1 ratio – as does human breast milk.

Which PUFAs?

It depends on which scientists you talk to. There is some evidence that the Omega 6 PUFAs in plant oils are potentially useful anti-cancer agents[38-40].

On the other hand, some animal experiments have shown that whereas the Omega 3 PUFAs in fish oil inhibit tumour growth, high levels of linoleic acid (an Omega 6 PUFA) can have the reverse effect[54-56].

The picture is not entirely clear, but some lipid specialists believe that the Omega 3 fish oils may be a better bet than the Omega 6 plant oils. Omega 3 oils have been shown to slow the growth of cancers in the lung, stomach, colon and pancreas[59, 223].

There is also some evidence of a decrease in cancer risk as the Omega 3/Omega 6 ratio in the diet increases (see Chapter 8, Essential oils) – although the data are not entirely consistent.

Remember to combine Omega oils with Vitamin E

Treat high doses of fish oils or plant oils with care. Animals fed a high PUFA diet long term have an increased risk of cancer, and a shorter life expectancy – **unless** they are given Vitamin E supplements as well[53]. Vitamin C should also always be taken.

THE PUFA STORY IN BRIEF ...

The story is a complex one, so let me recapitulate.

- PUFAs are not generally toxic to normal cells.

- Normal cells take up more PUFAs than cancer cells but don't oxidise them to nearly the same extent.

- Normal cells have less anti-oxidants than cancer cells, so they are somehow storing or compartmentalising the PUFAs in a safer and more controllable manner.

- Whereas normal cells are vulnerable to PUFA shortages, cancer cells are vulnerable to too much PUFA, as they cannot shield them from oxidation.

- When normal cells are irradiated, the degree of tissue damage is reduced by PUFA replacement therapy[49]. This is because much of the damage they suffer is due to PUFA shortage, caused by the radiation.

- When cancer cells are irradiated, more of them are killed after pre-incubation with PUFAs – because toxic free radicals are formed.

PUFAs in action

The vulnerability of cancer cells to PUFAs has been shown in a variety of experiments. For example, cancer cells in a Petri dish normally grow over and swamp normal cells. If you add high-dose PUFAs, the reverse happens[34], and the normal cells replace the cancer cells.

The next step is animal experiments and, fairly recently, GLA (one of the essential PUFAs) was shown to inhibit the initiation and growth of human cancers transplanted into mice[36, 37].

Even more recently, the first trials of high-dose GLA in human cancer produced some promising results.

In one study, involving cases of advanced and inoperable pancreatic cancer, increasing doses of GLA produced a significant increase in the length of survival of these terminally ill patients[38-40].

Other scientists have shown that the Omega 3 PUFAs in fish oil inhibit the growth of cancers of lung, stomach, pancreas and colon[141, 142].

Further work is in progress to clarify the role of PUFAs in cancer therapy.

Anti-oxidants – a two-edged sword?

Cancer cells, as we have seen, are very vulnerable to PUFA radicals. Any cancer cell which survives to multiply and become a tumour has, by definition, been able to survive such oxidative stress, by increasing its levels of anti-oxidants and decreasing PUFA uptake.

So what happens if you take massive doses of anti-oxidants? Could these help more early cancer cells survive?

In cancer cells, as we have seen, the levels of anti-oxidants, including Vitamin E, are often higher than normal. Cancer cells need high levels of anti-oxidants to keep levels of free radicals low. This may be partly because their high division rate makes their DNA very vulnerable to free radical damage, and partly because of their inability to store PUFAs safely.

So a cancer, once initiated, **might** do rather well on anti-oxidant supplements which offer it additional protection, particularly if the anti-oxidants used had no intrinsic anti-cancer properties (as the carotenoids and flavonoids do): or if the anti-oxidants are used inappropriately, ie Vitamin E or carotenoids **without** Vitamin C.

This alarming prospect cannot be entirely dismissed, and I believe it needs to be properly examined.

Before you throw away your supplements, bear in mind that certain anti-oxidants (beta carotene, Vitamins A, C and to some extent E) can be very effective in treating pre-cancerous conditions in the throat, larynx and the gut[7, 8, 140, 208]. Beta carotene can suppress the growth of cervical cancer cells, and cause them to self-destruct[9], although it is less effective than lycopene (see lycopene section on page 206). There is also evidence that an increased beta carotene intake is linked to a reduced risk of cervical cancer[10].

However, the optimal time to start taking most anti-oxidants is before a cancer has started. DNA damage caused by oxidation is an important cause of cancer and a recent study showed conclusively that supplements of Vitamins C, E and beta carotene (at 100mg, 280mg and 25mg a day respectively) reduce the amount of oxidised DNA in smokers and non-smokers alike[204].

Nevertheless, there is at least one small trial which suggests that anti-oxidant supplements may have a protective effect even after a cancer has started. In patients who had undergone surgery for bladder cancer, the cancer recurred in 80 per cent of the control group; but in only 40 per cent of those who took high doses of multivitamins including A, C, E, the B group vitamins and zinc[11].

Beta carotene – for non-smokers only

New work shows that if beta carotene is oxidised (as occurs in the lungs of smokers) it may become a pro-oxidant and a carcinogen[197].

Smokers should not take beta carotene.

On the balance of evidence, however, they should continue to take other anti-oxidants, including mixed carotenoids and Vitamin C.

Add anti-oxidants

High-dose anti-oxidants may make cancer treatments more effective[115-117].

DIETS WHICH FIGHT DISEASE : **Cancer**

The conclusion so far ...

Anti-oxidants can help reduce the risk of cancer if it has not already started[174].

But if there is a pre-existing (pre-clinical) cancer, high doses of some anti-oxidants **might** increase the chances of the cancer growing and becoming a clinical problem.

Not all anti-oxidants are the same. High-dose Co-enzyme Q10 or Vitamin K are more likely to kill or suppress cancer cells, by blocking cytokine synthesis[198, 212].

High-dose carotenoids and flavonoids also have well-documented cancer cell killing properties.

However high doses of Vitamin E or the carotenoids, both of which oxidise into damaging pro-oxidants, should be avoided – unless combined with Vitamin C, which recycles them.

At the time of writing, the picture is confused. There is simply not enough data to say whether anti-oxidants can encourage cancer growth or not.

Ongoing trials may help to settle the argument. In the meantime, it may be wise to assume that the relationship between anti-oxidants and cancer could be more complex than we thought.

If anti-oxidants are taken before a cancer has started, and perhaps also while the immune system is fully functional, most data suggests that this is a good thing, and will reduce the risk of cancer and other free radical mediated illness. But if anti-oxidants are taken later in life, it is conceivable that some of them may, under certain circumstances, increase the risk of cancer.

This suggests that it's fine to start taking anti-oxidants at any time up to your late 40s, or 30s if you are a heavy smoker. After this time it might be wise to add a little nutritional insurance.

If there is a possibility of a pre-existing cancer, it might be better to deal with it before beginning anti-oxidant therapy.

One (controversial!) way of doing this would be to take an immuno-stimulant and pro-oxidant package. This would combine broad-spectrum supplements with echinacea and high-dose PUFAs *without* anti-oxidants. It might even include an oxidising agent such as hydrogen peroxide or even hydrazine (the rocket fuel), both of which have been used by some practitioners. This should force some cancer cells to self-destruct. Of course, this approach is for professionals only, and *not* for self-medication.

After an initial oxidative phase, during which hopefully the cancer is knocked back, the logical next step would be PUFA replacement combined with anti-oxidants to replace the PUFAs which were destroyed in healthy tissues.

A Six Step Defence Plan against Cancer

The six-fold strategy below is progressive. The first two steps are preventative. The subsequent four steps 'manage' cancer. At each of these steps some cancer cells will be deactivated, neutralised or destroyed. The function of each subsequent step is to deal with any remaining cancer cells that the previous step did not overcome.

Cancer avoidance

Step 1 Reduce free radical damage to DNAs with anti-oxidants, and upregulate anti-oxidant enzymes with plant foods, ie increase fruits, nuts, vegetables and grain in your diet.

Step 2 Support the immune system with a broad spectrum vitamin/mineral supplement, plus Q10 and (occasional) echinacea.

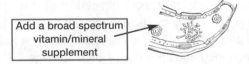

Add a broad spectrum vitamin/mineral supplement

Cancer containment

Step 3 Force the cancer cell to revert to normal ('redifferentiate').

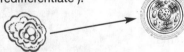

Soy isoflavones like genistein and daidzein, can do this, as can carotenoids like lycopene and alpha carotene, and flavolignans in flaxseed.

Step 4 Block the proteases that would otherwise activate the MMP enzymes that destroy healthy tissue (see page 93).

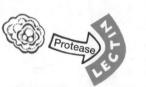

Inactive MMP

Protease LECTIN

Lectins found in beans and especially soy can achieve this.

Step 5 Block the activated and now highly destructive MMPs that breakdown the body tissue. Some flavonoids can do this directly.

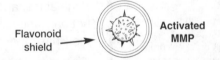

Flavonoid shield → Activated MMP

The flavonoids found in bilberry and grapeseed 'coat' and therefore shield the individual fibres of the body's cellular matrix against the MMPs (see Chapter 6, Flavonoids & isoflavones).

The MMP blockade will also choke off the blood supply to the cancer. Genistein, other flavonoids and cartilage extracts are all good angiostats – as are the drugs thalidomide and captopril.

Genistein

Cancer killing

Step 6 Kill the cancer cell by ultra high-dose Omega 3 possibly with a pro-oxidant. Very high doses of flavonoids can also kill cancer cells as can the carotenoid lycopene and the isoflavones (but see box on page 206).

The Anti-Cancer Diet

The anti-cancer diet is almost identical to the diets designed to protect against coronary artery disease, diabetes and obesity.

The ground rules for all three diets are:

- More fruit and vegetables
- More complex carbohydrates in grains, pulses and legumes
- Less fats, sugars, salt and smoked or pickled foods

There should be plenty of fruits, nuts, grains, legumes and vegetables on the menu, as all of these contain many different anti-cancer compounds.

Fruits are excellent sources of the anti-oxidant Vitamins A, C and the carotenoids and flavonoids. Grains and nuts are good sources of Vitamin E and the essential poly-unsaturated fatty acids and unique anti-oxidants such as avenanthramides[246-248]. Vegetables, and spices, such as rosemary and turmeric, provide not only anti-oxidant flavonoids, but also compounds which boost the Phase 2 enzymes which detoxify toxins and carcinogens.

Both fruits and vegetables provide flavonoids and carotenoids, and peas and beans, especially soy beans, are rich sources of lectins (the protease inhibitors). In addition, plant foods provide dietary fibres, which have an anti-cancer effect of their own (see Chapter 7, Pre-biotic fibre). Plant foods also provide the important B vitamins folic acid and niacin, which is important because folate and/or niacin depletion increases the risk of DNA damage[172, 178].

But which fruits and which vegetables should we eat to achieve optimal health?

The available data from in vitro work and from animal studies suggests that the following foods should be high on your shopping list[106]:

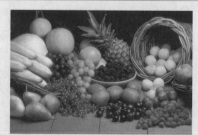

Fruit, vegetables and legumes are the top anti-cancer foods!

ANTI-CANCER FOODS

- cruciferous vegetables such as kale, cabbage, and Brussels sprouts[108, 112, 116], which may be particularly effective in protecting against colon and breast cancer
- broccoli
- citrus fruits
- tomatoes
- tea (green more than black)
- spinach
- rosemary, thyme, oregano, garlic[113-115]
- onions[117]
- soy products (which contain genistein and flavonoids)
- wheat or rice bran[122]
- walnuts
- raspberries, blueberries and blackberries[118, 119, 120]
- turmeric
- pears
- shiitake mushrooms[121]

Cutting colon cancer risk

An increased intake of pre-biotics (see Chapter 7, Pre-biotic fibre) together with calcium and Vitamin D [175, 176, but see also 177], will probably reduce the risk of colon cancer.

These foods will give you two out of the three important levels of protection against cancer[106], specifically:

1 Cancer avoidance

The first level prevents carcinogens from reaching their target sites (anti-oxidants, Phase 2 upregulators and vitamins and minerals to support the immune system).

AND

2 Cancer containment

The second level consists of compounds which suppress cancer cells directly (carotenoids and isoflavones); blocking or barrier agents (angiostats and matrix stabilisers); and the immuno-stimulants, which enhance the capacity of natural killer cells to attack tumours.

There are additional steps that help reduce the risk of certain specific cancers, if your family history suggests that you may be at a particular risk.

More herbs and spices

A surprising number of culinary herbs contain health-promoting substances. Rosemary is included in the good food guide

Folic acid – An anti-cancer vitamin

Researchers are now studying folic acid's role in reducing cancer risk – especially of the colon and cervix.

Many researchers now feel that a total folic acid intake of 400mcg a day – from food and supplements – is the least you need. Indeed, the RDAs are likely to be revised upwards.

Since the average intake is 252mcg, this indicates you need a supplement containing about 200mcg of folic acid.

Betaine is likely to be even more effective (see Chapter 11, Betaine).

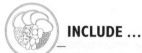

INCLUDE ...

A herb element –

- rosemary
- curcumin (the yellow pigment in turmeric and curry)
- thyme

Balancing act

Some food plants contain protective compounds and potentially harmful compounds. Basil (which contains estragole) was under suspicion as a possible carcinogen[243], but more recent work suggests that on balance, it is more likely to be cancer-protective[77, 105,106].

Cooking meat

Use olive oil and add wild rice to meat recipes.

Coat meat in powdered milk and breadcrumbs.

---

because it contains a number of ingredients, including carnosic acid, which inhibit cancer initiation and growth in animal studies[104, 107]. Curcumin, the yellow pigment in curry and a very powerful anti-oxidant, also has a number of powerful anti-cancer properties and anti-inflammatory properties (see page 92).

Less meat and dairy foods

A high intake of fat in the diet increases the risk of colon cancer[110, 111].

There are several reasons for this. A fatty diet increases the secretion of bile salts into the gut, which are taken up by gut bacteria and converted to carcinogens such as the aromatic polycyclic hydrocarbons. These are known to be linked to liver and other cancers[213].

A diet high in fats is often low in fruits and vegetables, and therefore low in the protective factors found in plant foods. And finally, fatty diets often contain high levels of meat products – and when meats are preserved and/or cooked in certain ways (ie browned) carcinogens are formed[99].

Meat also contains iron in a particularly bio-available form, and iron is something we should be careful with. Iron can be a potent source of free radicals, causing oxidative and genetic damage (see Chapter 14, Heart disease). We have complex systems to safeguard iron in the body, but these do not always work very well[162]. There is a disease called haemochromatosis, where iron accumulates in the body; which is linked to a 200-fold increase in the risk of liver cancer[163].

In people with high body iron (but not necessarily with haemochromatosis), the risks of lung and colorectal cancer are also increased[164,166]. And in patients with diagnosed cancer, high body iron strongly correlates with decreased survival time, suggesting that some tumours grow better in an iron-rich environment[165].

As ever, the evidence suggests that we reduce our intake of animal and dairy products, and increase our intake of plant foods. In addition, take basic precautions with fats and oils: do not overheat them when cooking, don't re-use, and don't use poly-unsaturates for cooking oil (see Chapter 8, Essential oils). Switch to mono-unsaturates such as olive oil; MUFAs may be less prone to encouraging cancer[109].

Die-hard carnivores could use amended cooking methods to reduce carcinogen formation. They could add ingredients such as wild rice to their meat recipes; wild rice is rich in phytates and polyphenols which bind iron, and reduce iron uptake[168].

Avoid roasting or grilling meats, because high protein foods produce carcinogens as the meat browns[99]. Steaming is fine, as are boiling, poaching, and microwaving. These cooking techniques aren't ideally suited to meats, but they are fine for fish, many of which contain Omega 3 fatty acids which have an anti-cancer effect[100-102].

If you can't bear to give up the Sunday roast, take some simple culinary precautions. Coat the meat with a mix of powdered milk and bread crumbs before cooking. This may sound odd, but the carbohydrates in milk and bread reduce the formation of carcinogens during the roasting and grilling process[103].

This is the nutritional basis for a healthy life. Supplement programmes do not replace this basis, but if you want to go further towards optimal health, supplementation should be considered.

Additional anti-cancer actions

More selenium

Selenium is essential for the immune system and has a number of potentially anti-cancer actions. The UK RDA is 70mcg/day – yet the average daily intake is 29-39mcg/day. This was highlighted in an editorial in the *British Medical Journal*, warning that the rise in cancer (which now affects four in every ten British residents!) might well be due to widespread selenium depletion[234, 235].

Larry Clark's study[234] showed that a supplement of 200mcg selenium a day (in a yeast preparation) reduced cancer of the prostate, lung and colon by around 50 per cent in a similarly selenium-depleted population in the USA. Further a recent study in London indicates that selenium can force cancer cells to commit suicide at 200mcg[250].

The PRECISE (Prevention of Cancer, Intervention with Selenium) study was set up to prove the case one way or another. Meanwhile selenium is safe at that level – so why wait?

Meat – a caution

Meat not only contains saturated fat, but iron that is easily absorbed.

High iron levels appear to be linked to a body environment that helps tumours to grow[165].

Increased iron in the gut produces free radicals – and is linked to colon cancer.

Do not consume iron oxide – often used to colour pills and supplements[69, 167].

Selenium

Selenium is essential for C43, the membrane proteins involved in cell contact inhibition and switching off cell growth. It should be combined with carotenoids for maximal effect.

TOP SELENIUM FOODS

Liver, seafood, lean meat, whole grains, oatmeal, brown rice.

Medicines

Oddly enough, aspirin may offer some protection against cancer. The data suggest that regular aspirin consumption reduces the risk of cancer of the colon, lung and breast[158, 227]. Aspirin can force cancer cells to commit suicide and anything that encourages cancer cell death will help to reduce the risk of a clinical cancer[206,228, 229].

Typical Western consumers could also take supplements of protective micro-nutrients such as lycopene, selenium and the non-digestible oligosaccharide prebiotics, all of which appear to reduce the risk of colon cancer (see Chapter 7, Pre-biotic fibre).

Finally they could switch from meat to soy substitutes, which are also protective against cancer (see Chapter 6, Flavonoids & isoflavones).

Reducing the risk of prostate cancer

In Japanese men who leave their home country and go to work in the USA, there is a statistical explosion of prostate cancer within the first few years of their arrival.

Some clinicians believe that this is because they are exposed to something in the American food or water which increases the risk of prostate cancer.

On closer inspection, this explanation falls down. It takes many years for a cancer to form, and it is highly unlikely that there is any ingredient in the American diet which could trigger so many cancers so fast. If there was, the incidence of prostate cancer in American men would be much higher than it already is.

It is more likely that the Japanese men had prostate cancer before they came West. While they remained in Japan, the cancers were held in check by naturally occurring growth inhibitors in the Japanese diet, probably in soy and green tea.

On relocating to the West, they lost this dietary protection and the cancers lurking in their prostates burst into malignant life.

Risk factors for this increasingly prevalent cancer are now being identified. Two recent studies indicated that Vitamin E might protect against prostate cancer[156, 224]; a third showed that selenium offered very significant protection[234]; a fourth that high calcium intake increased risk[249].

Vitamins E and D, genistein and selenium supplements, possibly combined with a low fat diet, are a good bet – and offer cardiac benefits too.

Processed tomato products are strongly recommended. A recent trial suggested that the risk of prostate cancer could be cut almost in half in men who ate 10 or more servings of tomatoes per week, or by a fifth in those who ate four to seven servings a week[192].

The carotenoid in tomatoes called lycopene has important anti-cancer properties, and is capable of making cancer cells re-differentiate[225, 226] (ie normalise) or commit suicide.

Lycopene inhibits prostate cancer cells in vitro[55-60, 325-330] and is now being tested in clinical trials, which are starting to show positive results[298].

Reducing the risk of breast cancer

Breast cancer is the most important non-tobacco-related cancer in women. It is a universal problem, yet in some countries (Canada, New Zealand, Hawaii) women are 10 times more likely to develop breast cancer than in others (Senegal, Korea, Nigeria).

A few dietary factors play a large part in determining the risk of post-menopausal breast cancer. For example, a high intake of dietary fibre reduces the risk of breast cancer, while a high fat content in the diet increases the risk. At the same time, post-menopausal cancers are known to be driven by oestrogen. Why is this?

High fibre lowers oestrogen levels

Oestrogen is removed from the blood by the liver, which links it with a molecule of glucoronic acid, and excretes it in bile, into the bowel. 'Bad' bacteria in the bowel unlink some of the oestrogen, and encourage its reabsorption into the blood.

A high concentration of fibre in the bowel slows the unlinking process, reduces the amount of free oestrogen that can be re-absorbed, and so lowers oestrogen levels in the blood[144].

Large amounts of fats in the bowel, however, increase the ability of the bacteria to free the oestrogen, increase the amount which can be reabsorbed, and increase blood oestrogen levels[145].

Eat a high fibre/low fat diet

The best way to reduce your risk of breast cancer is to eat a high fibre, low fat diet (ie: predominantly vegetarian)[205,207]; and to eat fermented milk products such as live yoghurt[146, 152] (see Chapter 7, Pre-biotic fibre).

The 'good' bacteria in live yoghurt displace the 'bad' bacteria which attack oestrogen. The end result is less unlinking, more oestrogen excretion and lower blood oestrogen. The same effect would be expected with pre-biotics, which increase the numbers of 'good' bacteria in the gut (see Chapter 7 again). There is evidence that pre-biotics do indeed lower the risk of breast cancer[149]. If you don't like yoghurt, a pre-biotic product is probably more effective.

Some fibres bind more oestrogen than others[148]. The best results have been obtained with wheat fibre, which reduces blood oestrogen levels significantly – oat and corn fibre had little effect[147].

Some scientists believe that reducing oestrogen levels could increase the risk of osteoporosis[157]. This can easily be countered (see Chapter 15, Bones).

Soy, tomatoes, melatonin – and selenium

Further nutritional protection against breast cancer is gained via a healthy intake of soy products. Soy contains compounds which block oestrogen receptors in the breast and elsewhere, which is one reason why a diet high in soy is linked to a greatly reduced risk of breast cancer[233] (see Chapter 6, Flavonoids & isoflavones).

If a cancer has been diagnosed, you might consider adding melatonin, the so-called 'dark hormone', to your anti-cancer regime. This compound (widely available in the USA, but restricted in the UK and in Europe), is an excellent sleep inducer[150]. It has also been shown to stop the growth of breast cancer cells[151, 169], and to have positive effects on established cancers[170] and other proliferative diseases[171].

Melatonin may explain why air stewardesses have twice the normal risk of breast cancer[179]. Each flight increases exposure to ionising radiation (London to New York = four whole body x-rays). And constant moving between time zones disrupts sleep patterns, and inhibits normal melatonin release patterns.

Female air staff and frequent flyers should take anti-oxidants and consider taking melatonin not just to get over jet lag, but also to help reduce the risk of breast cancer.

Lycopene (as with prostate cancer) is also strongly recommended[299, 301, 308-310, 325-330]. Alternatively, lutein may be considered[232], and also Q10[182-184]. Selenium supplements are also clearly indicated[234]. In one good study, 200mcg/day of selenium (in selenium enriched yeast) reduced breast cancer by around 50 per cent!

Reducing the risk of cancer

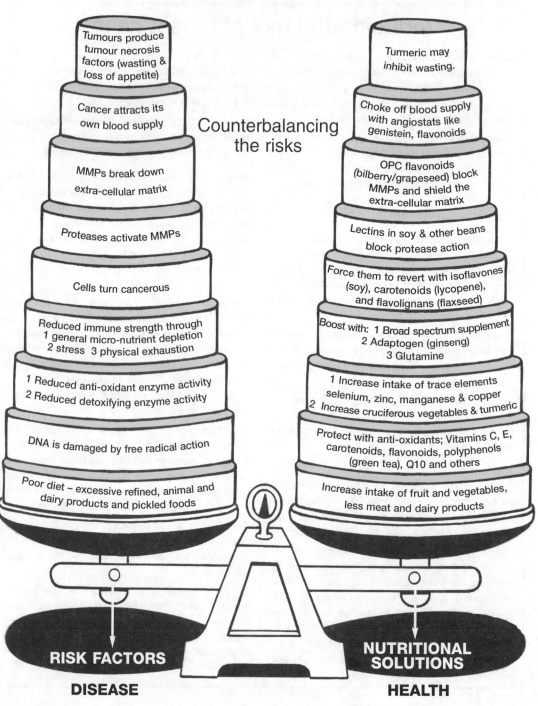

Counterbalancing the risks

Risk factors (left):

Tumours produce tumour necrosis factors (wasting & loss of appetite)

Cancer attracts its own blood supply

MMPs break down extra-cellular matrix

Proteases activate MMPs

Cells turn cancerous

Reduced immune strength through 1 general micro-nutrient depletion 2 stress 3 physical exhaustion

1 Reduced anti-oxidant enzyme activity 2 Reduced detoxifying enzyme activity

DNA is damaged by free radical action

Poor diet – excessive refined, animal and dairy products and pickled foods

Nutritional solutions (right):

Turmeric may inhibit wasting.

Choke off blood supply with angiostats like genistein, flavonoids

OPC flavonoids (bilberry/grapeseed) block MMPs and shield the extra-cellular matrix

Lectins in soy & other beans block protease action

Force them to revert with isoflavones (soy), carotenoids (lycopene), and flavolignans (flaxseed)

Boost with: 1 Broad spectrum supplement 2 Adaptogen (ginseng) 3 Glutamine

1 Increase intake of trace elements selenium, zinc, manganese & copper 2 Increase cruciferous vegetables & turmeric

Protect with anti-oxidants; Vitamins C, E, carotenoids, flavonoids, polyphenols (green tea), Q10 and others

Increase intake of fruit and vegetables, less meat and dairy products

RISK FACTORS — **DISEASE**

NUTRITIONAL SOLUTIONS — **HEALTH**

SUMMARY

The anti-cancer good food guide

A preventative strategy

▶ Low fat, high fibre, largely fruit and vegetable diet, organic if possible.

▶ Yellow and orange plant foods, dark green leafy vegetables, cabbage, broccoli, tomatoes, peas, onions and leeks, citrus fruits and rosemary.

▶ Add tomato concentrate and ketchup, preferably low salt.

▶ Grains (especially oats, wild rice and rye), plus nuts, pulses and fish oil for Vitamin E, PUFAs, phytates, anti-oxidants.

▶ Soy beans, soy products and/or a daily supplement with 40mg of isoflavones from soy.

▶ Anti-oxidants C, D, E, K, B group, Q10 and mixed carotenoids (at the levels recommended on page 338).

▶ Selenium, zinc, manganese and copper to ensure anti-oxidant enzymes are working well (levels on page 338).

▶ Rosemary and turmeric to upregulate Phase 2 enzymes.

▶ Pre-biotics and/or live yoghurt.

▶ Calcium and Vitamin D[175-177].

▶ Cut down on pickles and cured, grilled and fried meats.

A treatment strategy

▶ Soy beans and soy products to reduce tumour growth and metastasis.

▶ Shark cartilage as an alternative angiostat (but see box on page 197).

▶ Soy (again), lycopene and alpha carotene to induce cancer cells to revert to normal ('re-differentiation').

▶ Blackcurrants, elderberries and ginkgo as matrix stabilisers.

▶ Echinacea, Q10 and a broad spectrum vitamin/mineral supplement to boost the immune system (see page 338).

▶ Turmeric to block tumour necrosis factor alpha.

▶ Pre-biotics, especially for colon cancer.

▶ Omega 6 and Omega 3 oils, combined with iron and copper for increased killing of cancer cells (but very controversial).

Chapter 14

Heart of the matter

In the West, heart disease is the number one killer. In some other countries, however, coronary artery disease is almost unknown.

Why should this be so? It's now possible to say not only what causes it, but, more importantly, what will prevent it – and even reverse it.

This chapter outlines the lifestyle and diet which should, I believe, render you immune to heart disease.

Factors beyond your control

Let's start with those things you cannot change. There are not many, which shows just how much lies in your own hands.

Genetics

Apolipoprotein E is a molecule found in the blood. Which type you have is genetically determined. Apolipoprotein E4 contributes to increased blood cholesterol levels. More Finns have E4 than do Japanese, which may be one reason why the Finns have more heart disease. The E4 gene increases the risk of coronary artery disease (CAD), but by how much is not yet known[1, 2].

Low birth weight

Generally this is caused by foetal malnutrition, which in turn is caused by maternal malnutrition in the three to six months before conception and during pregnancy.

Low birth weight has been shown to increase the risk of hypertension, diabetes, obesity and CAD in later life[3].

Sex and age

Overall, men are about three times more likely to develop heart disease than women. Women's relative immunity may be due to their sex hormones, which are anti-oxidants and protect the blood vessels[50, 105]. This would explain why women are more at risk after the menopause. By age 80, the risk is the same for both sexes[4]. In the UK (one of the highest risk countries), CAD caused 170,000 deaths in 1992; killing 1 in 3 men, and 1 in 4 women[5].

Factors which you can change

OVERWEIGHT – avoid

A body mass index (see table on page 170) greater than 25 increases the risk of CAD nearly three times[6]. However, this statistic conceals more than it reveals; because the degree of risk associated with overweight depends on how you get there. Piling on the pounds on a diet rich in saturated fats and low in anti-oxidants (the British diet) is a recipe for CAD. Getting fat on a diet rich in anti-oxidants and mono-unsaturates such as olive oil, is probably not a risk – as the Mediterranean figures show[212].

SMOKING – stop

Men who smoke more than 20 cigarettes daily increase the risk of dying from a heart attack three-fold. Women who combine smoking with oral contraception increase their risk of a heart attack and/or a stroke by ten times[8].

ANTI-OXIDANTS – take them

A recent study of female nurses over an eight-year span showed that those who took Vitamin E capsules at a level of 400IU a day reduced their risk of CAD by 50 per cent[10]. In a parallel study, the risk in men was reduced by approximately 40 per cent[11]. The carotenoid lycopene may reduce the risk by 50 per cent[185].

It's never too late!

Within a year of stopping smoking, the risk of a fatal heart attack drops by about half. After three smoke-free years, the risk falls to that of a non-smoker[9, 185].

A reduction in the risk of lung cancer takes about three times longer.

Body shape

The 'apple-shaped' overweight – fat around the waist and abdomen – are more at risk[17].

Vitamin E

Recent intervention trials with Vitamin E were negative. Vitamin E should not be used as a single agent.

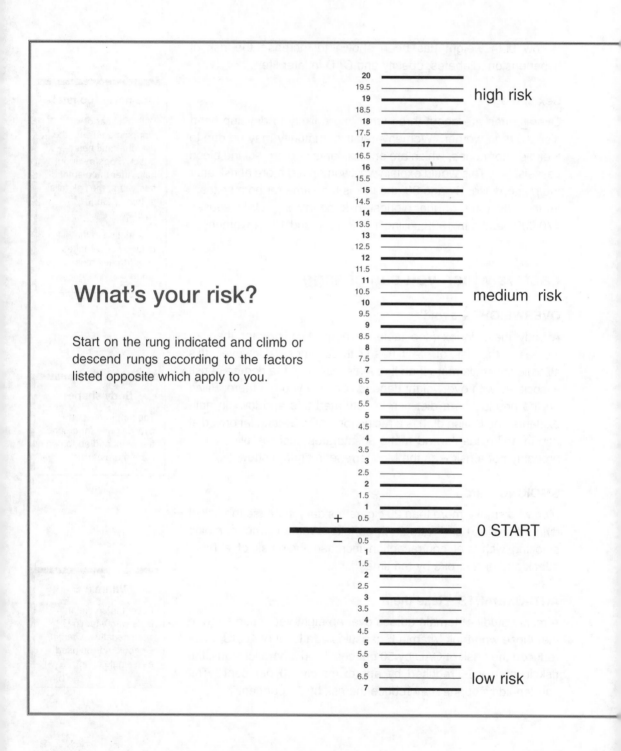

What's your risk?

Start on the rung indicated and climb or descend rungs according to the factors listed opposite which apply to you.

20
19.5
19 — high risk
18.5
18
17.5
17
16.5
16
15.5
15
14.5
14
13.5
13
12.5
12
11.5
11
10.5
10 — medium risk
9.5
9
8.5
8
7.5
7
6.5
6
5.5
5
4.5
4
3.5
3
2.5
2
1.5
1
+ 0.5
— 0 START
— 0.5
1
1.5
2
2.5
3
3.5
4
4.5
5
5.5
6
6.5 — low risk
7

Sex

Male: +1

Post-menopausal female: +1

Age

Men over 50: +1

Women over 60: +1

Birth weight

If significantly low: + 1.5

Genetics

If more than one member of your immediate family has or had CAD: +1.5

Weight

If overweight: + 0.5

If obese: +2

Smoking

More than five cigarettes a day: +1

More than 20: +2

Smoke and take the Pill: +4

Diet

Rich in oily fish: -3

Rich in anti-oxidants (fruit and veg): -3

Eat a lot of processed food: +2

Drink alcohol in moderation (especially red wine): -1

Drink excessively: +1

Eat a lot of meat and dairy products: +2

Exercise

Exercise vigorously for 20 minutes, 3 times a week or more: -3

Cholesterol levels

Men – cholesterol 5.5-7mmol: +1

Men – cholesterol over 7mmol: +2

Women – raised triglycerides: +1

Blood pressure

If diastolic blood pressure more than 92 mm Hg: +2

Diabetes

If diabetic: +2

Heart disease

If you have had angina or a heart attack: +2

Chlamydia or Helicobacter pylori infection

If positive: + 0.5

Personality type

Type A: + 1 (aggressive, ambitious, quick to anger)

Type B: -1 (calm, even-tempered, philosophical)

Chronic gum disease + 1.

Other anti-oxidants are also important. Low Vitamin C intake is a risk factor [181,182]. There are strong theoretical reasons to believe that an increased intake of the anti-oxidants Co-enzyme Q10 and the carotenoids lutein and lycopene may be even more effective against CAD than Vitamin E [12-14].

Selenium is another factor. A low intake of selenium is associated with an increased risk of CAD [183], and may even double it [15]. Phenolic anti-oxidants, such as those in black grapes and hence red wine, relax the coronary arteries [203], raise HDL cholesterol, reduce platelet stickiness) and confer considerable cardio-protection [16]. An oligo-proanthocyanodin (OPC) complex like grapeseed, pycnogenol or bilberry extract or isoflavones from soy [204] is also effective – see Chapter 6, Flavonoids & isoflavones.

OILY FISH – eat more

A recent Welsh study found that oily fish (salmon, herring, mackerel etc) eaten twice weekly resulted in significantly fewer deaths in middle-aged men who had already had a heart attack. The effect of eating fish became apparent as early as six months. After two years on the diet, total mortality was 29 per cent lower in the fish eaters [17, 164].

Fish oil reduces clotting and cardiac arrhythmias [17]. It reduces plasma triglyceride and LDL and increases production of HDL. In addition, it can lower blood pressure (slightly) [202]. Sadly, in the light of the obvious health benefits of fish, only a fraction of the Western population actually eat enough of this healthy food.

TRANS-FATS – avoid

Trans fats are the chemically modified (hydrogenated) fats widely used in processed foods. Higher intakes of trans-fats increase levels of LDL cholesterol (the 'bad' cholesterol), and decrease HDL (the 'good') cholesterol [18].

This helps to explain why epidemiological studies show that an increased consumption of trans fats from hydrogenated vegetable oils is linked to an up to 66 per cent increase in the risk of CAD [19-21].

50% reduction in heart attack risk with E alone

Vitamin E could slash CAD risks by 40% for men – 50% for women.

It has been calculated that Vitamin E taken at 400-800IU a day would save $578 million a year in US health care bills [186].

Additional protection is gained by adding more supplements – see box on page 239.

Vitamin E for better recovery

If you do have a heart attack, Vitamin E supplementers will probably suffer less damage to the heart muscle [112] – and are likely to make a better recovery. Remember to add Vitamin C!

EXERCISE – do it

Exercise reduces LDL (the 'bad' cholesterol), and raises HDL (the 'good' cholesterol), see Chapter 16, Diabetes. It can lower the blood pressure, and make the blood less likely to clot. A mere 20 minutes of exercise three times a week is reckoned to do the trick; and reduce the risk of CAD by up to 50 per cent[5].

ALCOHOL – in moderation

Alcohol consumption in excess of 21 units per week (men) and 14 units (women) is reckoned to increase the risk of hypertension and obesity – leading in turn to an increased risk of CAD. Moderate consumption, however, and particularly if it's red wine, is cardio-protective[31, 32].

B VITAMINS (INC BETAINE) – supplement

Supplementing with B vitamins and/or betaine reduces levels of the toxic metabolite homocysteine – which could, in turn, reduce your risk by half[143, 184].

Factors to check with your doctor

Blood cholesterol

As a rough guide, levels below 5.5 mmol are considered to be low risk. Levels between 5.5-7mmol denote a moderate increase in risk, and over 7 mmol is a zone of steeply increasing risk[159-161].

HOWEVER: the above relates mostly to men. In women, cholesterol levels are not an important risk factor – raised triglycerides and low HDL are thought to be more important[33]. Very high triglycerides increase the risk of CAD by up to five times[22, 23].

This means that a very low fat diet may not be the answer for women. Even in men, low fat diets don't bring cholesterol down by very much[24], although certain foods will. A more productive approach may be to raise levels of HDL, by de-stressing[26], exercise[5], lecithin or betaine; HRT[25] or menthol[168-170].

Varying your cholesterol levels

LDL cholesterol levels can be reduced by exercise or by consuming soy protein, citrus juice or a pre-biotic (see Chapter 7, Pre-biotic fibre).

HDL levels can be increased by exercise or by consuming lecthin and/or betaine (see Chapter 11, Betaine).

Finally, monoterpenes – these are a group of pungent compounds such as menthol, which gives mint its characteristic taste. 200mg of menthol a day, possibly combined with pinene (from pine needles), has the remarkable effect of raising the 'good' cholesterol by up to 40%[168-170,172,173,195] – which is very cardio-protective indeed.

Blood pressure

High blood pressure exacerbates any damage to the artery walls, making it more likely that atheroma will form. The MRFIT trial showed that in men with diastolic pressure over 92mm Hg, death from CAD more than doubled[27]. If you have hypertension, an immediate switch from table salt to a low sodium or, preferably, sodium-free substitute, could reduce it by up to 10mm Hg[200].

Chronic Infection

Not yet proven, but the data is persuasive. Some clinicians believe that eradication of chlamydia could reduce the risk of CAD[28, 29]. H pylori, the bacterium that causes peptic ulcers, is also under suspicion, as are the bacteria that cause gum disease.

How heart disease develops

One of the unsung successes in the field of CAD has been the recent and substantial progress in understanding how atheroma develops.

Along with this understanding has come a new idea of atheroma. It is seen no longer as an irreversible endpoint, but a dynamic entity which is constantly being built up and worn away; an entity, therefore, which can be treated by encouraging the body's own artery clearing systems.

These new ideas have freed us from our fixation with surgery and drugs, and have laid the ground for a far-reaching nutritional approach which offers the hope of achieving, even in old age, a young heart and blood vessels.

So just how does coronary artery disease start, and how does it end?

There are a number of links in the chain which culminate in a heart attack, but according to the evidence we have, one starting point is a tiny lesion in the inner lining of an artery.

How does this happen? Arteries experience considerable physical stresses as the blood is pumped through them. Like bone, which is continuously suffering micro-fractures and then being rebuilt, the lining of the arteries is also being continually

---

Vitamin C

Without Vitamin C, the tiny lesions in the arteries cannot be repaired.

Serious C deficiency (scurvy), now rare, causes bruising and bleeding as the blood vessels spring a leak.

Milder but chronic C deficiency is far more common. It doesn't cause gross bleeding, but in the long term it is just as lethal, because it allows heart disease to get started by damaging the extra-cellular matrix in blood vessel walls.

At these sites red blood cells may break down more easily – releasing iron which can cause local inflammation.

damaged and repaired. Additional damage is caused by turbulence in the blood stream and by toxic compounds in our diet, produced by a diet depleted in Vitamin C and/or flavonoids, and by bad eating habits and cooking techniques[37].

Under ideal circumstances the lesions are repaired by regenerating more collagen fibres in the area, the local extra-cellular matrix. If there isn't enough Vitamin C or flavonoids, however, repairs cannot be completed.

If the body cannot repair the arteries properly it puts a temporary 'sticking plaster' over the damage called apolipoprotein B – an extremely 'sticky' molecule. This solves the immediate problem, but it's not physically strong and it leaves the artery wall rough, with a tendency to promote thrombosis (blood clots).

This is when atheroma can start to form. Turbulence in the blood stream breaks up older red blood cells, releasing free iron – a powerful oxidant. The iron oxidises the cholesterol on the apolipoprotein 'sticking plaster', and produces Cholesterol Oxidation Products, or COPS[155, 190]. These are extremely toxic to arteries, and tear micro-holes in the lining of the artery – which attract more apolipoprotein, and more cholesterol[34, 37].

The tiny lesions draw in white blood cells which oxidise the COPS still further before dying off[191]. As they die, they create more inflammation and tissue breakdown[43]. This releases yet more iron into the site[42], attracts more apolipoprotein, more cholesterol, and more white cells, which turn into foam cells[191].

It is a vicious circle leading to yet more local oxidation, inflammation, and tissue destruction[43]. In other words, CAD can be thought of as a chronic inflammatory disease, rather like arthritis[37,42,43,131,165].

At this point we have to step back from the artery wall and look at events in the bloodstream.

Cholesterol vs anti-oxidants

All this time, LDL cholesterol has been circulating in the blood. If protected by fat-soluble anti-oxidants like Vitamin E, Q10 or lycopene, it remains in the circulation, and is delivered only where required.

Artery weak points

All arteries are subject to physical stresses caused by the abrupt changes in blood pressure as the heart beats. But looking at just where atheroma forms reveals that some sites are more at risk than others.

The coronary arteries are subject to additional physical stresses as they are squeezed flat by the heart muscle every time it contracts.

The other high risk sites are where turbulence occurs – at arterial junctions, where an artery divides.

Vitamin K

Oxidation in arterial walls causes the local (oxidative) destruction of Vitamin K. This is another link in the chain. K is essential for preventing unwanted calcification[205, 206], so a local K deficit leads to calcification (hardening) of the damaged arteries.

Paradoxically, many heart patients are given warfarin, an anti-K drug! While preventing blood clots, it is likely to make arterial calcification worse.

But if it is oxidised, it is taken up by white blood cells which migrate into damaged sites, attracted by the inflammation building up there. This additional source of COPS (Cholesterol Oxidation Products) makes the situation even worse.

As the inflammation builds, oxidation increases to the point where the immune cells break down, forming a thick, oxidising, gruel in the artery wall.

The atheroma grows and muscle cells in the artery wall multiply in a last gasp attempt to prevent a blow-out. The space through which the blood can travel steadily shrinks.

At the same time, the oxidative stress slows production of EDRF, a substance which normally relaxes the arteries[131]. This makes the arteries constrict, and encourages blood clot formation.

Angina may be an early warning, but if a blood clot forms on the atheroma site, the first symptom may well be the last – a fatal heart attack.

> ### B vitamins can cut heart attack risk by 50%
>
> High levels of an amino acid called homo-cysteine increase the risk of heart attacks.
>
> Folic acid, B6 and B12 work together to lower homocysteine. People with the highest levels of B vitamins (especially folic acid) have a 50% lower risk of heart attack – according to a study published in 1995 in the New England Journal of Medicine[94].
>
> It's possible to test your homocysteine levels.
>
> If it's above 14 micromoles per litre (14mm/l) for men and 8.5mm/l for women, you should take a B vitamin supplement.
>
> Not everyone responds to B vitamins, so betaine may be a better and safer alternative (see Chapter 11, Betaine).

THE STEPS IN HEART DISEASE

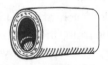

1 Normal artery.

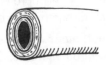

2 Minimal atheroma. Cholesterol builds up in the walls of the artery.

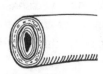

3 Advanced atheroma. The diameter of the artery becomes smaller and blood flow is restricted. Calcium deposits make the arteries 'harder'.

4 Severe atheroma. Blood clots can form and cause a complete blockage which may stop the heart beating.

Towards a unified theory of CAD

There are many links in the chain of events which culminates in a heart attack. These are also various defence mechanisms. It is the balance between the forces of decay and regeneration which determines whether atheroma builds, leading to a heart attack – or shrinks, leading to a renewal of the arteries.

One of the most important regenerative factors is HDL. HDL is the 'good' cholesterol, and its function is to remove cholesterol from the atheroma site and take it to the liver where it can be metabolised into, among other things, bile salts.

HDL cholesterol not only contains anti-oxidants[49] but also carries a rather specialised enzyme, paraoxonase, which may be involved in detoxifying the artery-damaging COPS and LOPS[145-147].

In addition to HDL, there is a wide range of cardio-protective anti-oxidants in our diet.

Risk factors

- Smoking[8] – this causes chronic mild Vitamin C deficiency. It also reduces plasma anti-oxidants such as E and lycopene, and increases the rate of LDL oxidisation.

- Hypertension[9] (high blood pressure) increases stresses on the blood vessel walls and increases the number of damage sites on the arteries.

- Diabetes[10] – the blood vessels are more vulnerable to micro-damage and anti-oxidants are depleted.

- Lack of exercise[11] not only leads to a fall in HDL levels, it also makes the blood more likely to clot.

- Saturated fats[12] – a diet high in saturated fat produces LDL cholesterol which is harder to oxidise: but it increases the rate at which inflammation develops in the artery walls; and it also tends to be low in anti-oxidants.

- Living in the developed West[13] – where people have a relatively poor anti-oxidant status and excessive cholesterol levels. If there aren't many anti-oxidant molecules in the blood then, as cholesterol levels increase, more of it will be unprotected and hence prone to oxidation, forming COPS.

- Excessive homocysteine – damages the blood vessel walls.

Protective factors

- HDL[3,4,5]
- Anti-oxidants[15]
- B vitamins or betaine
- Exercise
- Omega 3
- Vitamin K
- Flavonoids

Fat fit for a heart attack

There are two more major components in the risk equation – and both have to do with the fats we eat in our diet.

Trans-fats (which are labelled in margarines and processed foods as either vegetable fat, or hydrogenated vegetable oil), appear to be a substantial risk factor for CAD[35] and diabetes[34].

They lead to an increase in LDL cholesterol, but they also interfere with the body's ability to metabolise poly-unsaturated oils (PUFAs) such as fish oil, and vegetable oils[34, 36]. They can make a PUFA depletion worse, leading to an increased susceptibility to inflammation in the artery walls and elsewhere.

Trans-fats should be avoided, and are being phased out in some countries such as Sweden.

The other major sources of danger in our diet are COPS and LOPS. These – you may remember from Chapter 8, Essential oils – are Cholesterol and Lipid Oxidation Products respectively; and are produced by inappropriate food storage and cooking practices. Because they are formed outside the body and then consumed, anti-oxidants cannot protect you against them. (The flavonoid quercitin[180] or high doses of Vitamin B6 may be protective[148], but this is by no means proven.)

But that's just the start of a healthy eating programme ...

The Hearty Eating Diet

Oily fish

Oily fish (or fish oil) has a marked protective effect – so eat more herring, mackerel, sardines, salmon, etc. The effects of fish oil, which reduces inflammation of the arteries, cuts platelet stickiness and lowers triglyceride levels, can reduce the risk of a heart attack by around a third[55-62] (see Chapter 8, Essential oils).

Anti-oxidants

Vitamin E helps to prevent LDL cholesterol oxidation[154]. It also prevents the accumulation of inflammatory cells that contribute to tissue damage and atheroma[104, 197], and is a mild anti-clotting agent[168, 187, 188], which is why it reduces the risk of stroke.

Vitamin E at this level has been shown to reduce the rate of atheroma growth in patients by two thirds, and halt it altogether when combined with lipid lowering agents[70]. So Vitamin E supplements sound like a good idea, but there's a note of caution. If you don't have enough Vitamin C and Q10, the E can become a pro-oxidant and increase the rate of cholesterol oxidation[51, 67, 68].

So Vitamins E and C should always be taken together. C not only 'supports' Vitamin E[51, 52, 153] but it also prevents inflammation of the blood vessels[163, 178], is essential for their repair, and may help to raise levels of HDL in the bloodstream[47, 48].

Vitamin C [54] and the carotenoids[53, 127, 185] are also linked to a reduced risk of CAD, so add carotenoids to your anti-oxidant mix[152], starting with lutein, which is an extremely potent anti-oxidant[63, 64], and lycopene, which appears to be highly cardio-protective[190].

Co-enzyme Q10 may be the most effective LDL protector of them all[162] (see also Chapter 9, Co-enzyme Q10).

There are approximately 6-8 molecules of Vitamin E per LDL particle, making it the most common anti-oxidant in LDL cholesterol.

Beta carotene is less common – there is only 1 molecule per 2-5 LDL particles. This suggests that it is less important in preventing atheroma and this has been confirmed by recent work[93]. Q10 is in the middle of the range, with one molecule per 2 LDL particles, rising to 1 per particle after supplementation[66, 67].

Q10's importance is hinted at by the fact that when LDL is oxidised, Q10 is the first anti-oxidant to be sacrificed. After the Q10 has been used up, the LDL quickly starts to oxidise, even while much of the E is still there, and long before the beta carotene has started to go[66]. In fact, once the Q10 is gone the E is more likely to act as a pro-oxidant[67, 68, 177]. The best results are obtained by combining Q10 with E and C[68, 208].

Fruit and vegetables

The risk of CAD is considerably reduced by a diet rich in plant foods. Fruit and vegetables contain a wide range of anti-oxidant compounds, and many also contain compounds which stimulate the body into producing more of its own anti-oxidant enzymes.

Go for fresh, ripe (but not overripe) produce. Levels of anti-oxidants in fruit and vegetables increase as part of the ripening process, as the oxidisable sugar or lipid content of the plant increases[71]. Wash but don't discard the outer layers, which are likely to contain the highest concentrations of anti-oxidants (see Chapter 6, Flavonoids & isoflavones).

Walnuts, almonds and hazelnuts contain Omega 6 fatty acids, which lower blood cholesterol, and improve the HDL/LDL cholesterol ratio[107]. Onions, kale, broccoli, apples and cherries all

---

Combined defence

Considering that E alone reduces the risk of CAD by nearly half, a combination of E, C, Q10, lycopene and betaine is likely to do significantly better, and confer near immunity.

Lycopene

This carotenoid appears to be very cardio-protective; it lowers LDL and is a good anti-oxidant[207].

A high lycopene intake (over 20mg a day) has been linked to a 47% reduction in heart attacks[185].

If CAD already exists …

In cases of known and advanced CAD, it would be advisable to combine the E, C and Q10 with Omega 3 fish oil, ginkgo and, if you do not have high blood pressure, low dose aspirin.

These agents are highly effective in reducing platelet stickiness and the risk of thrombus formation[69, 129, 163].

contain, amongst other good things, quercitin, a flavonoid which may protect against COPS[180].

Dietary fibre

Eat more artichoke, or oats; alternatively take oligofructose or inulin supplements. Both strategies generate a wide range of cardio-protective effects. They lower post-meal glucose and insulin levels, LDL cholesterol and blood pressure; and can increase HDL cholesterol and levels of B vitamins which keep heart-damaging homocysteine in check (see Chapter 7, Pre-biotic fibre).

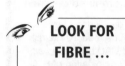

LOOK FOR FIBRE ...

such as an oligofructose supplement at about 8g a day.

Reversing heart disease

The right mix of nutrients should not only effectively immunise you against heart disease, it should also remove atheroma from furred-up arteries if atheroma has already developed.

Added ingredients

All the anti-oxidants we have discussed so far can be highly effective in protecting LDL from oxidation while it is in the plasma. But they cannot protect it once it has accumulated in the damaged arterial wall[72], because they do not enter the arterial wall in significant amounts.

Luckily there is another group of anti-oxidants in food sources which do. They are a group of flavonoids called the oligomeric procyanidins, found in grapeseed and skin, pine bark and tea, green more than black. Red wine is a particularly good source of these compounds.

Red wine

Wine contains a rich mix of cardio-protective nutrients. These include salicylates, which have an anti-platelet effect; and ethanol, which can cause the blood vessels to dilate and give a slight reduction in blood pressure[77] and may increase levels of 'good' HDL cholesterol.

Red wine also contains a mix of flavonoids that dramatically reduces free radical formation and the risk of thrombosis[75].

In particular red wine is a major source of the procyanidin flavonoids. They raise HDL cholesterol and inhibit LDL oxidation in the plasma so effectively[73, 76, 92] that some scientists believe that the habit of drinking a glass or two of red wine with every meal is the main cause of the low rates of CAD in France[74]. But they also get

The Wine List

Some wines have more flavonoids than others. As a rule of thumb, go for the deepest red colour and a good tannic structure.

High: Merlot, Cabernet Sauvignon, Chianti
Intermediate: Rioja, Pinot Noir
Low: Cotés du Rhone, Beaujolais, most rosé wines, whites

into the lining of the arteries, where they scavenge free iron, protect the extra-cellular matrix[198], prevent further oxidation of cholesterol already in the atheroma[78-87, 192], and help them open up[199].

Herbalists have known for years that both hawthorn and yarrow, plants exceptionally rich in procyanidins, can be used to treat angina and circulatory problems[88-91, 174-176].

Hesperidin, the major flavonoid in citrus fruit, also appears to be cardio-protective. Unlike the procyanidins, it doesn't seem to affect blood vessels but drinking a third of a litre of citrus juice a day lowers LDL cholesterol and triglyceride levels. The hesperidin, and perhaps other compounds in the juice, also increases the 'good' HDL cholesterol[156]; as does menthol[168-173].

Amino acids

The amino acids lysine and proline were a favourite of the late Linus Pauling. They are thought to act as a kind of arterial Teflon, stopping apolipoprotein B sticking to the artery wall. Used with high doses of Vitamin C and other anti-oxidants, they have reportedly achieved cures in patients with advanced CAD, relieving the symptoms of angina within a period of a relatively few months.

However, they don't protect the artery walls or prevent oxidation as the flavonoids do. I would only use them at the outset of an anti-atheroma programme, and replace them with the appropriate flavonoids within the first few days of treatment.

B vitamins (see Chapter 11, Betaine)

The most recent risk factor to be identified is hyperhomocysteinaemia[94,102,116,117,126]. This means having too much of an amino acid called homocysteine in the blood. Homocysteine is the opposite of an anti-oxidant – it is a pro-oxidant[103, 150]. This condition looks as if it may be a very strong risk factor indeed[108, 143, 184], but one that can be easily avoided.

Levels of the amino acid build up if there is a depletion of Vitamins B6, B12 and folic acid in the diet – and deficiencies are very common[110, 111, 115-119, 133]. All you have to do is to take a strong B complex preparation, which reduces levels of homocysteine[95, 96, 103,

Hawthorn

Hawthorn is amazingly cardio-protective. Its procyanidins calm inflammation in the artery walls[174]. They also inhibit angiotensin-converting enzyme and relax the blood vessel walls[175].

Finally, hawthorn strengthens the heart beat; unlike any other heart strengthener ('inotrope'), it does not increase the risk of cardiac arrythmias, but actually protects against them[176].

Folate and betaine

Low folate levels increase the risk of fatal heart attack by up to 69%[155].

Enriching basic foods with folate and Vitamin B12 would save thousands of lives[128,132]. Betaine would probably do even better – see Chapter 11.

Chapter 11, Betaine.

Chocolate

Chocolate contains flavonoids which protect LDL cholesterol from oxidation as effectively as red wine[167].

Green tea, which also contains similar flavonoids, is an acceptable alternative.

Homocysteine

Homocysteine not only increases certain clotting factors[149], but also the synthesis of the artery-toxic COPS and LOPS[150].

The B vitamins are prone to oxidation, which means that if you have a diet low in anti-oxidants or have factors which increase oxidative stress, such as smoking, this will lead to B depletion and elevated homocysteine[151] – another connection between poor anti-oxidant status and increased disease risk. Some people cannot metabolise folate[179], so betaine is often a better option - see Chapter 11, Betaine.

Folate deficiency is also linked to increased DNA damage, and an increased risk of cancer[130,136].

[115, 144] and should, by implication, reduce your risk of heart disease too[164]. Betaine is a better alternative at 500mg to 1g a day.

Minerals

Sodium and potassium

The modern diet, which contains too much sodium and too little potassium, is the prime cause of the age-related rise in blood pressure so common in the West. It is a major contributory factor to heart attacks and of stroke[193], particularly in the overweight.

Between 1972 and 1992 the Finns carried out a nationwide experiment, switching en masse from table salt to a mixed potassium and magnesium salt. The national average blood pressure fell dramatically, as did the incidence of heart attacks (55 per cent in men and 68 per cent in women), and strokes (62 per cent in men and women)[200, 209-211].

NB The Finnish product is called PanSalt.

TOP POTASSIUM FOODS

Potassium rich foods include:-

Baked potato	840mg	medium	Avocado	550mg	half
Lentils	730mg	1 cup	Carrot (raw)	232mg	medium
Kidney beans	700mg	1 cup	Orange juice	474mg	8oz
Prune juice	700mg	8oz	Milk	381mg	8oz
Tomato juice	652mg	6oz	Chick peas	470mg	1 cup
Banana	450mg	medium	Broccoli	224mg	1/2 cup

Magnesium

Magnesium salts are a major component in hard water, and people who live in areas where the drinking water is 'hard' have a reduced risk of heart disease[97]. Magnesium depletion causes atheroma in animals, and magnesium supplements clean the arteries out again[100]. This is thought to be because a depletion leads to an increased free radical synthesis and increased oxidation in the tissues.

The heart is uniquely sensitive to low magnesium levels and magnesium depletion is linked to a high risk of sudden cardiac (arrhythmic) death[101].

Magnesium supplements have also been shown to make the platelets less likely to form clots[98]. Although this would have little effect on atheroma formation, it would help to reduce the risk of thrombus formation, the last stage before the heart attack.

Calcium

Calcium intake is probably also important. A high calcium diet appears to lower the blood pressure[134, 135, 165, 166], which is a good idea in anyone at risk of a heart attack.

Copper

Copper may be involved too. Copper depletion is quite common, and has been linked to an increased risk of heart disease[99], possibly because one of the key anti-oxidant enzymes (SOD) depends on copper to work effectively.

Selenium

Selenium depletion is likely to have a similar effect. Veterinarians are familiar with heart problems caused by selenium depletion in cattle and other livestock. Humans are equally susceptible – although it is only in areas with an extremely low intake of selenium, such as Keshan in China, where cause and effect are relatively easy to single out. In the UK, the Scots are particularly likely to be low in this essential trace element.

Aluminium

Aluminium is intrinsically toxic to cells. It also displaces iron from its carrier molecules, and increased free iron could contribute to increased tissue damage in vessel walls.

Chronic aluminium exposure is likely, therefore, to be cardio-toxic.

Iron

Some scientists have suggested that too many iron supplements could increase the free radical load, and contribute to heart disease and other illness[113, 114, 121]. This is a difficult issue.

In most cases, and except for gross iron overload (as can happen after multiple blood transfusions, or in a genetic disease

Iron absorption

Iron in the diet or in supplements is best absorbed in the presence of Vitamin C, and meat. Absorption is reduced by phytates (in cereals), by calcium, and by flavonoids which occur in tea, coffee, red wine and some vegetables[122].

called haemochromatosis), most iron absorbed from the gut is safely bound to carrier molecules. Total body iron doesn't seem to be a common risk factor[106, 109]; but when tissue damage such as chronic inflammation leads to the release of free iron, problems are more likely to develop[125].

However, iron deficiency anaemia is widespread, especially in women. It's a common cause of fatigue and contributor to illness, and iron depletion during pregnancy may damage the brain of the growing foetus[123]. Iron supplements are therefore generally recommended for women of child-bearing age.

Men and post-menpausal women should be more cautious: there is some evidence that in men with very high iron levels in the blood, the risk of heart disease can be increased by as much as 100 per cent[113-114, 121]. Men should probably only take iron supplements if there is clear evidence of iron deficiency anaemia.

Herbs

Hawthorn, yarrow and grapes have already been mentioned, but herbal medicine has more to offer. Garlic is well-known as a cholesterol-lowering agent, and is almost as effective as some cholesterol-lowering drugs.

However, despite being a vital and much-loved element in southern and central European cuisine, many people dislike its pungent odour. If you are one of these, don't despair. There is at least one other herb which is probably more effective, and which has an array of quite well-documented properties which lower the risk of coronary artery disease dramatically.

The oddly named **Guggulipid** (an extract of Commiphora mukul) is already marketed in some countries as a lipid lowering agent. And although it does lower cholesterol and triglyceride levels, its more important effect may be to raise HDL (the 'good' cholesterol) by a highly significant 60 per cent[140, 141], via its phospholipid content. Guggulipid also has anti-clotting properties[142].

I have not yet been able to obtain safety data on Commiphora mukul, but the trial data, and its traditional use in Ayurvedic medicine, suggests that it is probably reasonably safe.

Avoid iron oxide

Iron oxide is not well absorbed and is a potent generator of free radicals in the gut – and could therefore increase the risk of gastrointestinal cancer.

It is slightly worrying that many pills and tablets still use iron oxide as a colouring agent, especially when other safer colours are available.

The new garlic?

Guggulipid seems able to raise HDL and lower LDL – perhaps even better than garlic.

Regime for a healthy heart

The information is all here. By combining these nutritional ingredients, I believe we can reduce the risk of CAD almost to zero.

We can do for coronary artery disease with nutrition what we did to cholera with public sanitation – banish it from the health statistics. And where arteries are already blocked, we can use the nutritional approach to open them again; to regain function, and health.

Levels of heart disease are already falling, because of lifestyle changes. Since 1968, the risk of dying from a heart attack in the USA, Australia and Finland has fallen by half, and in the UK the risk of heart attacks has dropped almost as dramatically in professional men – who are smoking less, and eating more fruit and vegetables. But smokers, diabetics (see Chapter 16, Diabetes) and those with chronic renal failure[157, 158], and indeed the rest of the population, remain particularly vulnerable.

If you or someone you love is carrying too many risk factors, why wait to take (or recommend) a nutritional insurance programme? Do it now!

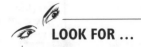

LOOK FOR ...

a daily supplement to reduce heart disease risk that has at least:

• Vitamin E	265mg
• Vitamin C	500mg
• Folic acid	200mcg
• Calcium	100mg
• Magnesium	50mg
• Mixed carotenoids	20-25mg
• OPC complex	100mg
• Q10	30-60mg
• B vitamins	300% of RDA
• Copper as a chelate	2mg
• Selenium	150mcg
• Betaine	450mg
• Vitamin K	50mcg

A COMPREHENSIVE CARDIO-PROTECTIVE ACTION PLAN

The Cambridge Heart Anti-oxidant Study (CHAOS) reported in *The Lancet* in 1996 that a Vitamin E supplement could be 400% more effective in reducing the risk of heart attack than the most common drug treatment. The overall risk reduction from Vitamin E supplementation was 75%[201].

The nature of such studies is that they seek to isolate the effects of a single variable – in this case Vitamin E.

If you want the most effective cardio-protective strategy, however, you would add Vitamin C, Q10, B vitamins and betaine (to reduce homocysteine formation), calcium, potassium and magnesium (to relax the muscle walls of the arteries), Omega 3 and Omega 6 (in flaxseed oil) and plenty of fruit and vegetables to increase your intake of potassium, flavonoids and carotenoids.

Avoid fried foods, salt, exercise regularly (20 minutes, three times a week) and don't smoke.

Result: your risk of heart disease should be near zero.

Preventing heart disease

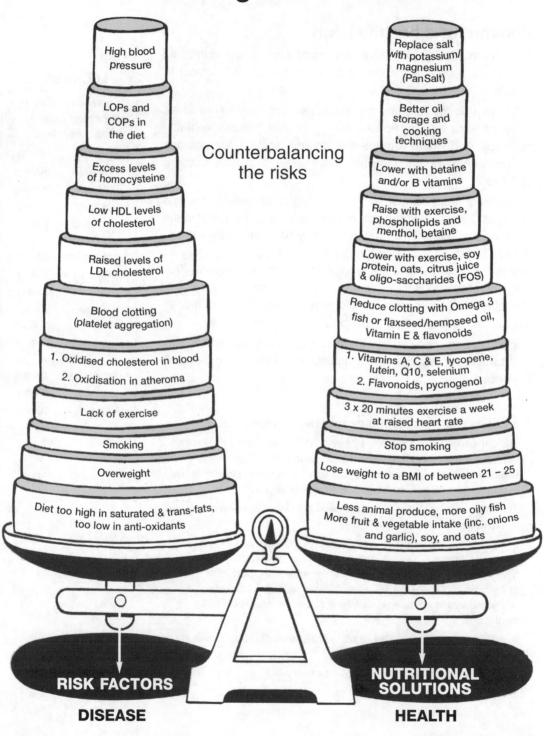

Counterbalancing the risks

RISK FACTORS

DISEASE

NUTRITIONAL SOLUTIONS

HEALTH

SUMMARY

The healthy heart guide

▶ Stop smoking.

▶ Exercise three times a week.

▶ Gradually lose weight to fit your ideal body mass index. Don't crash diet – rapid weight loss is usually soon regained, and yo-yo dieting <u>may</u> be associated with an increased risk of CAD[30].

▶ Eat oily fish twice a week.

▶ Incorporate plenty of ripe fruit and vegetables into your diet, including the flavonoid-rich plants (see Chapter 6, Flavonoids & isoflavones).

▶ Drink a third of a litre of citrus juice (orange, grapefruit, etc) a day.

▶ Take C, E, Q10, lutein or lycopene , B vitamins or betaine. Take Vitamin K in spinach, kale or broccoli.

▶ Top up with magnesium, calcium, copper and selenium.

▶ Cut back on saturated fats and avoid trans-fats in margarines and processed foods. They are usually identified on the label as vegetable fats, and hydrogenated or partly hydrogenated vegetable oils.

▶ Poly-unsaturated oils are fine for salad dressings, but not for frying.

▶ Keep margarines and oils in the fridge.

▶ Use mono-unsaturated oils such as olive or rapeseed oils for cooking.

▶ Substitute soy products for meat, and red wine for beer.

▶ Oat-based foods, and most types of bean, can help to reduce blood cholesterol levels; especially when combined with nicotinic acid (Vitamin B3), a supplement available in health food shops.

▶ Have regular blood pressure and cholesterol checks.

▶ If you have hypertension, switch from table salt to a low sodium salt or, if available, to a magnesium/potassium salt mix, such as PanSalt. It tastes identical, but gradually lowers your blood pressure.

- Osteoporosis is not confined to elderly women – it affects men, young women and even children

- It's a disease which leads to more deaths in women than cervical, ovarian and womb cancer combined. Early menopause, smoking, pregnancy, alcohol and steroids all raise the risk of osteoporosis

- Vitamin K is needed to build new bones – but pollution, anticoagulant drugs, antibiotics and laxatives all reduce the amount of K in our bodies

- A flavonoid product is used successfully in Japan and Italy to slow bone loss and encourage bone rebuilding

- Oestrogen slows down bone loss. Progesterone, however, may actually increase bone growth

- High doses of Omega 6 and 3 PUFAs increase the amount of calcium absorbed – and reduce bone loss

- The much-touted calcium supplements will do little to help if you're deficient in Vitamin K and other nutrients, such as magnesium and Vitamin C. Depletion in these nutrients is widespread

- Meat and dairy products are rich in calcium, but also in saturated fats, which block bone-building

Chapter 15

Skeleton in the cupboard

Dr Sheila Macrae was 35 when she started working out at the gym. She gradually became more involved in fitness training, and within two years was competing in triathlons.

She felt strong, self-confident, and slim. The only problem was that her periods became very irregular, and she and her husband wanted to start a family. She joined a research project at St Mary's Hospital in London, where they were studying irregular periods in women athletes. The researchers were shocked by what they found. This super-fit athlete had the bones of an old-age pensioner: so weak and fragile they were in danger of fracturing at any moment. She had osteoporosis, caused in large measure by her training routine.

Sheila Macrae's case is not uncommon. Osteoporosis, once a disease of the elderly, is striking younger victims.

A recent survey by the British National Osteoporosis Society found thousands of women in their 50s suffering from fractures, chronic back pain, loss of height and disability. More extreme is the relatively recently discovered osteoporosis of pregnancy, where fractures of the hip or spine occur late in pregnancy in women in their 20s and 30s[143].

Reports are coming in of ballerinas, athletes like Dr Macrae, and even children with fragile, osteoporotic bones. Men are involved too[200] – approximately a quarter of all fractured hips are male.

Fractured wrists and ankles, although painful and disabling, are the least serious clinical end-point. At the other end of the scale, fractured hips are a huge cause of disability and loss of mobility, with one in five progressing to death within 12 months[56].

Accumulating crush fractures of the vertebrae lead to stooping, weakness, pain, respiratory and other problems. They're another significant cause of immobilisation and premature death. Many women with stooping (kyphosis) suffer a severe loss of self-confidence and self-esteem, and become isolated. A combination of poor nutrition, lack of Vitamin D and insufficient exercise makes matters worse, and leads to a sad cycle of decline.

> **You have 2-3 lbs of calcium in your body!**
>
> The average adult's body is 2% calcium by weight.

> **BONE FRACTURES AFFECT 50% OF WOMEN**
>
> In the last 60 years the incidence of hip fractures has increased dramatically, six-fold in some areas[102, 192]. A third of women over 50 lose height almost certainly due to osteoporotic fractures of the spine, although the majority of these remain undiagnosed.
>
> By the age of 60, one woman in four has had a serious fracture. By the age of 70, it is one in two. One in two women will suffer a bone fracture at some time in their lives. And the latest studies indicate that as many as one in eight men will be similarly affected.

Shattering truth about fragile bones

The litany of injuries above are some of the reasons why osteoporosis is now killing more women than cervical, ovarian and womb cancer combined.

In the USA, osteoporosis costs $10 billion a year, and is set to hit $30 billion by the turn of the century[57]. In the UK, it will cost £3 billion by 2002. The situation in many other countries is broadly similar.

It used to be thought that the increasing tide of fractured hips was simply a reflection of an ageing society. Bone loss tends to increase with age, and the average age is increasing in the developed countries. But this is not nearly enough, in itself, to explain the growing problem.

> "I was devastated. All the training I did to make me fit and strong was on the point of crippling me. Thank God they caught it in time. I started HRT, and my bones are slowly recovering, although they're still not good.
>
> "These days the only exercise I get is swimming, and exercise bikes. I can't run any more because the osteoporosis affected my back. I shrank from 5'5" to 5'4"."
> *Sheila Macrae*

Clearly, there is some other growing environmental and/or dietary threat to our bones. The World Health Organisation recognises this, and has called for urgent action to prevent a worldwide epidemic of this silent, crippling disease.

Intensive research programmes are investigating why our bones are crumbling. Eventually the expert committees will reach a consensus position. But nutritional forms of protection are already available.

Bone loss can be 4% a year!

Until recently, doctors believed that bone mass was lost after the menopause at a rate of about 1 per cent a year.

But in May '95, scientists at the Nuffield Orthopaedic Centre in Oxford, England, showed that by the time a women reaches her late 60s, she will be losing bone at up to **4 per cent a year**.

That's 40% of the strength gone in a decade.

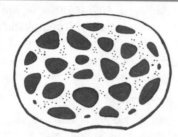

Bone micro-structure in a healthy bone. Note the thick, strong matrix.

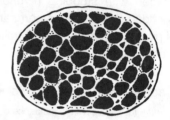

Bone micro-structure in osteoporosis.
The structure has become much thinner – it is fragile and easily fractured.

The warning signs are too late

In women over 40, wrist and ankle fractures are often the first indication of osteoporosis. After 50, loss of height, back pain and increasingly stooped posture are common symptoms, as is extensive tooth loss – an unfortunate combination of symptoms stereotyped in folklore as denoting a witch.

If you have one or more of the risk factors or symptoms outlined, or if one or more of your close relatives have or had osteoporosis, you should take a serious interest in early diagnosis and treatment.

Urine tests, which measure the rate of bone loss and therefore the risk of developing osteoporosis, are beginning to become available[27, 52-55], but are not universally accepted or widely used. Some doctors use hospital-based bone densitometry measurements (DXA scans) which take a 'snapshot' of bone density. Many, however, take a more passive role and do little until the first fracture occurs.

By then it's too late.

By the time a hip fractures as much as half of the mineral content of the skeleton (the calcium and magnesium salts which give it strength) may have gone.

There are no warning signs of this de-mineralisation until suddenly, the wrist breaks after a minor fall, or a bone in the spine or hip crumbles.

Why bones break

To understand how treatments work, we have to explain how the skeleton works.

Bones are metabolically very active. They're constantly being worn away and rebuilt. The entire skeleton is replaced about once every 10 years. This rebuilding is essential, because the forces transmitted through the bones when we walk, run or jump cause tiny stress fractures.

These have to be repaired before they can spread and cause serious disruption. This is done by an on-going, delicately balanced two-phase repair process. First the osteoclast cells move in, and remove the damaged bone. Then their opposite numbers, the osteoblast cells, arrive and rebuild new bone where the old bone used to be.

In healthy young people the rate of bone growth is faster than the rate of bone loss, and therefore the bones grow and strengthen through the first two decades. During the third and fourth decade the rates of bone loss and regeneration are in balance – so there is little net change. After 50 bone regeneration slows, while bone loss increases – so there is a progressive net loss of bone – see graph.

It's downhill all the way, particularly for women, who lose calcium more rapidly during the menopause, and who generally have smaller bones than men to start with[57]. The bones get thinner and weaker, until a fracture occurs. But although everybody is at risk, some people are more at risk than others.

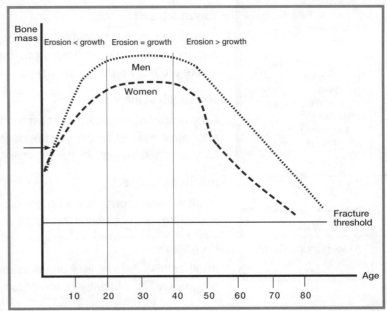

Hormones

An early menopause, whether natural or surgical, increases the risk of an osteoporotic fracture. So do anorexia and bulimia, both of which tend to cause dietary deficiencies and, in younger women, cessation of periods (a kind of mini-menopause).

Eating disorders are on the increase, in men as well as in women, and will add to our osteoporotic problems in the future. Endurance athletes and ballet dancers, who exercise excessively and may eat a wildly unbalanced diet, often have very low oestrogen levels and experience missed periods. They are another recognised high risk group: Dr Macrae was in this category.

Smoking

Passive smoking advances the menopause by two to three years. The smoker herself goes through menopause up to five years early – this is a definite risk factor. Smoking depletes the body of anti-oxidants including Vitamin C, essential for bone growth[17]. Smoking also suppresses the bone-building cells, so the current increase in cigarette smoking in young girls is particularly worrying. Combined with poor dietary habits, it confers a high risk of osteoporotic fractures to come.

Too much salt

Consumed in the quantities typically found in the Western diet, salt increases calcium loss from the body. Cutting down salt intake probably reduces the risk of osteoporosis[150-159].

Too much sulphate

Excess sulphate ingestion increases calcium loss. There is not much sulphate in the diet, unless you take high-dose glucosamine sulphate for your joints. This could, paradoxically, damage your bones.

Inactive lifestyle

Healthy bone growth is encouraged by weight-bearing exercise – ie walking, but not swimming. Lack of exercise is a risk factor.

Pregnancy

Another 'risk factor' in women is pregnancy. Osteoporosis of pregnancy is officially uncommon, but is almost certainly

---

Sweating it out

You can lose up to 500mg calcium in sweat during a single aerobic training session[160].

Don't smoke!

Cigarettes attack the bones and increase the risk of hip fracture by up to three times[17].

Soft drinks

These are not recommended, especially for children, if they replace milk drinks.

Colas are particularly bad: they contain phosphoric acid, which, when excreted in the urine, pulls calcium out of the body. Recently identified as a risk factor[201].

Walk!

A sedentary lifestyle causes bone thinning.

underdiagnosed. The main symptoms are pain in the back or hip, typically in the last trimester or while breast-feeding. This is easily missed, because so many women suffer back pain during pregnancy, which may also be due to postural change.

Symptoms such as loss of height (which can be as much as three inches) are easier to spot, and are caused by crush fractures of the vertebrae. The problems are caused when calcium is leached out of the bones to provide calcium for the growing foetus, and for the milk. Fortunately, bone mass generally recovers to some extent after weaning.

Drug use and alcohol abuse

Alcohol abuse and long-term oral steroid therapy both increase the risk of osteoporosis. Steroid therapy is implicated in up to 20 per cent of cases of osteoporosis; all the more reason for considering alternatives to steroids (See Chapter 6, Flavonoids & isoflavones).

Depression and stress

Depressive illness (which causes increased steroid synthesis in the body) is a risk factor[189]. Chronic stress, which also boosts levels of steroids, is therefore also a candidate risk factor.

Other risk factors

Some genes and symptoms have been identified which may increase the risk of osteoporosis[84-87] – but these are still hotly debated. Watch this space!

Digging up the past

Doctors can slow the progress of the disease with HRT, and prescribe painkillers; but to stem the tide of broken bones we need to know why Western women are twice as likely today to suffer hip fractures as their mothers were, and treat the cause of the problem.

A significant clue was unearthed by Dr John Stevenson at the Wynn Institute in London, who compared contemporary bones with those of people who died 200 years ago. He found that women's bones have become significantly more fragile.

Risk factors for osteoporosis

- **Excessive exercise**
- **Smoking**
- **Excessive salt intake**
- **Sedentary lifestyle**
- **Alcohol and drug intake**
- **Depression**
- **Chronic stress**
- **Excessive sulphate intake (rare, except in those taking glucosamine sulphate for their joints)**
- **Excessive intake of cola drinks**

This could be because we do more deskwork than our ancestors and less walking. Inactivity is bad for bones; astronauts, whose bones do little work under zero gravity, lose massive amounts of calcium.

Conversely, in patients who have osteoporosis, exercise programmes which increase stresses on the skeleton can help rebuild their thinning bones. But Dr Stevenson found that even the sedentary workers of 200 years ago had better bones than contemporary subjects. This suggests that the current epidemic of osteoporosis may be due to widespread micro-nutrient depletion.

Fibre-reinforced bones

Bone consists of two phases: organic and inorganic. The organic matrix, a mesh of biological micro-fibres built by the osteoblasts, provides a framework which is then impregnated and stiffened with inorganic calcium and magnesium phosphates.

The matrix is constantly being eroded and replaced; but if the rate of loss outstrips the rate of regrowth, there is a net loss of bone. If there is insufficient matrix, there is nothing for the minerals to latch onto – which explains why calcium (and magnesium) tablets have so little effect in treating osteoporosis.

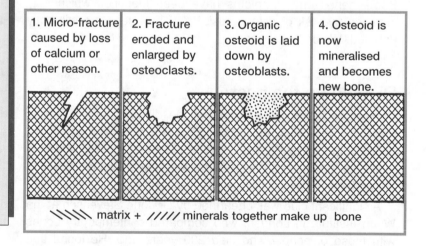

| 1. Micro-fracture caused by loss of calcium or other reason. | 2. Fracture eroded and enlarged by osteoclasts. | 3. Organic osteoid is laid down by osteoblasts. | 4. Osteoid is now mineralised and becomes new bone. |

\\\\\\ matrix + ////// minerals together make up bone

Vitamin K and other micro-nutrients such as Vitamins C, B6 and D, and the trace minerals zinc, copper and manganese are vital for matrix regrowth; without them calcium supplements cannot be effective, because there is no matrix for the calcium to latch onto. Most people are depleted in most of these micro-nutrients, but Vitamin K may just be the most important.

The calcium fallacy

Calcium intake during the early years, when the bones are growing, is important in contributing to peak bone mass. Young girls who eat more dairy products appear to have more calcium taken up into the bones[97]. But this may not confer much protection in later life.

There are plenty of communities with a low calcium diet and very little osteoporosis (such as Africa), and there are equally countries with a high calcium diet where osteoporosis is common (such as Sweden).

The fact is that we evolved with the ability to adapt to variations in our calcium intake. And although there is some correlation between high calcium intake during childhood and a reduced risk of osteoporotic fracture later in life (because you start off with more calcium in the bone bank), the clinical results of calcium supplementation in later life are disappointing[126-128, 148].

Bones are made of calcium, loss of calcium leads to osteoporosis, which can be easily measured – so let's throw calcium at the problem, runs the over-simplified thinking. But we've failed to see beyond the most superficial layer of evidence – and misread an effect as a cause.

Calcium in the diet or in supplements cannot be built into bone unless the other elements necessary for bone growth are also present.

One reason calcium is being lost in the first place is because the other necessary bone-building factors are not there at sufficient levels. It is these we should concentrate on putting right.

Special K

Vitamin K is well known as an essential co-factor for the carboxylation (and activation) of various blood clotting proteins, but it also activates at least three proteins made by the bone forming cells, the osteoblasts. These proteins are osteocalcin, matrix GLA protein and Protein S[119-121]. Although the function of these proteins is not understood, osteocalcin levels reflect osteoblast, bone-building activity[162, 164]; and it seems likely that activated osteocalcin is essential to the bone-building process.

Some scientists believe that low levels of activated osteocalcin predict hip fracture[124]; and have shown that reduced levels of activated osteocalcin correlate with reduced bone mineral density of the femoral neck[125].

> **K for Koagulation!**
>
> It was Danish researchers who discovered their Vitamin K was essential for blood to clot.
>
> The Danish for coagulation is 'Koagulation'.

With age, the proportion of inactive osteocalcin increases[4,5, 122-125]; bone mineral density decreases; and the risk of osteoporotic fracture increases markedly. Patients with osteoporosis[1-3, 134] and osteoporotic fractures[167] have particularly low levels of K. These pieces of evidence strongly suggest that the increase in inactive osteocalcin, the run-down in effective osteoblast activity, the loss of bone mass and the increase in fracture are all related to Vitamin K depletion.

This is supported by the fact that intensive nutritional support enhances bone mending in fracture patients[163]. More specifically, large doses of Vitamin K1 (1mg a day for 14 days) increased carboxylated osteocalcin to 'normal' levels[4]. This caused an improvement of bone metabolism, as urinary calcium and hydroxyproline excretion (bone-loss markers) both fell[4]. Even larger doses of K (45mg K1 a day for 48 weeks) resulted in improved bone health[161]; although at these doses K may be acting at additional sites, eg by inhibiting bone re-absorption[165, 166].

Scientists have recently found that post-menopausal women do indeed have very low levels of K activity with particularly high levels of unactivated osteocalcin[122-125]. This strongly suggests that in these women, a lack of Vitamin K is preventing osteocalcin activation, and hence slowing the building of new bone[4, 5]. This may in turn explain why post-menopausal women are particularly at risk of osteoporosis, and why they lose such large amounts of calcium in their urine.

These findings indicate that a Vitamin K supplement should slow, stop or even help reverse the disease process. By activating more osteocalcin, it should encourage the growth of new bone, and reduce calcium loss.

Dr Hodges' latest discovery concerns the way Vitamin K is stored in bone. Bones don't just thin with age – the bone marrow changes too. It becomes more fatty, and Vitamin K has a high affinity for fat.

When Dr Hodges analysed the bone marrow in elderly patients receiving hip replacements, he found higher than normal levels of Vitamin K inside their thinning bones[7].

This pool of Vitamin K was locked inside the fat, unavailable to help build bones, and therefore useless in warding off

---

Vitamin K

1mg of Vitamin K per day for 14 days reduced calcium loss and encouraged new bone growth[4].

K's other benefits

Dr Hodges' group has also shown that Vitamin K inhibits the production of Interleukin 6.

Interleukin 6, a messenger substance which triggers inflammatory changes, appears to be involved not just in osteoporosis[8] but also in rheumatoid arthritis[9], and cancer[11].

K supplements should, therefore, help in the treatment of all these disease conditions.

K – Kaution!

High-dose Vitamin K may exacerbate periodontal disease[10].

---

osteoporosis. It seems that as the numbers of fat cells inside the bones accumulate with age, they may 'steal' Vitamin K from the bone-building cells where it is most needed; and thereby contribute to the increased risk of osteoporosis with age.

This suggests that K supplementation should play an important role in the prevention of osteoporosis – and in treating it as well.

WARNING

People at risk from blood clots who are receiving anti-K coagulants such as Warfarin **must not** take extra Vitamin K, as it reduces the effectiveness of the anti-coagulant and may cause thrombus formation.

Everyone else, however, can take K supplements safely as they do not in themselves increase the risk of blood clots. In Japan, thousands of osteoporosis patients now take 45mg of Vitamin K per day prophylactically. The only side effect is that, at high doses, K acts as an anti-inflammatory analgesic – which makes it useful (but expensive) for treating toothache or arthritis!

Broccoli

Comfrey (traditionally known as knit-bone) is an old herbal remedy for broken bones – and a rich source of Vitamin K[6].

Comfrey also contains substances that may cause liver damage, so try broccoli, another excellent source of K, instead[6].

Evidence for the bone-protecting effects of broccoli is persuasive, but still circumstantial.

K clue to brittle bone epidemic

The K factor could explain the osteoporosis epidemic.

Industrial chemicals called PCBs, which were dumped in large amounts in the '60s, '70s and '80s, have a strong anti-K effect.

The dumped PCBs leaked into our water supplies and the food chain. As a result, we now all have traces of these toxic chemicals in our bodies.

Dutch research indicates that this is the cause of a 'new' disease, Late Haemorrhagic Disease of the Newborn, where month-old babies suffer from catastrophic and often fatal bleeding.

Vitamin K is routinely and safely[29] given to newborn infants to prevent haemorrhage, but in these babies the effects of the K injection were overcome by the high doses of PCBs they got from their mother's milk.

If exposure to four weeks' worth of PCBs via breast milk can kill newborn babies, what damage would 20 years of exposure to these toxic chemicals do to the bones of a middle-aged woman?

The new 'organo-phosphate' pesticides (OPs) may also be strong K blockers, which is a serious worry; and modern medicine is implicated too.

Anticoagulant drugs like Warfarin were introduced in the '50s to prevent blood clotting in at-risk patients. These drugs are powerful Vitamin K blockers, and long-term use could interfere with Vitamin K's bone-building activities, leading to thinning of the skeleton.

Antibiotics and laxatives are further candidates. Some Vitamin K is made by intestinal bacteria, and anything that disturbs these bacteria could cause a Vitamin K deficiency. Laxatives became very popular in the '50s, and antibiotics were prescribed in enormous numbers through the '60s and '70s.

The wide spectrum antibiotics, in particular, have been shown to cause severe K deficiency states[101]. Here is yet another possible cause of crumbling bones.

Additional therapies

Although Vitamin K is vital for skeletal health, there are four other powerful nutritional weapons in the fight against osteoporosis – flavonoids, hormones, PUFAs and minerals. These can be used in conjunction with K.

You may be surprised that minerals – particularly calcium – don't top the list. Calcium (and magnesium, and phosphorus, etc) can only be deposited in bone if the overall nutritional state is favourable. If it is, a low calcium diet is unlikely to harm you. If it isn't, all the calcium you can swallow won't help much.

1 Flavonoids

As long ago as the early '70s, the flavonoid ipriflavone was found to limit bone loss in rats, chickens and sheep. Scientists realised that they might have a useful anti-osteoporosis agent on their hands, and went on to use it to treat experimental osteoporosis in animal models, with great success[31-33].

As a result of these and other studies, ipriflavone is now licensed for use as an anti-osteoporosis medicine in Italy, Hungary and Japan. In Britain, the USA and elsewhere, patients are denied access to this safe and effective nutritional remedy. Doctors to whom I spoke dismissed it as 'unknown, untested, irrelevant'. These views are a sad reflection of the current state of medical education.

In fact, ipriflavone has been intensively studied, and there is a fair degree of consensus as to its multiple bone-building effects. It enhances the effect of oestrogen on preventing bone loss[35, 36]. Ipriflavone also slows down the bone-corroding osteoclasts and increases the growth of the bone-building osteoblasts[44-49]. This last effect makes ipriflavone look more like a progesterone mimic than the oestrogen mimic it is sometimes thought to be[71].

A well-designed dose-response study in Japan with assessment of bone mass increase and a safety profile evaluation showed that a daily oral dose of 600mg of ipriflavone was the optimal treatment for osteoporosis. Other clinicians have used a 1200 mg dose without problems.

Bone stimulants

A combination of micro-nutrients including Vitamins K, D and B6 has been shown to be effective in stimulating bone regeneration in post-menopausal women[147].

Ipriflavone

The flavonoid ipriflavone reduces bone loss and promotes bone rebuilding.

There have been **60** clinical studies, including 16 randomised controlled human trials, showing significant benefit: but it's not available in the US or UK.

The overall assessment of scientists who have worked with ipriflavone is that it reduces bone resorption and enhances bone formation in an entirely physiological way[37].

In a series of studies of post-menopausal women with low bone mass, ipriflavone produced a significant increase in total bone mass within 12 months[38-41, 94, 114, 115, 149, 168, 193]. It also reduced bone pain[42, 43, 114].

Ipriflavone is also effective in treating thinning bones caused by osteogenesis imperfecta, an inherited disease which causes multiple fractures in men and in women[91-93].

No abnormalities have been found in the structure of the new bone that is encouraged to form by the flavonoid, and no side effects have been noted. However, in patients with renal problems, ipriflavone should be used with caution, as there is a theoretical, if slight, possibility of flavonoid build-up in the body[34].

Natural sources
Ipriflavone is found in alfalfa and various types of beans.

2 Proteins and hormones

The recently discovered Bone Morphogenic Proteins (BMPs), which stimulate new bone growth, hold considerable promise but are still at the research stage.

There are several hormones which play an important role in creating a favourable climate for bone growth. Oestrogen (in HRT) and calcitonin are both used to reduce calcium loss, but cannot replace lost bone.

Testosterone, growth hormone and some of the anabolic steroids have been used to promote bone formation in men, but are not suitable for all patients.

In any case, you won't get any of these hormones without a prescription, and you won't get a prescription unless you can persuade your physician that you are at significant risk of developing osteoporosis, or already have osteoporosis.

HRT is the easiest of the hormone products to obtain. Calcium loss accelerates during the menopause, and for many years doctors assumed this was because of the fall in levels of the sex hormone oestrogen which occurs at the menopause.

HRT may not reduce bone loss
HRT is often prescribed at too low a dose to prevent bone loss[51].
A recent study found that the bones of older women, who had been on long-term oestrogen therapy, were no better than the bones of women who had not received oestrogen treatment[58].

The good news about being fat!

Adipose tissue continues to make oestrogen. In obese post-menopausal women, the adipose tissue keeps oestrogen levels high enough to give partial protection against osteoporosis, but not enough to protect against heart attacks.

Eroding bone

Oestrogen slows down erosion by encouraging the osteoclasts, cells that erode bone, to commit suicide[189].

Saturated fats

Cut down on animal (saturated) fats. These reduce progesterone synthesis in the body. Switch to mono-unsaturated oils when possible.

The logical response was to prescribe oestrogen replacement therapy, but this was found to increase the risk of breast and uterine cancer, so they added progestogens to the mix and called it Hormone Replacement Therapy, HRT.

Women on HRT live an average three to four years longer than women not on HRT. In women after the menopause, who take HRT for five years or more (which is longer than most women remain on HRT), the risk of fracture is reduced[149, 150].

Unfortunately, HRT is linked to a variety of problems and side effects which make it unsuitable for many women. And although it reduces the risk of osteoporosis for a while, it doesn't give anything like as much protection as it should if oestrogen really were the key to the problem[133].

Could it be progesterone? At the menopause, levels of oestrogen fall to well below the levels needed to prepare the lining of the womb for pregnancy, but not to zero. Other tissues, like the adrenal glands, liver and adipose tissue continue to make oestrogen.

Levels of progesterone, however, fall away to nothing. And the fascinating thing about this is the timing. Levels of progesterone start to fall a year or so before the menopause, and there is evidence that the rate of calcium loss also begins to increase just before the menopause[80].

Progesterone is produced during the second half of the menstrual cycle by the group of cells left behind in the ovary after an egg has been released (the corpus luteum).

The ovulation process is complex and easily disturbed. If the egg is not released, progesterone is not produced.

Excessive exercise and weight loss both block ovulation and lead to so-called anovulatory cycles, where oestrogen levels are normal but progesterone falls away almost to nothing. A recent study of young women athletes with normal oestrogen levels found many with anovulatory cycles, very low progesterone levels and all the biochemical signs of developing osteoporosis[62].

These findings have stimulated clinicians to take a new look at the workings of the sex hormones. It turns out that although oestrogens reduce the rate at which bone is eroded[64], there is a compensatory decrease in bone formation. So, although there are some benefits[139], the end result is little more than a temporary slowing of the rate of bone loss[59].

Although progesterone is a similar molecule, it seems to have a different mode of action. There is evidence that it binds to, and activates, the bone-building osteoblast cells[63, 81], in a way that resembles the effects of Growth Hormone[99]. And there is evidence that, like growth hormone, progesterone can help build stronger bones[69,103-108].

The American general physician John Lee has used progesterone to treat many women with apparent success[65-68]. His bone density studies showed increases of up to 30 per cent after a few years of treatment, with women of 60 and 70 (treated for osteoporosis) developing bones resembling those of a woman of 35, the age when the skeleton is at its peak. These are dramatic results. But sadly, Dr Lee's trials are poorly designed and documented. They may be very important – but we cannot be sure until they are duplicated. However …

The progesterone molecule is very similar to the male sex hormone testosterone, which has long been known to be vital to bone health in men. Osteoporosis frequently occurs in men who are deficient in testosterone[60]; and when testosterone is given to these men, it prevents and even reverses their osteoporosis[61, 72,145].

As well as post-menopausal osteoporosis, other clinical conditions where there is rapid bone loss have also been shown to respond to progestogen therapy. In patients taking high-dose steroids for asthma[109-110], and in certain other conditions progestogens stop and reverse the otherwise unremitting loss of bone[111-112].

Why the menopause can cause osteoporosis

It is probable that both oestrogen and progesterone contribute to bone health. Oestrogen slows down bone loss, and progesterone may increase bone growth. When progesterone levels fall, before the menopause, the body starts to lose calcium possibly because it can no longer be built so

Growing bone

Progesterone may halt osteoporosis, by encouraging new bone growth[82].

Bone loss and the menopause

It may be the dual effect of lower progesterone **and** lower oestrogen at the menopause that triggers accelerated bone loss.

efficiently into the skeleton. Then oestrogen levels fall, and now the rate of bone loss accelerates too. Slower bone building and increased bone loss is a recipe for osteoporosis – and explains why these menopausal changes result in post-menopausal problems.

Hormones without Prescription

In many countries such as the UK progesterone is an 'unlicensed medicine', only available on prescription.

In the USA, 'progesterone cream' can be bought in health food shops. Alternatively, try yams, which contain the compound diosgenin. (Edible yams contain less diosgenin than medicinal yams, as it is quite bitter.) Diosgenin increases calcium uptake by certain cells[88-90]: and is metabolised in the body NOT to progesterone (as often claimed), but to DHEA[6, 175].

DHEA is an important anti-ageing 'parent' hormone with a considerable 'feel good' effect[160]. It appears to offer protection against diabetes and coronary artery disease[169,170,185]; obesity[182,183]; cancer[174,181,188] and osteoporosis[173,184,187]. In one study, DHEA given as a topical cream for 12 months led to a significant increase in bone density at the hip[180].

DHEA exerts a number of different osteo-protective effects, including:

- anti-corticosteroid actions[173, 177-179, 184, 186];
- anti-inflammatory actions[168, 171, 172, 176]; and
- a direct stimulation of the bone-building osteoblasts[191].

This may be why in countries where yams are a staple food, osteoporosis is thought to be relatively uncommon. However, other variables such as higher activity levels and lower life expectancy must also be considered.

---

3 PUFAs

A third group of nutrients which play a role in maintaining bone health are the Omega 3 and Omega 6 fatty acids. These are found in fish oil, and evening primrose (or starflower/borage) oil respectively. Oils that contain **both** Omega 3 and 6 in a near ideal ratio include hemp and flax oils.

In large doses these oils increase the absorption of calcium from the gut[12], rather like Vitamin D does. In this way they can make up for a low calcium diet, and are a more efficient way of increasing calcium uptake than simply taking huge calcium supplements. (A high calcium intake interferes with iron absorption in the gut, and increases the risk of anaemia[50].)

Not only do the PUFAs increase calcium absorption, they also reduce calcium loss. Excretion of calcium in the urine is

> **Importance of PUFAs**
>
> A diet which contains normal amounts of calcium, but is deficient in PUFAs, increases the risk of osteoporosis[20, 21].

significantly reduced, as is the risk of kidney stones[13, 14].

This double effect increases the amount of calcium stored in the body. Some doctors were concerned about whether the extra calcium is going into the bones, or elsewhere. However high-dose PUFAs actively prevent the abnormal deposition of calcium in soft tissues, where it is not wanted[19] and increase the calcium content of the bones[16, 17, 190].

And because they are doing all these good things, it should come as no surprise to find that high-dose PUFAs slow the bone loss that otherwise comes after the menopause[15], or even that they stimulate the growth of new bone[16, 18, 190].

4 Minerals

If I were still at medical school, I would be very concerned that there had been no mention of minerals. Well, here they are. And they are important, because even if the bone-building environment is positive, you still need the right minerals to make new bone – they are, after all, the inorganic construction materials. But they can only be used by the body if the other hormonal or nutritional factors are already in place.

- **CALCIUM** ✔

  A reasonable amount of calcium in the diet is important, together with Vitamin D which is essential in improving calcium absorption from the gut, and promoting its uptake into new bone.

  It's important to start early in life. By encouraging children to eat calcium-rich foods and take plenty of exercise, their bones grow thicker and stronger. They're building up a calcium reserve, so that even if they do start to lose calcium later in life, they're starting off from a stronger position. But is what is good for children necessarily good for adults?

  One problem is that many of the richest sources of calcium are meat and dairy products. And for many reasons, we're encouraged to cut back on these, due to their high content of saturated fats.

Omega 3 & 6 build bone

Many studies show that the combination of Omega 3 and 6 fatty acids has a positive effect on bone metabolism.

To obtain clinical benefits, however, they must be taken in high doses (up to 10g a day) in conjunction with the other micro-nutrients recommended for osteoid formation.

Calcium RDAs

Current RDAs for calcium and magnesium are 800mg and 300mg respectively.

These are excessive. Based on the misconception that mineral supplements alone are an appropriate treatment, they may increase the risk of prostate and breast cancer[202-204].

When combined with appropriate micro-nutrient support for osteoid formation, I believe the daily requirement for calcium and magnesium could be cut dramatically.

These fats block progesterone synthesis, and compete with the vital, bone-building PUFAs in fish oil and plant oils, and interfere with their bone-building properties.

One answer is to switch to soy products, which are a good source of calcium in a highly digestible form. They also supply the essential PUFAs, are a good source of dietary fibre (see Chapter 6, Flavonoids & isoflavones), and have anti-cancer properties (see Chapter 13, Cancer).

TOP CALCIUM FOODS					
Yoghurt	415mg	8oz	Broad beans	128mg	1 cup
Milk	300mg	8oz glass	Broccoli	122mg	1 cup
Cheddar cheese	200mg	1oz	Almonds	80mg	1oz
Tinned salmon	200mg	3oz	Sardines	90mg	3oz
Tofu	260mg	1 cup			

- **MAGNESIUM** ✔

An adequate magnesium intake is just as important as getting enough calcium. It may even be more important, because magnesium is not just a major structural element in bone, it also regulates the active transport and metabolism of calcium. Magnesium depletion could be another contributing factor to the current osteoporosis epidemic.

In a recent two-year study, high-dose magnesium supplements given to post-menopausal women prevented fractures, and resulted in a significant increase in bone density. The optimal ratio of calcium to magnesium in the diet, or in supplements, is approximately 2 to 1. Very large doses of calcium may actually reduce magnesium absorption from the gut.

TOP MAGNESIUM FOODS

Beans	121mg	1 cup	Peanuts	52mg	1oz
Tofu	118mg	½ cup	Oatmeal	56mg	1 cup
Almonds/cashews	84mg	1oz	Yoghurt	40mg	8oz
Lentils	70mg	1 cup	Bread	23mg	1 slice
Potato	55mg	1 medium	(wholewheat)		

When you have insufficient levels of magnesium (and calcium) in your blood, your body pulls them from your bones, precipitating osteoporosis.

- **BORON AND MOLYBDENUM** ✔

These are also thought to be essential for bone formation. They are not built into the bone as calcium and magnesium are, but are needed in tiny amounts to help the enzymes which take part in bone growth.

For example, boron depletion results in excessive urinary calcium loss and abnormally low levels of the sex hormones – which are both risk factors for osteoporosis[30]. Conversely, boron supplements reduce calcium loss in the urine, and raise oestrogen and testosterone levels[98].

The bones of people who take boron supplements are reported to be harder than average. In other respects, too, boron appears to be essential for healthy bones. A boron deficiency may increase the risk of arthritis, and in areas where there is a high boron intake, due to geographical factors, the incidence of arthritis is much lower than average[100].

- **ALUMINIUM** ✘

Aluminium is also involved in bone building, but in an entirely negative way. This highly toxic metal is taken up into growing areas of bone[22], where it damages the bone building process[23]. One of the many appalling symptoms of aluminium poisoning, which occurred quite

LOOK FOR ...

an anti-osteoporosis supplement that includes at least 600mg of calcium, 300mg of magnesium, 8mg of manganese, 2mg of boron and 2mg of copper a day, together with Vitamins K, D and B6.

Add ipriflavone at 600-1200mg a day.

Magnesium and boron help build bones

You need magnesium to ensure calcium is absorbed; and Vitamin D and boron (probably) for the enzymes that encourage bone growth.

> ### Silicates
>
> Aluminium interferes with bone growth. Silicic acid binds with aluminium to neutralise this effect[194-199].
>
> Silicates in bone may also initiate the deposition of calcium salts and magnesium.

> ### Cut down on salt and sulphates
>
> A high intake of sodium leads to increased calcium loss.
>
> Switch to a salt substitute, eg PanSalt, which is based on potassium and magnesium, and which is also cardio-protective.
>
> If you take glucosamine sulphate for your joints, switch to glucosamine hydrochloride.

> ### New hormones
>
> Parathyroid hormone may become a medical treat[132] – but is not yet proven.

frequently in kidney patients during the early days of dialysis, was bone fragility and breakage[24, 25].

Our exposure to aluminium is increasing for a variety of reasons, and it could be that this is another contributory factor underlying the increase in osteoporotic fractures. For this reason, anyone keen on warding off osteoporosis should take silicic acid (see Chapter 17, A healthy brain). This natural compound binds to any aluminium in the gut and turns it into harmless sand.

A silicic acid supplement has been shown to reduce the absorption of aluminium by 85 per cent or more[26], and should be a part of any anti-osteoporosis regime.

- **SODIUM (AS IN TABLE SALT)** ✗

Excessive salt intake leads to increased calcium losses in the urine. There has been one report[28], that calcium loss can be reduced by large doses of potassium bicarbonate – but this is not yet proven.

- **MANGANESE** ✔

The trace element manganese is essential for the formation of osteoid (the precursor for bone) [140].

5 Other treatments

- **GROWTH HORMONE**

Growth hormone is known to increase bone growth, but is expensive, must be taken as an injection, is **not** risk free, and is generally unavailable without a prescription.

The amino acid arginine stimulates the formation and release of growth hormone in the body, with resulting tissue-building effects[118]. This should logically help to combat osteoporosis.

This is still only theory[113], but as arginine is cheap, non-toxic and widely available, it seems to be worth trying.

- **FLUORIDE**

Fluoride salts have been tried, with only mixed results[130,131].

- **VITAMIN D**

Vitamin D is essential for calcium uptake and distribution in the body. Dairy products are fortified with Vitamin D, but, although the RDA is 5mcg per day, many people eat only half of this or less. Vitamin D depletion is very prevalent[117, 135-138], particularly in the winter when the skin isn't exposed to much sunlight[141].

In conjunction with a calcium/magnesium supplement it may reduce the risk of other health problems[202-204], therefore Vitamin D may be helpful[116, 137]. Doses as high as 17.5mcg per day have been shown to reduce bone loss in post-menopausal women[96, 129, 142] but doses of D higher than 20mcg/day are not recommended without medical supervision.

D for bones

A 1997 study showed that men and women over 65 can cut the risk of bone fractures by 50% with a simple supplement of 18mcg of Vitamin D (700IU) plus 500mg of calcium.

A more comprehensive supplement would have given even better results.

TOP VITAMIN D FOODS

Sardines	25mcg	in 3oz	Milk	2.5 mcg	in 8oz
Cod liver oil	11mcg	in 1 tsp	Salmon	9mcg	in 3oz
Mackerel	23mcg	in 3oz	Egg	0.6mcg	each

Preventing osteoporosis

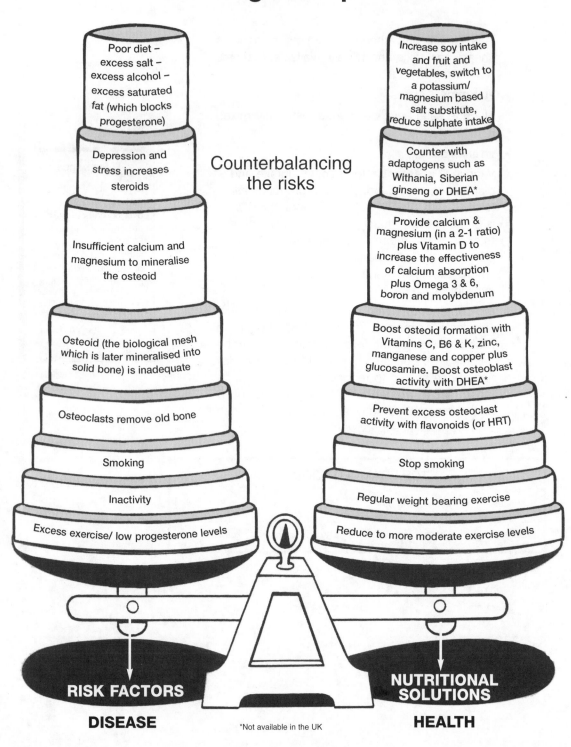

Counterbalancing the risks

Left side (RISK FACTORS / DISEASE):

Poor diet – excess salt – excess alcohol – excess saturated fat (which blocks progesterone)

Depression and stress increases steroids

Insufficient calcium and magnesium to mineralise the osteoid

Osteoid (the biological mesh which is later mineralised into solid bone) is inadequate

Osteoclasts remove old bone

Smoking

Inactivity

Excess exercise/ low progesterone levels

RISK FACTORS

DISEASE

Right side (NUTRITIONAL SOLUTIONS / HEALTH):

Increase soy intake and fruit and vegetables, switch to a potassium/magnesium based salt substitute, reduce sulphate intake

Counter with adaptogens such as Withania, Siberian ginseng or DHEA*

Provide calcium & magnesium (in a 2-1 ratio) plus Vitamin D to increase the effectiveness of calcium absorption plus Omega 3 & 6, boron and molybdenum

Boost osteoid formation with Vitamins C, B6 & K, zinc, manganese and copper plus glucosamine. Boost osteoblast activity with DHEA*

Prevent excess osteoclast activity with flavonoids (or HRT)

Stop smoking

Regular weight bearing exercise

Reduce to more moderate exercise levels

NUTRITIONAL SOLUTIONS

HEALTH

*Not available in the UK

SUMMARY

The Good Bones Guide

To prevent osteoporosis:

▶ Regular exercise, from childhood, builds stronger bones. Excessive exercise may weaken them.

▶ Smoking suppresses bone-building cells, so quit!

▶ Take 60mcg Vitamin K, together with 15-20mcg Vitamin D3, 7.5mg Vitamin B6, 500mg Vitamin C, 10mg zinc, 4mg manganese, 2mg copper and 500mg glucosamine. This will help build osteoid and encourage calcium absorption.

▶ Take up to 600mg calcium and 300mg magnesium.

▶ Add traces of boron and molybdenum, plus a silicic acid supplement to protect against aluminium.

▶ My specific anti-osteoporosis recommendation is on page 259.

▶ Switch to soy products rather than meats and dairy produce for calcium.

▶ Cut down on saturated fats. When these are metabolised in the body they reduce the ability to make progesterone.

▶ Cut down on salt and sulphates (ie glucosamine sulphate) which increase calcium excretion, as do cola drinks.

▶ If you already have other risk factors (such as a smoking habit), a shift to mono-unsaturates, such as olive oil, may be a wise decision.

Chapter 16

How you can avoid and treat diabetes

Juvenile diabetes

When you understand how complex and sophisticated breast milk is, even the best infant formulae look primitive – and potentially hazardous. There is growing evidence that infant formulae based on cow's milk may be an important risk factor for Type 1 diabetes, also known as juvenile or insulin-dependent diabetes[1].

One of the proteins in cow's milk, Bovine Serum Albumen (BSA), is found in most infant milk-based formulae[7]. Many insulin-dependent diabetics have raised levels of antibodies against BSA in their blood[1, 2].

When adults eat protein foods, the molecules are broken up in the gut and do not normally enter the blood and trigger antibodies. Infants are less well protected: they produce fewer digestive enzymes and their guts appear to let more protein molecules, like BSA, enter the bloodstream. Once there, they are recognised as foreign molecules and the immune system begins to produce antibodies against them.

By an unfortunate coincidence, part of the BSA molecule bears a strong resemblance to molecules on the membranes of the beta cells in the pancreas which produce insulin[1, 6]. This probably means that antibodies raised against BSA molecules can also attack the beta cells, leading to their eventual destruction, and therefore diabetes. (Beta casein, another protein found in cow's milk, has also been implicated[117].) Cow's milk has been found to trigger diabetes in animals too[3, 4].

In babies, cow's milk may trigger antibodies that attack insulin-producing cells. Wheat and soy are also under suspicion[115].

AUTO-IMMUNE DISEASE?

Scientists have long suspected that insulin-dependent diabetes might be an auto-immune disease – that is, one caused by the immune system attacking its owner. And the evidence is getting stronger.

A recent Finnish study showed that babies who were older than four months when first given formula milk had lower rates of diabetes than babies who received formula from an earlier age[5].

In children who were exclusively breast-fed, the risk of diabetes was the lowest of all[8].

Breast-feeding reduces risk of diabetes

Children who are exclusively breast-fed have the lowest rate of Type 1 diabetes.

Adult-onset diabetes

The majority of diabetics (over 50 million worldwide) develop the disease later in life, typically in middle age. This form of diabetes is called Type 2 diabetes, adult-onset or non-insulin-dependent diabetes, and the risk of developing this condition is increased by obesity, inactivity, high saturated fat intake, alcohol consumption, smoking and a poor anti-oxidant intake[98, 109, 110].

Insufficient insulin (Type 1) or insulin resistance (Type 2) both lead to excessive blood sugar levels (hyperglycaemia). The long-term complications of hyperglycaemia are potentially very serious[18]. Intensive treatment to normalise blood sugar (in Type 1 diabetes) slows the onset of these problems, but does not avoid them completely[19, 26, 27].

One of the ways in which hyperglycaemia contributes to all these diseases is because of the high oxidative load it imposes on the body[20, 21, 99, 100]. To make matters worse, copper and zinc levels are usually low in diabetics[22, 23, 103], probably because of increased urinary losses. This is damaging, because the important anti-oxidant and anti-ageing enzyme, Superoxide Dismutase (SOD), needs both copper and zinc to function properly.

The results of diabetes:

- **Increased free radical load**

- **Damaged anti-oxidant defences**

- **25 times the risk of blindness**

- **20 times the risk of kidney failure**

- **20 times the risk of gangrene**

- **Up to six times the risk of heart disease**

Oxidation and anti-oxidants

Hyperglycaemia also damages tissues directly. Excess glucose molecules bond directly to proteins, damaging them and impairing their normal function. The destructive combination of oxidation and glycosylation causes the accelerated ageing that occurs in diabetic arteries, kidneys, blood vessels and other tissues

Prime targets for free radicals in the body are the poly-unsaturated fatty acids (PUFAs) in cell membranes. The body finds it hard to replace PUFAs which have been oxidised. If the oxidised PUFAs are not replaced with fresh PUFAs, cell membranes begin to deteriorate and this impairs their normal functions.

In addition, when PUFAs are oxidised, they form lipid peroxides. In diabetics and pre-diabetics, levels of peroxides in the blood are abnormally high[17, 30, 39]. These peroxides cause serious damage to the lining of blood vessels[31, 32]. At the same time, high blood glucose levels block Vitamin C uptake into vessel walls, causing further local breakdown of the extra-cellular matrix and tissue damage[76, 77, 123, 131-133]. This explains why the course of diabetes can be modified by high-dose anti-oxidants and other supplements[128].

Lipid peroxidation in diabetics is reduced by high-dose Vitamin E[12, 81, 101, 108, 112]. In diabetes-prone rats, anti-oxidant therapy delays the onset and reduces the incidence of diabetes[24, 25]. Even more excitingly, some (perhaps most) of the complications of diabetes, such as the degeneration of the nervous system that causes loss of sensation and impotence in male diabetics, can be reversed with high-dose Vitamins E and C, and other anti-oxidants such as alpha lipoic acid[74, 116, 127, 128].

Glycosylation and anti-glycosylants

Moving from nerves to blood vessels, nutritionists have long known that anti-oxidant flavonoid preparations (such as pycnogenol) can strengthen the fragile capillaries which are characteristic of diabetes. The flavonoids can also stabilise diabetic retinopathy, the main cause of diabetic blindness by normalising blood vessl function[43, 44, 74] (see Chapter 6, Flavonoids & isoflavones).

Double Whammy

Diabetes hits us with a left and a right, because at the same time as it increases free radicals in the body, the illness also damages our anti-oxidant defences[22, 23, 29, 103, 125].

Anti-oxidants against diabetes

Anti-oxidant therapy appears to reduce and even reverse some side effects of diabetes.

Diabetes and ageing

When a molecule of glucose ('blood sugar') bonds to another molecule such as a protein, this is termed 'glycosylation'. As blood sugar levels increase, this increases the rate of glycosylation.

Excessive glycosylation of proteins is another cause of accelerated ageing in diabetes[29].

Glycosylation of crystallins (proteins in the eye) leads to cataract. Glycosylation of elastin and collagen in the blood vessels can cause hardening of the arteries and kidney damage.

Diabetic retinopathy, cataract and renal disease are caused by the glycosylation of proteins, whereby sugar molecules bind to proteins, disrupting their normal function. High-dose Vitamins E and C can reduce this somewhat[113, 114] – but there is a more appropriate nutritional response.

The flavonoids in red wine protect cholesterol and other lipids from oxidation and increase levels of 'good' HDL cholesterol[36].

But the salicylates and flavonoids in red wine also prevent glycosylation, as does curcumin, the flavonoid in turmeric[101, 130]. Flavonoids, are, therefore, strongly recommended for **all** diabetic patients.

Anti-glycosylants

1 Flavonoids in red wine, pine bark extract or turmeric.

2 Salicylates, including aspirin.

3 Low G.I. diet (see page 271)

ANTI-OXIDANTS AND PREVENTION

High-dose anti-oxidants such as Vitamin E reduce the rate of PUFA oxidation, and the levels of peroxides in diabetics[12, 81, 101, 108, 112] and protect against blood clots[71].

More surprising are studies which show that high doses of Vitamin E (900 mg/day) improve blood sugar control and reduce platelet stickiness and 'bad' LDL cholesterol levels in Type 2 diabetics[34, 35, 108], a combination which should be highly cardio-protective. Vitamin C appears to offer different, but equally significant, benefits[97, 111, 113].

Even more surprisingly, recent work suggests that E depletion may be a risk factor for developing diabetes[68, 98]. Low carotenoid status is another[69].

This implies that oxidative stress, and lipid peroxidation, may be causes of diabetes, as well as important exacerbating factors.

Red wine and grape juice

Red wine contains compounds which counter the effects of diabetes.

Excess alcohol is not recommended – so grapeseed extract may be preferred. Grape juice, although a good source of flavonoids, may contain too much sugar.

Fat factors

The dietary content of fats and oils is important, and can be manipulated to produce health benefits.

As well as having excessive levels of sugar in the blood (hyperglycaemia), diabetics also have abnormally high levels of triglycerides.

Post-prandial hypertriglyceridaemia (having very high levels of triglycerides – or fats – in the blood after a meal) is inevitably found in diabetics. This is also found in many of the (apparently) healthy relatives of diabetics, which has lead some scientists to conclude that this may be the forerunner of hyperglycaemia[40].

Vitamin E

In human diabetics 900mg Vitamin E a day significantly improved peripheral nerve function[128], while alpha lipoic acid (600-1200mg a day) improved blood sugar control[74].

As levels of triglycerides increase, they begin to interact with LDL and HDL cholesterol. Cholesterol enters the triglyceride particles, making them more likely to cause coronary artery disease; and the LDL/HDL ratio increases, which has a similar effect.

Diabetics have excessive levels of triglycerides because, although triglycerides are normally removed from the blood by an enzyme called LPL, LPL depends on normal levels of insulin, and the LPL enzyme is therefore generally defective in diabetics.

A diet rich in fat, and especially saturated animal fats, decreases the activity of LPL, leading to an increase in triglycerides, and an increase in the risk of coronary artery disease.

Regular exercise, on the other hand, makes LPL in the muscles more active, and so lowers triglycerides, and reduces the risk of heart disease.

Although this is an oversimplification, it helps to explain why our lack of exercise and undue fondness for junk foods high in saturated fats and low in anti-oxidants and micro-nutrients has led to insulin resistance and hypertriglyceridaemia in 25-30 per cent of middle-aged adults.

Regular exercise, plus lower calorie, predominantly vegetarian diet can often help reduce the severity of Type 2 diabetes – and may even bring it under complete control.

Family matters

One study of diabetics and their non-diabetic relatives may eventually change the way we think about coronary artery disease.

Among the non-diabetic relatives, there were two distinct types. One group, who were probably not prone to diabetes, had normal insulin, normal triglycerides, and normal LPL activity. The other group, who were likely to develop diabetes, had high insulin, high triglycerides (especially post-prandial triglycerides), and grossly sub-normal LPL activity. This pre-diabetic combination is termed ALP and is probably genetically determined[63, 64].

ALP types can benefit from losing weight and taking more exercise. Additionally, they should eat more oily fish, because the

---

Anti-oxidants & prevention

Diabetes during pregnancy increases the risk of birth defects. High-dose Vitamin E may give some protection against this[72].

ADD ...

Omega 3 fish oil or hemp or flaxseed oil and Vitamin E, and a glass of red wine!

PUFA supplements, together with anti-oxidant support (such as evening primrose oil and high-dose Vitamin E) restore nerve function in animal models of diabetes[33].

The right combination

PUFA supplements should always be combined with anti-oxidants[10, 124], particularly Vitamins E and C, and Co-enzyme Q10[24].

Weight loss and exercise are also essential elements in any self-help programme for Type 2 diabetes.

Omega 3 PUFAs in fish oil increase LPL activity, and bring the triglycerides down[9, 41, 42, 65-68]. They also lower insulin levels in healthy subjects and in Type 2 diabetics: and improve the HDL/ LDL ratio[9].

ALP types should definitely increase their intake of Vitamins E and C. Chromium supplements are also strongly recommended. Not only do they reduce triglyceride levels in Type 2 patients[45], they can also improve many ALP symptoms such as sugar craving[55, 62] and excess insulin levels[82].

Mineral deposits

A survey carried out in 1993 by the US Department of Agriculture showed that the average diet is very low in chromium. Chromium supplements may therefore be a good idea, especially for dieters, athletes, the elderly, the overweight and diabetics.

Some scientists believe that chromium depletion can lead to insulin resistance[105], the primary symptom of Type 2 diabetes. Chromium is probably part of the Glucose Tolerance Factor (GTF), which is needed for the normal metabolism of sugar and other carbohydrates[46, 47], although not everyone agrees[84-87, 89].

Chromium and/or GTF deficiency is thought to occur particularly after pregnancy[48, 49], and in the elderly[50], but chromium depletion is probably much more widespread[16, 37, 57, 59-62].

So what are the likely benefits of chromium supplements?

- There are reports that the glucose tolerance curve, which often deteriorates with old age, can be normalised by chromium-containing yeast supplements[51-54, 90, 107]. Even a slight improvement should confer considerable health benefits[107].

- Transient hypoglycaemia, a condition characterised by erratic glucose tolerance, mood swings, sugar craving and weight gain, and which may be a form of latent diabetes (see ALP above), may respond well to chromium supplements[55, 62].

Are you an ALP? Early warning signals for diabetes

- **Weight gain**

- **Cravings for sweet foods**

- **Spells of cold, tiredness and irritability**

- **Raised levels of insulin and serum triglycerides**

Preventative chromium

Hexavalent chromium compounds are toxic and should be avoided. Go for the organic trivalent chromium – about 120mcg a day.

TOP CHROMIUM FOODS

Apples, eggs, nuts, mushrooms, broccoli, tomatoes.

Have your oats

Diabetics and pre-diabetics should try eating oat-based foods. Beta glucans in oats reduce the absorption of sugar and fats from the gut, and as a result lower levels of blood glucose, LDL cholesterol and triglycerides.

They have extra benefits for blood sugar and lipid levels. Even a slight reduction in post-prandial glucose may have significant benefits[102].

Beta glucans are technically pre-biotics, like inulin or FOS (see Chapter 7, Pre-biotic fibre). These compounds will likely have similar benefits in diabetes.

... And exercise too

Weight loss and exercise are essential elements in any self-help programme for Type 2 diabetes.

Vanadium?

This trace element may have a therapeutic role[70] – not proven yet.

In healthy but possibly pre-diabetic subjects with raised insulin levels, there is evidence that chromium supplements can lead to a normalisation of insulin levels[82].

- Finally, in diabetic animals, chromium supplements reduce blood sugar, water consumption and weight loss[56, 58]. Human diabetics seem to respond equally well. Work carried out at London's King's College has shown that chromium supplements improve the condition of many Type 2 diabetics, and enable some diabetics to come off their medication altogether[38, 104, 123].

There may be other reasons to take chromium, as some studies find that long-term chromium supplementation increases levels of HDL (the 'good' cholesterol) in the blood[13, 14], and reduces levels of triglycerides[45], which would reduce the risk of heart attacks.

It must be said that not all trials have found such positive results[88]. Nevertheless, the trivalent chromium compounds have little toxicity, and worth trying if you suffer from adult-onset diabetes, hypoglycaemic episodes, sugar cravings and weight gain.

NB: Chromium-enriched yeast or chromium polynicotinate may be better than chromium picolinate, which has been linked with psychiatric problems[106].

Magnesium

Low magnesium levels in diabetes are associated with insulin resistance and an increased risk of late complications of the disease. Magnesium supplements have been used with good results in diabetic patients[75, 91, 92], and it has been suggested that they might help to minimise the late complications of diabetes[11, 93].

The evidence for this is not very extensive, but magnesium supplements do have an effect on improving plasma lipid levels[93], and reducing platelet stickiness[39] – which would help reduce circulatory and heart problems. Accordingly, a multi-mineral product combining magnesium (50mg) with chromium (120mg), together with zinc (10mg) and copper (2mg), which are also low in diabetics, should help to reduce the risk of late complications. Chitosan, a lipid-absorbing fibre, may also be helpful[118-122].

Herbs

Herbal medicine may also have much to offer the diabetic. How they work isn't known, but there is some clinical and traditional evidence for bitter aloes[94], bitter melon[95] and fenugreek[96] as potentially safe anti-diabetic agents. Further studies are in progress, and I hope to report on these in the next edition of this book.

Glycaemic Index (GI)

When carbohydrate foods are eaten they increase blood sugar levels. Refined carbohydrates cause large increases (they are high GI foods), while unrefined carbohydrates (whole grain products, pulses, legumes) cause smaller increases (they are low GI foods). Switching to a low GI diet improves many aspects of Type 2 diabetes, reduces the risk of developing the condition and is strongly recommended.

Anti-diabetic drugs

The alternative to an anti-diabetic nutritional programme is, of course, oral anti-diabetic drugs like sulphonylurea and tolbutamide. But, while the nutritional approach described here reduces the risk of heart disease, oral anti-diabetic drugs have been linked to an increased risk of fatal heart attacks[107].

Anti-diabetic diet

Reduce the amount of sweets, sugary drinks, white flour products and potatoes eaten, and increase the consumption of wholemeal foods, particularly oat-based foods, pulses and legumes.

This lowers the surges in blood sugar, lipids and insulin, which occur after meals and which are substantial risk factors for coronary artery disease[102].

The anti-diabetic diet should also include:

- Less meat and dairy products
- More Omega 3 and 6 fatty acids (oily fish and grains/nuts respectively)
- Up to three glasses of red wine or black grape juice every day – or grapeseed extract, or other source of flavonoids, such as turmeric

- Olive oil, which helps the circulation[80]
- Vitamins E and C (high-dose)
- More vegetables

For best results add Co-enzyme Q10 and an organic chromium supplement, which many people say they find helpful in reducing their cravings for sweet foods. Magnesium, copper and zinc should also be considered.

This diet should help to ensure a degree of weight loss, which is in itself a good thing. It should ideally be combined with an exercise programme of at least 20 minutes brisk walking, three times a week.

And please stop smoking!

Preventing diabetes

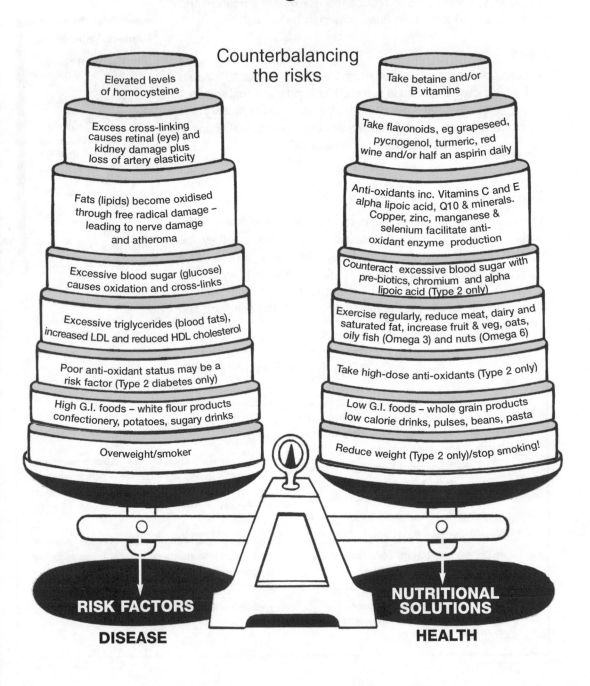

Counterbalancing the risks

RISK FACTORS

Risk (left side)	Nutritional solution (right side)
Elevated levels of homocysteine	Take betaine and/or B vitamins
Excess cross-linking causes retinal (eye) and kidney damage plus loss of artery elasticity	Take flavonoids, eg grapeseed, pycnogenol, turmeric, red wine and/or half an aspirin daily
Fats (lipids) become oxidised through free radical damage – leading to nerve damage and atheroma	Anti-oxidants inc. Vitamins C and E alpha lipoic acid, Q10 & minerals. Copper, zinc, manganese & selenium facilitate anti-oxidant enzyme production
Excessive blood sugar (glucose) causes oxidation and cross-links	Counteract excessive blood sugar with pre-biotics, chromium and alpha lipoic acid (Type 2 only)
Excessive triglycerides (blood fats), increased LDL and reduced HDL cholesterol	Exercise regularly, reduce meat, dairy and saturated fat, increase fruit & veg, oats, oily fish (Omega 3) and nuts (Omega 6)
Poor anti-oxidant status may be a risk factor (Type 2 diabetes only)	Take high-dose anti-oxidants (Type 2 only)
High G.I. foods – white flour products confectionery, potatoes, sugary drinks	Low G.I. foods – whole grain products low calorie drinks, pulses, beans, pasta
Overweight/smoker	Reduce weight (Type 2 only)/stop smoking!

RISK FACTORS

DISEASE

NUTRITIONAL SOLUTIONS

HEALTH

SUMMARY

Avoiding and treating diabetes

▶ Anti-oxidants:

Vitamins E and C, Q10, alpha lipoic acid, copper, zinc, selenium and manganese

▶ Anti-glycosylants:

Grapeseed extract, half an aspirin, a tablespoon of turmeric or 2-3 glasses of red wine a day. Choose the deepest red in colour with good tannic structure (see The Wine List on page 234).

▶ Minerals:

Magnesium, chromium, copper and zinc supplements.

▶ PUFAs:

Omega 3 and 6 PUFAs, but only when combined with anti-oxidants.

▶ Avoid fats, particularly saturated, which raise triglycerides – whereas exercise reduces them.

▶ Switch to low G.I. foods, ie oat-based products, whole grain foods, pulses, legumes, pasta.

▶ If you can, breast-feed your babies to give them the best chance of avoiding juvenile diabetes.

Chapter 17

Building and maintaining a healthy brain

Good nutrition builds better brains. And nutritional depletion threatens those brains in later life. This chapter looks at both aspects – but we'll start with the older brain.

Alzheimer's

Use it or lose it

This chapter outlines a nutritional approach to defending yourself against brain degeneration.

Equally importantly, brain scientists have found that keeping mentally active – through work, hobbies and even activities like crossword puzzles – is a key element in retaining mental acuity.

As long as we keep making new **connections** between brain cells we can maintain our alertness – provided there is no underlying physical deterioration. That is where nutrition comes in.

Alzheimer's is one of our most feared diseases – and in an ageing society, it is becoming ever more prevalent. It affects two in every 100 people over the age of 65. In those of us who reach our eighth decade, it will hit an alarming one in five.

The victim is, in a way, the least affected. Consciousness of the growing darkness soon fades as self-awareness recedes, but the gradual loss of faculties and the slow disintegration of the personality impose terrible burdens on the carers (typically daughters or younger sisters), and generate huge social and economic costs.

The disease is even more tragic when it occurs in otherwise healthy individuals, robbing them of their retirement, grandchildren, wisdom and memories.

Until very recently there has been no light in this darkness; no therapeutic strategem or device that could stop or slow the descent into unreason. But that is changing.

New evidence shows that the condition, though age-related, is not caused by the ageing process per se[65].

Nutritional and preventative approaches may be able to halt the disease process – and even put it into reverse, if the illness is diagnosed and treated early enough.

Aluminium – one of the usual suspects

It's been known for over 100 years that aluminium is extremely neurotoxic. In the early days of renal dialysis, kidney patients died of brain damage caused by aluminium in the dialysing water getting into the brain.

In 1991, an MRC research group in Newcastle, England, found aluminium in the 'plaques' and 'tangles' in the brain that characterise Alzheimer's disease. And in 1994, a study of patients exposed to aluminium during renal dialysis found Alzheimer-like changes in their brains[35].

In 1992, Professor McLachlan's group in Toronto, Canada published the first account of a treatment which stabilised Alzheimer's, and slowed the otherwise rapid and irreversible decline into dementia and death. This treatment involves removing aluminium from the bodies and brains of their patients. It's a difficult and expensive chemical leaching process, unsuitable for extensive clinical use.

The aluminium-silicon link

In nature, aluminium and silicon nearly always occur together, welded into some of the most stable, insoluble and long-lived compounds known. Clays, quartz, sand, mica and sandstone are major components of the Earth's crust. And on a building site, you'll find aluminium silicate in cement, concrete, bricks and glass. These are all safe, neutral and, importantly, **in**soluble compounds.

But although aluminium's public image is efficient, clean, cheap, safe – think of baking foil, cooking pans and double glazing - aluminium is *not* intrinsically safe.

Soluble forms of aluminium are highly toxic. They chew up cell membranes, degrade DNA, poison most of the enzymes

Aluminium and acid rain

Acid rain kills fish in rivers and lakes. Adding lime to neutralise the acidity doesn't help – because it is the aluminium washed out of the soil by the acid rain that kills the fish[116, 117].

Silicic acid poured onto the water binds to the aluminium to form sand – and prevents any further loss of life[118, 119].

Where does your water come from?

Surface water (ie from rivers) tends to have more aluminium than silicon.

Deep water (ie from wells) tends to have more silicon.

Intake of aluminium and silicon in foods also contributes to your overall silicon/aluminium ratio. If this is too low, consider a silicic acid supplement.

essential to cellular function; and destroy the proteins which give the cell structure and organisation.

Aluminium – the 'lead' of the 21st century

Some eminent scientists believe that chronic accumulation of aluminium in the brain may contribute to, or accelerate, damage in the brain such as is found in Alzheimer's[120-122].

Early studies suggested that areas where the water had the highest content of soluble aluminium had the highest incidence of Alzheimer's Disease[123, 125]. Further investigation indicated that it was in areas where water was high in aluminium and low in silicon that the incidence of Alzheimer's was high. In areas where the water was silicon-rich, and aluminium-poor, Alzheimer's was relatively uncommon[124].

The evidence linking aluminium to Alzheimer's has been disputed, and it is fair to say that even if aluminium is a contributory factor, it is clearly not the only one.

But what is indisputable is that aluminium in the body causes cell damage, dysfunction and death. Aluminium in the brain causes brain damage. Furthermore, aluminium in the brain is concentrated in the senile 'plaques' and 'tangles' that are characteristic signs of Alzheimer's[126, 127].

Where does it come from?

Drinking water is one source of aluminium. In many areas it's added to drinking water as a clearing agent. But there are other sources. Aluminium is widely used by the food processing industry, in medicine and in cosmetics.

Although industrialists knew how potentially dangerous aluminium compounds were, they felt it was safe to use them in our food and water because they believed our defences against aluminium were good enough. They thought that aluminium compounds could not be absorbed from the gut. Unfortunately, we now know that some aluminium compounds are absorbed.

Our defences are fine at dealing with the aluminium compounds which occur in nature, but they can't cope with some of the new aluminium compounds which industry is now producing.

Some of these are highly soluble, such as aluminium maltolate, an additive used in America by the food processing industry. So are the aluminium salts of various fatty acids, which are used in the EC. (The E number for this latter group is E470b.)

Then there is aluminium hydroxide, an ingredient used in many antacids. It's insoluble, but unfortunately the passage of aluminium through tissue barriers, such as the gut wall, is dramatically increased by the presence of other compounds such as citrates or sugars. And these are present in many foods and drinks[130].

Citrates are also used by the pharmaceutical industry to produce dispersible and effervescent medications, such as aspirin or paracetamol.

The combination of aluminium-containing antacids and citrate-containing medicines produces levels of aluminium in the blood which if sustained, lead to brain damage, dementia and death[131, 132].

The British Royal Society of Medicine responded in 1993 by recommending that aluminium-containing antacids should not be taken by pregnant women, who have a tendency to suffer from heartburn[134]. (They may have been influenced by unpublished work which found aluminium in the brains of aborted human foetuses.)

The silicon solution

At this point, you may be beginning to wonder what can be done to reduce exposure to this hidden hazard. There are several possible strategies. You could filter all your water, wash your food in filtered water, check the E numbers on all processed foods, throw out your aluminium cookware, stop using pharmaceutical products and cosmetics.

Alternatively, you could increase your zinc intake, together with Vitamin B6 which improves zinc absorption.

Some of the signs of aluminium toxicity are very similar to signs of zinc depletion. This isn't surprising because aluminium competes for zinc in the body (as well as iron, magnesium,

---

Daily aluminium intake

Our daily intake of aluminium is estimated to be between 10 and 30mg. It is ingested in so many forms that contact with the metal is unavoidable.

Increased aluminium intake

In 1993, Professor James Edwardson's group published the results of a series of crucial experiments[133].

Radioactively labelled aluminium was given to five healthy volunteers, in orange juice which contained citrates and sugars. Edwardson measured the amount of aluminium that was absorbed into their blood.

Then he gave the volunteers the same drink, but with added silicic acid. This time the amount of aluminium absorbed into the bloodstream was reduced by a massive 85 per cent.

He concluded: "A long-term increase in the dietary intake of silicic acid could prove to be of therapeutic value by reducing the gastro-intestinal absorption of aluminium in those at risk".

The positive effects of silicon

Animals fed a silicon rich diet have lower levels of aluminium in their brains[137].

High levels of brain aluminium correlate with mental impairment.

The conclusion seems to be that a silicon rich diet should be one of the protective strategies against aluminium intoxication and mental deterioration.

You find silicon in oats, cereals and hops.

INCLUDE ...

More oats and cereals in your diet.

If you are especially concerned use a silicic acid supplement. Tablets are relatively ineffective; colloidal silicic acid is preferable.

Also ensure your diet is rich in Vitamin B6 and zinc.

---

manganese and other metal ions), and blocks its physiological actions[135, 142]. But even this would not offer complete protection.

Another answer is to take supplements of the essential trace element silicon in the form of silicic acid. The silicic acid binds with the dietary aluminum to produce aluminium silicate (sand!), which passes harmlessly through the body[133].

The richest food sources of silicon are the cereals, with oats in particular containing very high amounts[136]. We eat less cereals, especially oats, than ever before. Could this be contributing to the current increase in neurodegenerative disorders such as Alzheimer's or Parkinsonism?

ESSENTIAL TRACE ELEMENTS

Trace elements like silicon have been largely ignored by medicine, due to the common belief that trace element depletion is rare. Evidence to the contrary was never taken seriously, because it comes from the humble vet.

Veterinarians have known for years that trace element depletion is extremely common in domestic and farm animals, and that mineral supplementation can often result in improved health.

Humans are unlikely to be exempt and recent trends in food processing and eating habits increase the probability of trace element depletion.

	Average Intake	Optimum Intake
Fe (iron)	13.2mg	15mg*
Mg (manganese)	4.6mg	10mg
Zn (zinc)	11.1mg	20mg
Cu (copper)	1.5mg	3.5mg
Se (selenium)	35mcg	100-200mcg
Cr (chromium)	30mcg	100-150mcg
Si (silicon)	10-100mg	100-1000mg

*In women of child-bearing age. Men and post-menopausal women require rather less.

One disease – many causes

All of the above research suggests that aluminium may be a contributory factor to Alzheimer's; but it is not the only one. In fact, there seem to be several different ways of getting Alzheimer's.

Genetic susceptibility has been demonstrated in a small proportion (about 5 per cent) of cases. Head injury, depressive illness and late first pregnancy are also associated with a higher risk of the disease.

However, none of these factors – and certainly not the genetic factor[66] – are enough to explain the 15 or more millions of people worldwide who have been diagnosed as having Alzheimer's disease. When a (non-infectious) disease occurs on this enormous scale, it is often more fruitful to look for an environmental and/or nutritional cause.

There is evidence that some degenerative brain diseases of old age, such as Alzheimer's and Parkinson's disease, which are both on the increase, may be caused by long-term exposure to low levels of environmental toxins. Aluminium compounds could conceivably fit the bill, but there are other potential neurotoxins such as organic solvents and agrochemicals.

Even more persuasive is the evidence that depletion of micro-nutrients – vitamins, minerals and trace elements – leading to excessive free radical damage, is the most important cause of most cases of Alzheimer's.

> ### Different causes – common mechanism?
>
> Head injury, depressive illness and late first pregnancy may seem unrelated, but all are thought to cause brain cell damage; and anything that causes brain cell loss brings dementia closer.

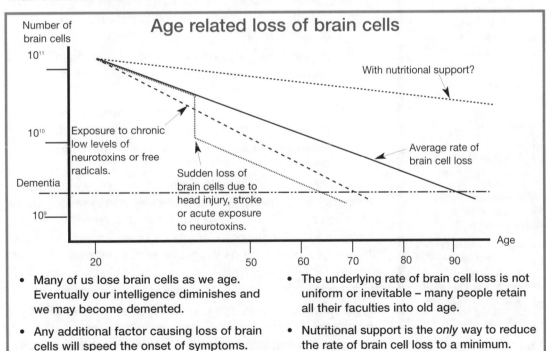

Age related loss of brain cells

- Many of us lose brain cells as we age. Eventually our intelligence diminishes and we may become demented.

- Any additional factor causing loss of brain cells will speed the onset of symptoms.

- The underlying rate of brain cell loss is not uniform or inevitable – many people retain all their faculties into old age.

- Nutritional support is the *only* way to reduce the rate of brain cell loss to a minimum.

A free radical disease

Most medical scientists accept that oxidative stress, an excess of free radicals, is a prime cause of coronary artery disease; and they are happy to recommend anti-oxidants to reduce the risk of heart attacks. But they have not yet made the glaringly obvious connection to diseases of the ageing central nervous system, including Alzheimer's. Even more than the heart, the brain and related tissues are a prime target for oxidative damage because ...

1 Brain nerve cell membranes contain high levels of poly-unsaturated fatty acids (PUFAs), which are extremely vulnerable to free radical attack.

2 There is a lot of oxygen used in the brain. (The brain receives 25% of the cardiac output even though it is only 3% of the body's weight.) The more oxygen, the more likely that oxidation may take place.

3 The brain's anti-oxidant defences are poor. Levels of glutathione, catalase, Vitamin E, etc. are low[101, 109-112]. Levels of iron (a potential pro-oxidant) are high.

4 At least one compound found in the brain (dopamine) forms breakdown products which create free radicals[108].

5 The elderly's eating habits leave them progressively more at risk of being depleted in micro-nutrients and especially the anti-oxidants.

It's hardly surprising therefore that the incidence of the neuro-degenerative diseases is high in the elderly, and increasing as the population ages. Older brains have suffered more cell loss due to chronic oxidative damage; and this could be enough to explain why we lose brain cells as we get older. It's probably little more than cumulative oxidative damage leading to progressive nerve cell loss.

This may show up as age-related cognitive decline (ARCD), a gradual loss of mental processing power which occurs commonly with age; or its end stage, which is Alzheimer's disease. Oxidative

---

Brain protection

Lipids account for 60% of the brain's dry weight, and the bulk of these are poly-unsaturates.

Poly-unsaturated fats are very vulnerable to free radical attack.

Any brain fitness programme must therefore include anti-oxidants.

More anti-oxidant data

Free radical damage is strongly implicated in loss of memory and cognitive function during ageing.

Anti-oxidant supplements (Vitamins C and E) given to elderly rats improved some cognitive parameters[83].

Anti-oxidant intake is important in reducing the risk of age-related cognitive decline in elderly humans[78-80, 105, 106, 113]; and in Alzheimer's patients[81, 82, 114].

In a very recent study it was found that elderly subjects who took Vitamins C and E were largely protected from developing Alzheimer's[104].

neurone loss may, if exacerbated by specific metabolic, genetic or other environmental factors, manifest itself as Parkinsonism, Huntingdon's disease or Amyotrophic Lateral Sclerosis.

These diseases have much in common. They are all characterised by slowly progressive brain cell death. Their onset is often subtle, beginning in mid-life and slowly becoming symptomatic in later life. And there is a great deal of evidence that oxidative damage, leading to brain cell suicide, is involved in all these conditions[37, 106-108].

Anti-oxidant supplements should therefore have a role to play in reducing the risk of neuro-degenerative illness, as they do in heart disease[85, 113]..

The choice of anti-oxidant is determined by the types of molecules we wish to protect. In the brain, the main targets of free radical attack are the Poly-unsaturated Fatty Acids (PUFAs) in the brain cell membranes. And here the pioneering work of Dr Stanley Deans at the SARC Institute in Auchinruive, Scotland, shows the way forward.

Dr Deans found that as lab animals age, levels of PUFAs in their brains gradually fall[96]. The numbers of viable brain cells and the animals' 'brain power', ie their ability to learn and run through a maze, fell away more or less in parallel[29].

But was the decline in PUFAs the cause of the loss of brain cells, or was it merely a consequence?

In Dr Dean's next study, the animals were given anti-oxidants in the form of thyme oil which entered the brain, and stopped the oxidation of lipids. As these animals aged, there was no reduction in brain PUFA levels; no loss of viable brain cells; and no age-related fall-off in memory[29-32].

The implication is clear. Oxidative damage to brain cells causes cumulative brain cell loss, and is likely to be a prime cause of the age-related loss of brain cells which manifests itself as age-related cognitive decline, and other conditions such as Alzheimer's disease.

The logical route to reducing the risk of these conditions is, therefore, via appropriate anti-oxidant supplementation.

LOOK FOR ...

a supplement that includes anti-oxidants like Vitamins C and E, flavonoids such as the soy isoflavones, and thyme oil.

Alpha lipoic acid is an interesting alternative. And as glutathione peroxidase is important in protecting lipids from oxidation, its co-factor selenium should also be included; together with riboflavin, the co-factor for glutathione reductase.

Spice of life

PUFA levels in elderly brains are almost equally well preserved with clove, nutmeg and pepper oil[29-32, 207-211].

Add these to your diet!

More anti-oxidant evidence

More anti-oxidant evidence

Beta amyloid, which is found in other brain disorders[33-35] is not the only source of the destructive free radicals which contribute to Alzheimer's disease.

Aluminium (in the form of aluminium silicate) found in the tangles in Alzheimer's brain tissue, is another generator of free radicals[46].

This is another very good reason to take a comprehensive anti-oxidant supplement.

Anti-oxidants block a part (perhaps the most significant part) of the whole disease process.

Some laboratories have concentrated on the problem of plaque, a characteristic micro-lesion found in the brains of subjects with ARCD and Alzheimer's.

The main component of plaque is a peptide called beta amyloid. There are good reasons to think that this peptide may be involved in causing Alzheimer's.

In Down's Syndrome, for example, an excess of amyloid is produced and the incidence of early onset Alzheimer's is very high[24]. More recently, beta amyloid has been shown to be toxic to nerve cells[25, 26]. Interestingly enough, it kills them by producing free radicals, which oxidise PUFAs in the nerve cell membranes and more or less tears them apart[27, 28, 43, 68-72].

The neurotoxic effects of beta amyloid can be blocked by anti-oxidants such as Vitamin E[26]. So if beta amyloid is a cause of Alzheimer's, then, once again, lipid-soluble anti-oxidants such as Vitamin E, thyme oil or the herb rosemary should be useful in slowing the progression of the disease.

In support of the anti-oxidant hypothesis, a recent study showed that high-dose Vitamin E (2,000IU/day) slowed the progress of Alzheimer's very significantly[81]. But Vitamin E is not the optimal anti-oxidant to treat brain hyper-oxidation, as it takes months to enter the brain at high levels[84-87].

It would be more logical to examine the potentially therapeutic role of thyme oil[29, 32] and other natural anti-oxidants which enter the brain more rapidly such as the soy isoflavones: labs in the UK and elsewhere are already doing this.

Additions to anti-oxidants

The basic anti-oxidant strategy attempts to protect the PUFAs that are such important components in brain cell membranes. But there are other, complementary strategies.

The cell membrane is a dynamic entity; PUFAs are constantly being lost, via oxidation and other routes, and being replaced by new PUFAs derived ultimately from the diet. Combining the appropriate anti-oxidants with appropriate PUFA supplements should therefore reduce the deficit, enhance the replacement rate, and give supra-additive effects.

There is one proviso. For optimal replacement, it is very unlikely that the usual PUFA supplements will be sufficient. Free PUFAs hardly exist in the brain; they are largely incorporated into molecules called phospholipids. Phospholipids are simply fatty acids (lipids) combined with phosphates and other groups. It is these phospholipids which form the basis of all cell membranes, and which are the main target of free radical attack in the brain.

Phospholipids – a key to brain function

Phospholipids, because of their molecular structure, are surfactants; a category of compounds which includes soaps and detergents. If you add soap to water, and mix it, bubbles form; and if you add phospholipids to water, they naturally form into membranes which in turn become micro-bubbles. These are the prototype cell membranes.

Like all tissues, the cell membranes are dynamic; they are constantly being damaged and repaired. Phospholipids in the

> **Membrane ageing**
>
> I don't underestimate the importance of nuclear and mito-chondrial ageing.
>
> However, I think that phospholipid-related ageing of the membranes is also very likely to be a major contributor to the overall rundown in cellular and organ function that constitutes the ageing process (see Chapter 20).

membranes are broken down to form neurotransmitters and other messenger substances that transfer information between brain cells. In addition they may simply be oxidised.

If these phospholipids are not replaced, membranes deteriorate and the cell becomes progressively more dysfunctional and eventually dies. So, the rate of phospholipid replacement is critical in keeping the brain cells and brain functioning.

We obtain phospholipids from our diet, and we can synthesise them in the liver. But there are problems. Our dietary intake of phospholipids is at an historic low, thanks to trends in food processing[90], and specifically to our increased use of refined oils. Levels of phospholipids may reach 3 per cent in virgin oils, but in refined oils they are virtually undetectable.

Production of phospholipids in the liver may be sub-optimal too because it is complex, slow and energy intensive. It is slowed even further by multiple micro-nutrient depletion, which surveys show is extremely common in the elderly. Anti-oxidant depletion simultaneously increases the rate of phospholipid oxidation. This combination of reduced production and accelerated breakdown leaves the elderly doubly vulnerable to phospholipid depletion.

This is why levels of phospholipids in cell membranes, such as in brain cell membranes, decline with age. This is a major component in the ageing process in many tissues[30-32, 91, 96, 102], where increased oxidation of phospholipids, and the resulting accumulation of the oxidation end-product, lipofucsin[30-32, 97, 102], leads to a progressive loss of membrane and other cellular functions.

The fact that the elderly are doubly at risk of phospholipid depletion – their poor micro-nutritional state leading to reduced rates of phospholipid production **and** increased rates of phospholipid oxidation – means they are logical candidates for anti-oxidants **plus** phospholipid supplements. But which phospholipid?

An important new brain supplement

Here is where it pays to know a little biochemistry.

A phospholipid typically consists of two fatty acids, linked to a 3-carbon 'collar', which is linked to a phosphate group and one other group. This last group may be choline, making phosphatidyl choline (PC); or serine, making phosphatidyl serine (PS).

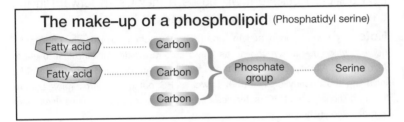

The make–up of a phospholipid (Phosphatidyl serine)

Fatty acid .... Carbon
Fatty acid .... Carbon   Phosphate group .... Serine
Carbon

Although phosphatidyl serine is much scarcer than phosphatidyl choline, it is particularly important in keeping the brain cells' membranes healthy. Because of its surface charge, PS has the unique ability to bind to protein molecules such as the ion pumps. (These pumps, which sit in the cell membranes, are essential for keeping the cells alive, and for maintaining their electrical functions, which are especially important in nerve cells.)

If PS is in short supply, the binding action weakens. The ion pumps slow down, and then drop out of the cell membranes altogether[88]. The nerves become dysfunctional, swell up and burst. But if levels of PS can be restored to normal or near-normal values, nerve cell death may be averted and function restored.

PS supplements have been used on their own to improve membrane, and particularly nerve cell membrane function. In elderly animals, many of the symptoms of an ageing brain (including failing circadian and estral rhythms, memory loss, and the loss of nerve cell connections in the brain), can be prevented or reversed with PS[88, 98, 99] – but **not** with other phospholipids.

Does this apply to humans? There are 42 clinical studies of PS used to treat Alzheimer's, and its pre-clinical precursor Age-Related Cognitive Decline (ARCD). These trials, although most are small and/or poorly designed, show improved learning and memorising of information; enhanced recall of frequently misplaced objects; better recall of telephone numbers; recognition of names and faces; and maintenance of concentration while reading, conversing and performing various tasks[93, 94, 95, 100].

Sadly, the fundamental flaw in all these trials is that phosphatidyl serine was used alone; and as we can now see, it should ideally have been combined with anti-oxidants. This combination is shortly to be tested, and will be reported on in the next edition. I believe it will be be a major step forward in the prevention and treatment of Alzheimer's.

Note: The role of phosphatidyl serine (PS) may help to explain why cholinergic nerves, which use acetyl choline as their neurotransmitter, are the first to die in Alzheimer's. All the nerve cells in the elderly brain are depleted of phospholipids, including phosphatidyl choline (PC) as well as PS; but in cholinergic nerves, there is an additional loss of PC molecules from the membranes as the cell uses them to make acetyl choline.

When levels of phosphatidyl choline in the membrane are critically low, the cell attempts to replenish them from wherever it can; and if there is insufficient PC in the diet, or being made in the liver, the nerve steals from its much smaller store of PS molecules. If levels of PS are already low, this additional drain may be enough to dislodge the ion pumps; leaving the cholinergic nerve exposed to a uniquely lethal combination of oxidative, osmotic and electrical stresses.

Some cholinergic nerve cells also contain high levels of iron. When these cells die the iron is released and causes more free radical damage. This also may contribute to the fact that cholinergenic nerves are more likely to be lost in Alzheimer's.

Low B vitamins and nerve cell damage

Depletion of the B vitamins folic acid, B6 and B12 has been linked to nerve cell damage via excessive homocysteine levels.

Homocysteine is a pro-oxidant.

B depletion is common in the elderly, and a B supplement should therefore be combined with the anti-oxidant/PS regime for additional protection[195].

In recent studies, Vitamins B6, B12 and folic acid supplements improved some aspects of intelligence in the elderly[167, 205].

Alternatively, a betaine supplement is recommended.

When should prevention begin?

It is not universally agreed that age-related cognitive decline (ARCD) is the pre-clinical form of Alzheimer's, but it seems increasingly likely that it is. The behavioural changes, neurochemical changes, and even the histological signs of Alzheimer's (the plaques and tangles thought to be the hallmark of the disease), are all found to a lesser extent in ARCD. And, although some doctors still maintain that ARCD is a middle-aged condition, Professor Tom Crook at NIMH Bethesda has shown that if sufficiently sensitive instruments are used, the first signs of mental decline appear in the 40s and become progressively worse with each subsequent decade; a decline which starts well before the routine tests notice anything wrong[94].

Nutritionally, prophylaxis should therefore ideally begin in the 40s, but should still help even if started later in life.

Other strategies for reducing risk

Nerve cells may be killed off by causes other than oxidative stress. Accordingly, other nutritional factors may have something to offer. Cell suicide in the brain may, for example, be triggered by hormonal changes which occur with age.

Normally, nerve cells are sustained by a range of nerve growth factors. If the growth factors dry up, the nerve cells switch on their suicide programme. This could be why women who take HRT have a lower risk of developing Alzheimer's[75, 76]. It's reckoned that the oestrogen in HRT may function as a nerve growth factor[77] and, like a cellular Samaritan, encourage the neurone not to switch on its suicide (apoptotic) programme.

If true, a high intake of soy products (which contain oestrogen-like compounds) should also be protective. Resveratrol in red wine is another potential protector.

Another factor which can trigger apoptotic cell death is a sustained reduction in the oxygen supply. The sudden and complete lack of oxygen caused by a stroke or strangulation leads to uncontrolled cell death (necrosis). But a long-drawn-out reduction in the oxygen supply to the cell, which is what happens when the cerebral arteries gradually fur up, is known to switch on the apoptosis sequence.

This means that bad circulation is another possible cause of Alzheimer's, which is probably why hypertension increases the risk of the disease[67].

In this case, and particularly if there is evidence of arterial disease in other organs such as the heart or legs, a crash course of anti-atheroma nutrition is in order. At the very least this approach will reduce the likelihood of cerebral infarcts, or mini-strokes, which can add to and exacerbate the underlying Alzheimer's; and reduce the loss of brain tissue if a stroke does occur[103].

Stroke

Only one third of dementia is due to Alzheimer's, another third is damage from multiple strokes, and the rest are mixed. Anti-stroke nutrition will, therefore, greatly reduce the risk of dementia, as well as the damage caused by the stroke itself.

Oestrogen anti-oxidant

Oestrogen may be a nerve growth factor; but it is also certainly an anti-oxidant, and a lipid-soluble one at that[77].

This is just what is needed to protect brain cell membranes – so oestrogen may be acting primarily as a membrane protector.

The isoflavones in soy, which not only mimic oestrogen but also act as strong anti-oxidants, and are known to enter the brain quite rapidly, are almost certainly protective.

Stroke prevention

Stroke is a loss of blood supply to an area of the brain, caused either by an artery rupturing (generally due to high blood pressure), or becoming blocked from atheroma or blood clots.

Blood pressure is lowered by cutting down on salt intake or by changing to a low sodium or sodium-free salt substitute (see page 319). Atheroma and platelet stickiness are reduced by flavonoids [91,115], which thus decreases stroke risk[212].

The high speed anti-atheroma programme

This would include the Vitamins C and E, Q10 and lycopene. It could also initially contain the amino acids lysine and proline, switching to grapeseed, bilberry or hawthorn flavonoids after about a week, plus a good fish oil.

It should also contain ginkgo, which has been shown to increase the resistance of nerve cells to hypoxia[12, 13], and reduce oxidative damage to the nerve cells[17].

The Tau theory in a nutshell

If axonal flow is blocked, the brain cell dies. This could be another route to Alzheimer's, so preventing such blockage is vital.

Blockages are caused when proteins called Tau proteins stick together in the tubelets that carry the axonal flow.

Manganese appears to return the Tau protein to normal and thus may help to restore or maintain axonal flow and hence brain cell function[7-10].

Go with the (axonal) flow

A relatively new idea is that Alzheimer's may be triggered in certain cases by depletion of the trace element manganese. This concept was introduced by Dr Iqbal at the New Institute for Basic Research in Developmental Difficulties, New York, and hinges on the concept of 'axonal flow'.

The next page shows how axonal flow in the brain works. Essentially, the constant activity involved in the transmission of information between brain cells creates wear and tear at the dendrites – the end of the cell containing the synapses where information is transferred from one brain cell to another.

To repair this damage involves transporting 'broken parts' from the dendrites along an axon to the nucleus. Then 'replacement parts' are sent from the nucleus back out to the dendrites. If this transport loop is blocked the brain cell dies. Preventing such disruption may be another way to defend against Alzheimer's.

You can see that the internal transport system ('the axonal flow conveyor belt') for each brain cell is built of Tau proteins.

In a healthy cell, the Tau proteins remain separate. Dr Iqbal's work suggests that, under certain circumstances, Tau proteins stick together, and build up into the helical filaments found in the brain 'tangles', in a runaway reaction. But what makes those first few Tau proteins stick together?

Some studies have shown that in Alzheimer's, Tau proteins in the filaments have too many phosphate groups attached to them[1-4, 21] – known as hyper-phosphorylated Tau, or Hyper-T.

Dr Iqbal's group believe that Hyper-T is what makes the Tau proteins stick together. They found that Hyper-T disrupts axonal flow[5]. They also showed that in Alzheimer's disease, the nerves die back in a pattern of retrograde degeneration[6], which is exactly what happens when axonal flow is blocked.

So if the phosphorylation of Tau proteins could be reduced, this might restore axonal flow and help to slow the course of Alzheimer's disease.

Dr Iqbal's lab has discovered two groups of enzymes: the Tau kinases, which attach phosphate groups onto Tau protein, and the Tau phosphatases, which strip them off again.

AXONAL FLOW

A blockage in 'axonal flow' leads to brain cell death and may be involved in Alzheimer's disease. Restoring axonal flow could help stop brain nerve cells from dying back.

1 The structure of a brain cell

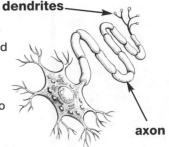

dendrites

axon

A brain nerve cell typically consists of a rounded cell body or nucleus, and a long trunk reaching out from the nucleus called an axon. The axon ends in a spray of nerve endings called dendrites. These dendrites are highly active sites because at the end of each dendrite is a synapse. Neurotransmitters are the chemicals that allow the electrical impulses of thoughts to 'jump' across the synapse. There appears to be a substantial degree of tissue wear and tear at these dendrites.

2 Axonal flow

The workshop where replacement parts for dendrites are made is back in the cell nucleus. To get the broken-down parts from the dendrite nerve endings back to the nucleus, and to send replacements back out again to the dendrites, involves 'axonal flow'.

This is a sort of conveyor belt which runs the length of the axon. One lane ferries new components from the nucleus to the nerve endings, and the return loop brings debris back from the nerve endings to the nucleus, where they can be recycled.

axonal flow

3 Retrograde degeneration

If the flow of materials along the conveyor belt is blocked the nerve endings die first, and then the axon starts to die back in a slow process of decay, called retrograde degeneration, which eventually reaches back to the cell body. Up until this moment the decay is reversible, but once the degeneration reaches the cell body the nerve cell is irretrievably dead.

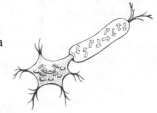

4 Cross section of axon conveyor belt

The axon's conveyor belt is built out of micro-tubelets, which in turn are made from smaller components, including one called Tau protein.

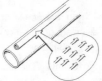

5 Plaques and tangles

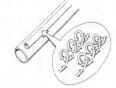

There are two characteristic lesions in the brains of Alzheimer victims, plaques and tangles. The tangles consist of Tau proteins stuck together in long, paired helical filaments. In this form they can no longer contribute to axonal flow.

Preventative manganese?

More work needs to be done before the manganese hypothesis can be proven.

However, a manganese supplement added to the anti-oxidant regimes described elsewhere in this chapter, seems like a good insurance policy for anyone who thinks they might be at risk of developing Alzheimer's disease.

Smart drug

The so-called 'smart drug', hydergine, which may mimic nerve growth factors[38, 39] may be helpful in the early stage of Alzheimer's[40, 41].

Unsurprisingly, it's less effective in the later stages[42].

TOP MANGANESE FOODS

Tea, spinach, broccoli, orange juice, nuts, beans, wholegrains and blueberries.

This suggests two ways of restoring axonal flow, and therefore the health of the brain's neurons.

1 Slow down the Tau kinase enzymes, which attack the phosphate groups. However, there are several enzyme groups involved and inhibiting all of them would almost certainly cause severe toxicity problems.

2 Encourage the Tau phosphatases, and increase the rate at which excess phosphate groups are stripped off the Tau proteins. This seems a more likely proposition, because these enzymes are underactive in Alzheimer's brain tissue[7]. Furthermore they can be activated by the trace element manganese[8, 9, 10].

This leads to two tentative conclusions. Firstly, chronic manganese depletion might increase the risk of Alzheimer's. This would also explain why the Tau phosphatase enzymes are underactive in the disease. Secondly, a manganese supplement might be able to stop or slow the disease process in some cases, although it would not confer anti-oxidant protection, which remains essential.

A manganese supplement might help to return the Tau protein to normal, which would restore axonal flow, stop further degeneration of the affected neurones, and permit regrowth of the damaged axons and nerve terminals – if there is also adequate anti-oxidant and membrane support.

MANGANESE LEVELS

How much manganese should one take? There are no clinical guidelines, but 50 mg per day of manganese gluconate gives enough manganese in the brain to achieve maximal activation of the Tau phosphatases[11].

This dose is inside the safe dose range of this essential trace element. However, manganese supplements should not be taken by patients with severe liver disease, as the resulting build-up of manganese in the body could cause toxicity problems[62-64, 73, 74].

For a preventative, rather than therapeutic manganese level, 4-10mg a day may be sufficient.

Aluminium, manganese – and zinc

The manganese story may prove to be an object lesson in how science develops. Many non-scientists believe in a confrontational model of science, where old theories hold sway until they are destroyed by new evidence, and replaced by different and better ideas.

This sort of conceptual coup d'état does occur, but is not as common as evolutionary change, where an old idea which previously seemed complete is revealed by new knowledge to be part of a larger whole.

Although there were always gaps in the evidence for aluminium being the sole cause of Alzheimer's, there is too much evidence linking aluminium to brain damage to allow the hypothesis to die away altogether.

Manganese depletion may prove to be a better candidate than aluminium excess, but the manganese theory doesn't replace the aluminium theory so much as update it and expand it.

Aluminium is not only extremely toxic to nerve cells, but it also competes with manganese. If someone was low in manganese, exposure to aluminium could tip them into serious manganese depletion, which could also lead to Alzheimer's. Anyone eating a manganese-rich diet, on the other hand, might be less vulnerable to aluminium.

Zinc can also compete with manganese, and extra zinc given to Alzheimer's patients, who are probably manganese depleted (as many of us are), would tend to make manganese depletion, and their condition, worse, as has recently been shown.

So the manganese theory may update the aluminium story. What's more, the manganese hypothesis is easily testable.

It is only fair to say that not all scientists agree with Dr Iqbal's work. Some say that most Tau proteins in the paired helical filaments are not over-phosphorylated[22, 23]. And some say that hyper-phosphorylated Tau might discourage, rather than encourage filament formation[23]. So the debate continues.

Dangerous skins?

If you eat potatoes or aubergines, be cautious. Potato and aubergine skins contain the tropane alkaloids, calystegine A3 and B2[12].

This group of compounds causes degenerative neurological diseases in cattle[13, 14, 18], and may be implicated in causing anencephaly and spina bifida in humans[19].

They may not be a significant cause of Alzheimer's, but anything which kills large numbers of brain cells will exacerbate the disease, and speed its onset.

Tropane alkaloids are soluble in water, so if the potatoes or aubergines are to be boiled or stewed the toxins will leach safely into the cooking water. If, however, the potatoes are roasted or baked traces of the alkaloids may remain in the skins.

LOOK FOR ...

a supplement that includes anti-oxidants, carotenoids, a flaxseed oil or grapeseed oil and also OPC flavonoids (oligo-proanthocyanidins) like grapeseed/bilberry extract – at about 100mg.

To that add isoflavones at about 30-40mg. These all have anti-oxidant and anti-inflammatory properties and make a good preventative strategy against Alzheimer's.

Oxidation – Inflammation

The processes of oxidation and inflammation are very closely intertwined. Significant oxidation cannot exist without inflammation and vice versa.

Flavonoids

The flavonoids' abilities to reduce platelet stickiness and improve vascular health should protect against strokes[91, 115].

Additional help for Alzheimer's

Q10

Another factor which may contribute to Alzheimer's disease is mitochondrial ageing. Mitochondria become less efficient with age, and old, burned-out mitochondria can't make enough ATP (the energy compound) to fuel the body cells[44]. This is another well-established cause of cellular suicide.

In cases of Alzheimer's caused largely by mitochondrial inefficiency, high-dose Co-enzyme Q10, which can improve mitochondrial output, is the theoretical remedy of choice[57].

The scientific reports, however, are confusing; some find sub-normal levels of Q10 in the brains of Alzheimer's victims[14], while others find increased Q10[45]. This may be yet another indication that you can end up with Alzheimer's via a number of different routes.

Flavonoids

There is good evidence that Alzheimer's is, at least in part, an inflammatory condition. The disease was classically described as having some of the appearances of inflammation, and it has been described by some contemporary researchers as 'arthritis of the brain'.

Other experts disagree, but it is an interesting fact that in people with rheumatoid arthritis, and who were treated with anti-inflammatory drugs, the incidence of Alzheimer's is rather lower than in the general population. When this was first discovered, further work revealed that the reduction of risk occurred mostly in the sub-group of arthritic patients who were treated with indomethacin, one of the few drugs of its type which penetrates the brain in large amounts.

Indomethacin is a powerful drug with potentially serious side effects, and is not recommended for long-term prophylactic use except under medical supervision. However, there are various flavonoids, derived from food crops, which do much the same thing as indomethacin.

The oligomeric procyanidins (OPCs), found in bilberry extract and grapeseed extract, for example, enter the brain, are potent anti-inflammatory agents and, remarkably, have the additional ability of preventing the hyper-phosphorylation of proteins such as the Tau proteins[15, 16].

This combination of therapeutic actions, and their well-attested safety, makes the oligomeric procyanidins excellent candidates for long-term prophylaxis against Alzheimer's (see Chapter 6, Flavonoids & isoflavones).

Rosemary

Rosemary contains flavonoids which are anti-inflammatory and powerful lipid-soluble anti-oxidants. They have another valuable property: they bind to iron, preventing it from generating free radicals[54]. This herb, combined perhaps with thyme, would be a very good bet in the treatment not only of Alzheimer's, but also of Parkinson's disease and Amyotrophic Lateral Sclerosis.

Light at the end of the tunnel?

Screening for a lethal disease that cannot be cured raises difficult ethical dilemmas. At the time of writing, conventional wisdom says, "There is no drug which can prevent Alzheimer's, and there is very little that can be done, other than to slightly delay the progress of the disease."

I am no longer convinced that we have to be so pessimistic, or as passive. In all the neuro-degenerative diseases (Alzheimer's, Parkinson's and Amyotrophic Lateral Sclerosis) free radicals have been strongly implicated in causing brain damage[55].

As we get older, and as our diet becomes depleted in micro-nutrients, more and more of us are developing the so-called neuro-degenerative diseases, and these are eating up an ever-growing share of the health-care budget.

Anti-oxidant therapy would appear to be a logical response. Vitamin E is probably an important anti-oxidant in the brain under normal circumstances[56], but is not necessarily the best form of therapy, as it takes a very long time to get into the brain and may become pro-oxidant in existing disease states.

I prefer to combine Vitamins C and E with OPC flavonoids, and isoflavones as a preventative strategy. I would add a thyme oil

---

'Rosemary for remembrance'

An alternative to rosemary is hawthorn.

This plant also contains flavonoids which are anti-oxidant, bind iron, and enter the brain where they are needed.

The only side effect is mild sedation. Herbal practitioners sometimes use hawthorn to help sleep (see Chapter 6, Flavonoids & isoflavones).

and phosphadityl serine supplement in cases where actual mental decline is suspected, with B vitamins or betaine and optional manganese.

AN ALZHEIMER'S TEST?

When a solution of tropicamide (a drug used by opthalmologists) is applied to the eye, the pupils of Alzheimer's patients dilate by 13 per cent or more; whereas the pupils of healthy subjects don't.

This finding is being checked, but it may provide us with a relatively cheap and hence accessible early warning system.

Increased levels of Tau proteins in spinal fluid, although more difficult to measure, may be an alternative. Preliminary findings indicate that these are not only raised in Alzheimer's patients, but also in people with genes predisposing them to Alzheimer's, before they develop the illness[36].

Stress and Alzheimer's

It may be possible to reduce the risk of Alzheimer's with a life-style change. There is evidence that depressive illness is a risk factor for Alzheimer's[47-50]. This may be due to the fact that during depression, levels of the stress hormones (glucocorticoids) increase in the body to the point where they become neurotoxic, and cause brain damage[51], a process which tends to worsen with age[52, 53].

Chronic stress leads to the production in the body of the same neurotoxic hormones and this could be one of the reasons why under-educated people have a higher risk of developing Alzheimer's. It has been suggested that this is because their brains are 'less exercised', but it could equally well be because the under-educated are likely to be lower down the social ladder, and living more stressful lives. And it may be another reason to take one of the ginsengs which reduce the stress response.

A more potent and more specific antidote, however, could well be the hormone dehydroepiandrosterone (DHEA). This has been described as an anti-ageing hormone. Levels of DHEA in the blood peak by the end of the second decade and then go into a long decline, falling to a third or less of peak values by the age of 60[58, 139].

DHEA has many interesting properties, but the one which appears particularly relevant here is its powerful anti-glucocorticoid action[59, 138-140].

The glucocorticoid blocking effect means that DHEA could protect brain cells from stress or depression-induced injury. The fact that DHEA levels are very low in the elderly could be a significant factor in predisposing to Alzheimer's disease.

For this reason, a DHEA supplement is also worth considering as part of a risk reduction programme. The side effects of DHEA appear to be entirely positive: they include enhanced immune function[60, 61], a marked increase in feelings of wellbeing[20], and probable improvements in weight control and diabetes[20]. (See Chapter 15, Bones).

Food for thought?

So far we have been looking at ways to prevent mental deterioration in later life. But what about building brains at the *beginning* of the life cycle? Can micro-nutrients make children more intelligent?

This apparently simple question has been fiercely debated ever since 1988 when Gwilym Roberts, a science teacher in Wrexham, Wales, found that vitamin and mineral supplements increased the (non-verbal) intelligence of children in his school.

They also became better able to concentrate and less disruptive. The teaching staff were delighted, as were Larkhall, the nutrition company that supplied Mr Roberts with the supplements.

It didn't take long, however, for the opposition to muster. The seemingly innocent Wrexham study sparked off a period of fierce infighting, industry lobbying, lawsuits and dirty tricks which led, ultimately, to the end of Mr Roberts's career in Britain.

Initially academics and doctors rejected Roberts's findings out of hand, probably because he was a 'mere' schoolteacher.

Dr David Benton, however, could not be so easily dismissed. A psychologist at Cardiff University in Wales, he repeated Roberts's trial with equally positive results[157]. In the USA, Dr Stephen Schoenthaler reported similar findings[158, 159].

These studies, together with Gwilym Roberts's school trial, were included in QED, a BBC television programme, which generated an enormous amount of publicity.

The 'lost' generation

Professor John Garrow, Head of Nutrition at London's Bart's Hospital and former Chairman of HealthWatch, was one of the scientists who initially argued against Mr Roberts' findings. Subsequently he was prepared to admit the possibility that he may have been wrong. But then again, the evidence against him was overwhelming.

Professor Garrow is famous in nutritional circles for claiming that the only thing supplements do is create expensive urine. Not long after he said this, research carried out in his own and other

---

33% of children risk nutrient deficiency

As many as one in three schoolchildren are nutritionally depleted. Even the anti-supplement lobby now admits that giving these children extra nutrients means their behaviour and school performance improves.

Poor diet – poor marks

The unhealthier the child's diet, the worse his or her behaviour and achievement levels.

Research shows that a good supplement can help improve matters.

Sceptics confounded

Only one study attempted to refute Benton and Roberts's work[160]. This study was subsequently revealed to be so fatally flawed as to be effectively worthless[161].

hospitals proved that supplementing with folic acid and other micro-nutrients during pregnancy reduced the risk of low birth weight[209] and disorders such as spina bifida[177, 178], cleft palate, hare lip, and urinary tract malformations[189, 190, 192].

The real victims in this hotly debated case, however, are the many schoolchildren (as many as one in three, even in the 'developed countries'!) who are considered to be eating such deficient diets that their non-verbal IQ, and school performance, could be improved by supplements.

A generation of these children could have been helped if 10 years of medical infighting had not squandered that opportunity.

Admittedly, the children of the academics and doctors who opposed vitamins may not have needed them, because they were probably eating a relatively good diet. But if the establishment had read Gwilym Roberts's report more closely, they would have found that their children were not the most at risk.

Roberts had noticed that it was the children who ate the unhealthiest diets, and who were often underachievers, who seemed to benefit most from the supplements.

Cautious in advocating vitamins, he concluded that, although it would be better to improve their general diet, supplementation could have an important part to play in enabling them to perform better at school. And this is where, for the moment, the issue rests.

The science suggests that for parents concerned about their children's diet (and how many children do you know who eat a sensible diet?), a properly designed vitamin and mineral supplement can help in IQ tests and in the classroom[162-166].

It's hardly a new concept. The idea that eating fish is somehow good for the brain has been around for many years. The medical profession dismissed it as an old wives' tale – and yet, the emerging science of nutrition and IQ has proved that this old tale is largely correct.

Bringing up baby

It's important for children and adults to eat the right nutrients to optimise their mental functions. But it's even more critical for infants.

Poly-unsaturates and birth defects

A lack of the right poly-unsaturates in pregnancy is linked to an increased risk of babies with cerebral palsy, sight problems and learning difficulties.

Pre-term babies appear to be most vulnerable – and most responsive to Omega 3 supplements.

The growing brain has a high requirement for certain poly-unsaturated fatty acids (PUFAs). Large amounts of these were present in our diet as we evolved as a species[187], and are secreted in mother's milk. But some formula milks still don't contain the right PUFAs. As a result, they can impair the normal growth and maturation of the bottle-fed baby's brain.

This has been demonstrated in a number of studies. In one typical trial, formula-fed infants scored significantly worse in tests of brain and nerve function than breast-fed babies. The authors considered this was because the bottle babies were PUFA-deficient[219]. Bottle-fed babies tend to grow more slowly, and suffer more illnesses. At one year they weigh less[143], their IQ is lower[144, 229], and their coordination is not as good as their breast-fed siblings[145], these differences appear to be life-long[230].

As a result of studies like these, the influential European Society for Paediatric Nutrition decided in '94 that all infant foods should contain the PUFAs essential for brain function.

It's surprising that the formula manufacturers didn't think of this first, because logic tells you that any formula should resemble mother's milk as closely as possible[132].

We don't know how much damage has been done to the brains of how many children, but at least this unnecessary nutritional depletion is being stopped. But, although it's a good idea to supplement baby foods, this is like bolting the stable door after the horse (or in this case the baby) has left.

ESSENTIAL FATTY ACIDS IN PREGNANCY

PUFAs critical to brain growth and function include DHA (docosahexanoic acid) and AA (arachidonic acid)[152, 201]. The best source of DHA is a good fish oil, and AA is formed in the body from vegetable oils. So eat oily fish two or three times a week, plus a helping or two of walnuts or brazil nuts (see Chapter 8, Essential Oils).

A good multi-vitamin and mineral supplment including Omega 3 and 6 (or flax or hemp oil) is also strongly recommended; the PUFAs and other nutrients essential to your baby's growth are absorbed into your blood stream, cross the placenta, and supply the baby with everything it needs to develop its potential to the full[192, 202].

Folic acid

Folic acid supplementation is now a universal recommendation in pregnancy to reduce the risks of low birth weight, spina bifida, hare lip and malformation of the urinary tract.

To this add a well-designed pregancy supplement and a 1000mg capsule of a good Omega 3 fish oil – or a 1000mg flaxseed or hemp oil capsule.

Avoid high doses of Vitamin A in pregnancy

Although most nutritional supplements are very safe, high doses of Vitamin A should be avoided by women of child-bearing age.

Doses as low as 10,000IU (four times the RDA) have been linked to an increased incidence of birth defects[197].

Beta carotene is a safe substitute but must always be combined with Vitamin C and never with smoking. (Pregnant women shouldn't be smoking anyway!)

Delicate balance

Throughout pregnancy, the developing foetal brain is highly dependent on a good supply of a number of key nutrients. At the pioneering Institute of Human Nutrition in East London, Professor Michael Crawford, Wendy Doyle and co-workers have been publishing papers linking maternal dietary deficiencies (including PUFAs and a range of vitamins and minerals) to birth problems such as cerebal palsy since the mid-'80s[147, 148].

Studies at other labs have shown similar results. PUFA intake is absolutely crucial for the normal growth of the retina and the brain, which contains very high levels of PUFAs in the membranes of brain cells[149, 240]. If the mother eats a grossly deficient diet in the three to six months before the pregnancy, or during it, the lack of PUFAs means that the baby's growing brain will take up the wrong fatty acids, incorporating saturated fatty acids instead of the poly-unsaturated ones[150, 151].

This is the best that nature can do to compensate, but it is not good enough. It may lead to premature, low birth-weight babies with brain damage such as cerebal palsy[152, 153, 219], or in lesser cases, visual problems and learning deficits[153, 154].

As a result, Crawford's team (and most of their international colleagues) now recommend that all pregnant women, and indeed any woman planning to become pregnant, should eat a diet containing portions of oily fish, as well as green leafy vegetables.

However, for the many women who can't or won't eat such foods, supplementation is an obvious option.

Breast-feeding and the infant brain

The human brain continues to grow after birth, as does its need for the essential PUFAs, so nursing mothers should continue taking the supplements until weaning.

But although fish oil improves infants' brain development[179, 190] and learning ability[176]; resist the temptation to feed supplements directly to your baby. Fish oil, for example, contains another PUFA called EPA, which does not occur in breast milk. There is a good reason for this: EPA competes with DHA and makes it less available for the baby's brain. This means that while fish oils are fine for adults, and especially pregnant and nursing mothers, they should not be given to infants.

The best formula manufacturers now enrich their formulae with DHA not from fish oil but eggs, which is a step in the right direction; but the best food for babies remains mother's milk.

In fact, mother's milk is a beautiful example of human adaptability. Because PUFA intake is so crucial for the normal development of the growing brain, the breast tries to maintain a constant ratio of Omega 3 and Omega 6 PUFAs in the milk, despite large fluctuations in the mother's diet.

The PUFA content of breast milk in women living in fish or vegetable eating communities is very similar, despite a very different dietary intake of Omega 3 and Omega 6 PUFAs[146].

If the mother is not eating enough of one or the other type of PUFAs for her baby, her body will cannibalise her own resources to give the baby what it needs. It is only in extremis, or when an abnormal diet is eaten, that safety mechanisms fail and foetal brain damage ensues.

The evidence that common micro-nutrient deficiencies before conception and during pregnancy can adversely affect the developing foetal brain, is increasing. And it's not just the exotic micro-nutrients. The most common depletion, that of iron, is now also suspected of contributing to impaired intelligence in childhood and in later life also[192, 193].

Keeping in mind that many pregnancies are not confirmed until after the first three months, this is another potent argument for improved nutrition for all women of child-bearing age. Widespread food fortification programmes, and/or supplementation are the only answers.

Not just a problem for the poor

Infant brain damage caused by foetal malnutrition, which is caused in turn by maternal malnutrition, is a well-known pattern in areas of the world where food shortages and starvation are common.

Premature birth risks

Fish oils can prolong pregnancy without any detrimental effects. So Omega 3 PUFA supplements can be tried if you are prone to premature labour[155].

Another good reason for pregnant women to take fish oil supplements during pregnancy is that they may reduce the risk of the dangerous rise in blood pressure which can complicate the last three months and birth[156].

Fish oil should always be taken with anti-oxidants, which, especially Vitamins C and E, may reduce the risk further[204-207].

Iron and intelligence

Iron levels in pregnancy are often depleted and can lead to lower intelligence in children[192, 193].

TOP IRON FOODS

Liver, meat, chicken, whole grain, peas, beans, spinach, nuts.

Iron – caution

Iron supplements are not advised for men or post-menopausal women unless iron-depletion anaemia has been diagnosed.

In the West, too, low birth-weight, cerebral palsy and related problems are strongly associated with social deprivation. And even in wealthy and well-nourished communities, many pregnant women are deficient in a range of vital micro-nutrients.

This has been shown by recent studies where multi-vitamin and mineral supplements reduced the risk not only of babies with congenital neural tube defects such as spina bifida and oro-facial clefts[177, 178], but also congenital disorders of the urinary tract[188, 189, 190, 192].

Are the roots of schizophrenia in the womb?

The developing brain is uniquely sensitive to malnutrition. The psychoanalytical and viral theories of schizophrenia have been discredited. Some forms of schizophrenia have now been linked to faulty development of the brain during growth in the womb, probably during the second trimester[193-197].

Studies have suggested that maternal dietary deficiency, leading to foetal deficiency, is a cause of schizophrenia which may not manifest itself until 20 or more years later in the affected child's life[198, 199].

It is not known which micro-nutrients are involved, but folic acid and Vitamin B12 are likely candidates. Both of these vitamins are important for nerve function.

B12 deficiency in adults leads to nerve damage, and a deficiency in either or both of these vitamins during pregnancy has been linked to neural tube defects such as spina bifida[177, 178, 213].

It may be no coincidence that in certain communities (such as Ireland) where there are specific problems with B vitamins, a high incidence of both spina bifida and juvenile onset schizophrenia have been reported.

However, there is probably more than one way of contracting schizophrenia. There is evidence for a genetic causative factor in some cases of schizophrenia[190, 191, 199] which may interact with the nutritional factors.

Food and mood

The brain communicates with the body – and vice versa – through electrical signals, through neuro-transmitters (chemicals) and via hormones. The proper function of neuro-transmitters and hormones depends upon correct nutrition. So we shouldn't be surprised if mental function improves with optimum nutrition (or that the immune system suffers through stress and grief).

In some cases patients with mental problems have responded as well, if not better, to nutraceutical treatment than to pharmaceutical treatment.

For example, some patients with depression have responded well to Vitamin B complex, magnesium, the amino acid tryptophan and DMAE (see box below).

Generally, the nutritional supplement programme, recommended on page 338, should not only help maintain a good state of mental health, but act preventatively against the risk of degenerative disease.

Depression – some answers

Depression is the most common psychiatric illness. The World Health Organisation estimates that as many as five per cent of the world's population suffer from depression, and numbers could be on the increase.

Temporary depressive states are even more common and affect as many as one in five of us.

Prozac is the drug of choice to treat depression, but a herbal equivalent has been around for centuries – St John's Wort (*hypericum perforatum)*.

This herb was known in the Middle Ages as 'Fuga daemonum', or 'flight of demons'. Its common name, Walpurgis Herb tells a similar tale: this was a herb which could drive out the devils of melancholy.

It is only in the past few years that the herb has been systematically studied. The results indicate that the medieval herbalists were right. St John's Wort contains compounds with a powerful anti-depressant action – and fewer side effects than most anti-depressant drugs.

In two fairly typical trials Hypericum significantly reduced the symptoms of depression, and effected a complete recovery in many cases[180, 181]. Symptoms of insomnia and fatigue responded particularly well. Unlike some anti-depressants, Hypericum doesn't cause drowsiness[105, 182]. Dependence or addiction does not develop.

Nutrients are just as important, and may be more effective. Methyl groups are needed to make the crucial (monoamine) neurotransmitters involved in mood, so methyl depletion (surprisingly common) predisposes to depression. This explains trials which show that strong Vitamin B complex[196], S-adenosyl methionine[231-236] and DMAE (di-methyl-aminoethanol) [183-186], all have anti-depressant activity. However, the clinicians clearly didn't understand the biochemistry; because the best source of methyl groups is betaine (see Chapter 11).

Logic dictates that betaine must be as or more effective than standard anti-depressant drugs in cases where methyl depletion is involved – and this is reflected in my personal experience.

Betaine is contra-indicated in bipolar illness (manic-depression), as it may trigger episodes of mania[235]. For these patients, fish oil is the nutrient of choice. When Omega 3 fatty acids are built into nerve cell membranes they act as damping or modulating agents[237] and have been shown in two studies to lead to marked improvement in symptoms[238-239].

My preferred anti-depressant regime begins with betaine, and then adds Hypericum and the amino acid tryptophan, if needed.

Preventing mental deterioration

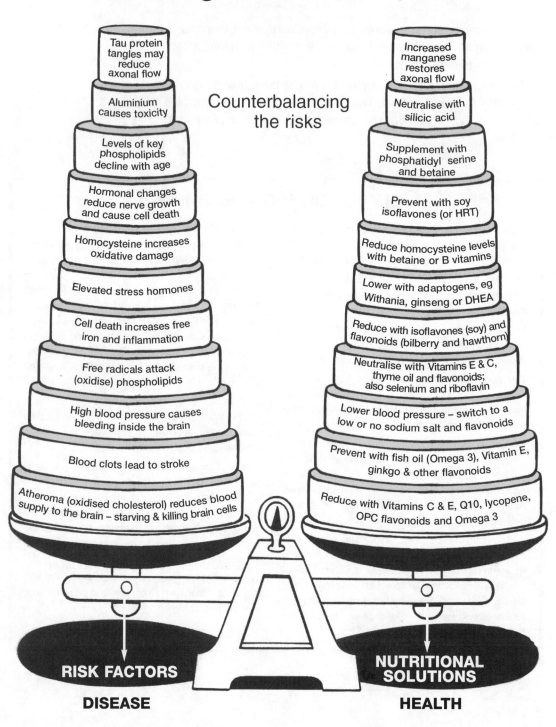

Counterbalancing
the risks

RISK FACTORS

Tau protein tangles may reduce axonal flow

Aluminium causes toxicity

Levels of key phospholipids decline with age

Hormonal changes reduce nerve growth and cause cell death

Homocysteine increases oxidative damage

Elevated stress hormones

Cell death increases free iron and inflammation

Free radicals attack (oxidise) phospholipids

High blood pressure causes bleeding inside the brain

Blood clots lead to stroke

Atheroma (oxidised cholesterol) reduces blood supply to the brain – starving & killing brain cells

NUTRITIONAL SOLUTIONS

Increased manganese restores axonal flow

Neutralise with silicic acid

Supplement with phosphatidyl serine and betaine

Prevent with soy isoflavones (or HRT)

Reduce homocysteine levels with betaine or B vitamins

Lower with adaptogens, eg Withania, ginseng or DHEA

Reduce with isoflavones (soy) and flavonoids (bilberry and hawthorn)

Neutralise with Vitamins E & C, thyme oil and flavonoids; also selenium and riboflavin

Lower blood pressure – switch to a low or no sodium salt and flavonoids

Prevent with fish oil (Omega 3), Vitamin E, ginkgo & other flavonoids

Reduce with Vitamins C & E, Q10, lycopene, OPC flavonoids and Omega 3

RISK FACTORS

NUTRITIONAL SOLUTIONS

DISEASE

HEALTH

SUMMARY

Alzheimer's aid box

Protecting yourself against Alzheimer's is another example of a multi-layered defence strategy

Level 1

▶ Anti-oxidant nutrients (at the levels recommended on page 338) to prevent free radical damage to the fatty acids in the brain – especially the phospholipids;

▶ Flavonoids (eg bilberry/grapeseed extract) to help prevent inflammation;

▶ B vitamins and betaine to prevent nerve damage caused by homocysteine.

Level 2

▶ A thyme oil supplement.

Level 3

▶ Supplement with phosphatidyl serine to boost levels of this key phospholipid in the nerve cell membranes.

Level 4

▶ A manganese supplement which may help prevent Tau protein tangles and hence disruptions of axonal flow.

Additional action

▶ A Q10 supplement to help delay mitochondrial ageing.

▶ Silicic acid in a colloidal form.

Level 1 defence action would be an appropriate strategy for anyone over 40.

Level 2 action for anyone over 55.

Levels 3 and 4 strategies would be appropriate in cases where the onset of Alzheimer's is actually suspected.

Caution with alumininium

▶ Don't use aluminium based antacids, especially if you're pregnant.

▶ If you think you are at risk, use a silicic acid supplement.

▶ Don't cook acid foods (ie fruit) in aluminium cookware.

▶ Avoid foods containing E470b.

Brain food in childhood

▶ If your child has problems at school, look at his or her diet. A good, all-round supplement could help.

▶ Breast is best for many reasons, but if you are bottle feeding, check the formula contains the right poly-unsaturated fatty acids. (Often referred to as LCPs.)

▶ Pregnant and breast-feeding women should take folic acid, B12, Omega 3 as fish oil, evening primrose oil, plus a good multi-vitamin and mineral supplement.

▶ Be careful with Vitamin A if pregnant – mixed carotenoids are safer.

Chapter 18

Saving your skin

The effects of gravity and slack facial muscles creep up on us so slowly, it can be hard sometimes to see just how much the face has been marked by the passage of time.

To find out what has happened, lie on your back on your bed, lower your head over the edge, and look at your face in a mirror. For anyone past the age of 35 or so, this can be a very disconcerting – and motivating – experience.

To exercise and tone the facial muscles, try to bring that upside-down face back into its normal shape. These muscles, if properly exercised, can help to rejuvenate the face once you're upright again. But they can't improve skin texture, and many people find the exercise programme hard to maintain. So what else can be done to slow the hands of time?

How to avoid cosmetic surgery

I'm not in favour of cosmetic surgery as a first line anti-ageing treatment, although it can be effective in removing some of the signs of ageing.

Before considering surgery, there are a number of strategies which can be used to block or slow down the ageing process. We should stay away from doctors – and especially surgeons – as long as we can, and only use them when they're really needed.

So, instead of saving up for a face-lift in five or ten years' time, reach for the supplements now. An anti-ageing programme begun today should mean you could delay surgery for many years.

What makes skin look old?

Much of the damage we think of as due to ageing – thinning skin, loss of elasticity, the appearance of lines and wrinkles – is nothing to do with age at all.

These changes typically appear in ageing persons, but ageing doesn't cause the changes. The fact that the skin changes as we get older is really no more than a coincidence. Even 70- and 80-year-olds generally have smooth, unlined skin on parts of their body. And this is the clue, because those are the parts which are not often exposed to the sun.

As much as 80 or even 90 per cent of skin ageing is extrinsic, caused by exposure to sunlight (known as 'photic ageing'), and other sources of free radicals. Intrinsic ageing, which occurs eventually even in sheltered skin, accounts for a mere 10-20 per cent.

Intrinsic ageing, as the skin gradually thins and becomes less robust, can be treated to some extent. Think of the well-documented effects of HRT in women: the oestrogen stimulates the fibroblast cells to produce more collagen and elastin, micro-fibres which give skin its strength and resilience, with a resulting improvement in skin texture. Growth hormone treatment and testosterone replacement therapy are reported to have similar effects in elderly men.

Extrinsic ageing too can be slowed, and perhaps stopped or even reversed. Here, free radicals are the key. Reducing exposure to sunlight and other sources of free radicals can have a dramatic age-retarding effect.

Boosting the exposure to free radicals has, as you might expect, exactly the opposite effect. This is why the face of the sun-worshipper is more lined than average for his or her age. The face of the smoker, too, is generally more heavily lined than the face of a non-smoker of the same age.

This is largely because of free radicals generated by sunlight, and tobacco smoke respectively.

Additional creases in the smoker are caused by squinting through the smoke, and there is also thought to be a 'curing' effect, rather like the smoking of a kipper. Crowsfeet round the

---

The sun is to blame!

Your skin doesn't age so much where the sun doesn't reach.

Sunlight causes up to 90 per cent of the thinning and wrinkling of the skin we think of as ageing. This is called 'photic ageing'.

Tanned skin is **not** healthy skin, but skin that is showing signs of UV damage.

A good UV filter is the first step to slowing ageing effects on the skin – and could slow skin ageing by up to 80 per cent.

eyes, tiny wrinkles spreading around the upper and lower lips, and lines on the cheek and lower jaw are particularly noticeable. Tobacco induced changes to the blood supply to the skin make the matter worse, by giving the skin a greyish tinge.

The ageing effects of tobacco are clearly quite complex, but it is the free radicals formed by the interaction of smoke and biological tissue that cause the bulk of the damage; not just to the skin, but the lungs and other parts of the body too.

Reducing free radical damage in the skin by stopping smoking, and avoiding excessive exposure to sunlight, is important in slowing the ageing process. But to stop ageing, and reverse its effects, we must look under the skin.

Movement under a still surface

All biological tissues (skin, bone, muscle, arteries, etc) are in a state of constant flux. Their apparent constancy conceals the twin processes of tissue breakdown (catabolism), and repair (anabolism), both of which run constantly and in parallel throughout life. During childhood, tissue growth and regeneration generally predominate, and there are net tissue gains. In later life, and in certain disease states, breakdown predominates; leading eventually to ageing and loss of function.

This picture may seem depressing, but it is the key to skin and tissue rejuvenation. In adults, if the rate of tissue decay is ten units/day, the rate of tissue repair is typically nine units. This net change, the loss of one unit per day, is so small it cannot be seen; but if continued over years, it gradually brings on the signs of ageing – rather like the slow erosion of a landscape.

Slow the process of decay by a mere ten per cent, and increase the rate of tissue repair by ten per cent, and the net change shifts from minus one to plus one unit /day. The ageing process is now in reverse; from slow erosion to slow rejuvenation.

This general principle applies equally to the formation or removal of thrombus in an artery; the erosion or regeneration of bone and cartilage, the loss or stabilisation of brain cells; and the decay or the regeneration of the extra-cellular matrix which lies under the skin, supporting it and giving it firmness and elasticity.

How ageing happens

Now we can begin to understand how skin ages – and how to stop it. When ionising radiation (sunlight) strikes biological tissue such as the skin, it triggers a burst of free radicals. Free radicals may cause acute cell death, leading to sloughing of skin and the loss of generative cells in the lower dermis. They may cause DNA damage, leading to cellular dysfunction, loss of skin structure or cancer. They also damage cell membranes, triggering the release of a group of highly destructive enzymes known as the matrix metalloproteases (MMPs) (see Chapters 6, Flavonoids & isoflavones, and 10, Amino sugars).

In the inflammatory reaction which follows, the MMPs break down the extra-cellular matrix, the mesh of microfibres which provides a 'soft skeleton' for the skin (and all soft tissues). This results in thinning and wrinkling of the skin, loss of firmness and elasticity, strength and moisture-holding capacity. In short, it causes most of the cosmetic elements of ageing skin[27, 28].

The micro-fibres which make up the matrix are the proteins collagen and elastin, and a range of amino-sugar polymers. They are constantly being broken down; and replaced by generative cells in the dermis such as the fibroblasts.

Normally, the rate of breakdown exceeds the rate of renewal by a small margin, or a larger one if there is extensive exposure to sunlight. This deficit, if sustained over time, causes a growing loss of the microfibres in the matrix, and gradual skin ageing.

If the rate of tissue loss can be reduced by a small amount, and the rate of repair enhanced, it should allow repair to predominate, causing a net gain of micro-structural elements, and slowing or even reversing the ageing process.

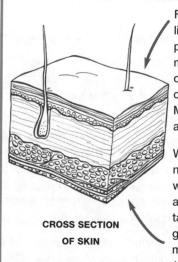

The inside/outside skin care plan

Fat-soluble anti-oxidants, like Vitamin E, can help to prevent damage to cell membranes, and the release of MMPs. These compounds, and some MMP blockers, can be applied topically.

Water-soluble micro-nutrients such as Vitamin C, which is an anti-oxidant and a matrix builder, can be taken orally. So can glucosamine, another key matrix builder (see Chapter 10, Amino sugars).

CROSS SECTION OF SKIN

From loss to profit

This explains why some people have skin which ages less rapidly than others; the net rate of matrix loss in their skin has been slowed down, due to reduced exposure to sunlight, and enhanced nutrition.

Matrix breakdown and repair are both profoundly affected by the presence or absence of various micro-nutrients. Basically, the rate of repair is increased by one group of micro-nutrients; while the rate of decay is slowed by another group. Unfortunately, as we saw earlier, the vast majority of people suffer from multiple micro-nutrient depletion. The resulting slight slowing of repair, and equally slight acceleration of tissue breakdown, is enough to speed the ageing process unnecessarily.

By supplying the right micro-nutients topically and orally (reaching the skin directly and via the sub-cutaneous blood vessels), healing can be enhanced and damage slowed – only slightly – but enough to move from a net loss to a net gain. If the regime is continued, long-term improvements in skin structure and appearance must ensue[14-17].

As the mechanism of ageing involves so many components, commercial products which rely on basic anti-oxidants can never be very effective.

Vitamin E – use with care!

For example, the one anti-oxidant in most skin care products is Vitamin E. Vitamin E is an anti-oxidant, it's lipid soluble so you can get it into the skin, and it's a moisturiser, so it seems a logical choice.

But it isn't that simple, because when a molecule of Vitamin E is oxidised it becomes a free radical itself, and can cause great damage by oxidising lipids (fats) in the cell membranes. Oxidised Vitamin E must be recycled to make it safe again, and in the body, oxidised Vitamin E is recycled by Vitamin C plus carotenoids[13]. This is known as the Vitamin E cycle (see page 63).

Vitamin C is an important anti-oxidant in skin, particularly in the fluid between the cells. One of its key roles there is to refresh

---

Balancing the books

"Annual income twenty pounds, annual expenditure nineteen pounds, nineteen and six, result happiness. Annual income twenty pounds, annual expenditure twenty pounds nought and six, result misery."

Mr Micawber in 'David Copperfield' by Charles Dickens

Under the skin

Lose 10 units/day and gain 9 = -1 unit/day = -365 units/year = ageing

Lose 10 units/day and gain 10 = no change

Lose 9 units a day and gain 10 units = +1 unit/day = rejuvenation

---

Liposome care

If you're buying a sun lotion with Vitamin E, flavonoids or alpha lipoic acid, make sure it's a liposome or phytosome formula which will give better skin penetration.

oxidised Vitamin E. If you take too much Vitamin E and not enough Vitamin C and carotenoids, you could end up worse off than if you hadn't taken E at all, because the skin may be full of oxidised Vitamin E, which would accelerate skin ageing.

Vitamin C has at least two other roles in preventing skin ageing, which are distinct from its anti-oxidant properties. It helps build the extra-cellular matrix by stimulating collagen synthesis, and blocking aryl sulfatase B, an enzyme that would otherwise damage it[22].

This underlines the importance of a co-ordinated micro-nutritional approach.

The nutraceutical approach outlined below is designed to modify nearly every significant component of the ageing process; and to tip the balance away from ageing, towards regeneration.

Dual anti-ageing approach

The strategy consists of two basic components. The first reduces the destructive effects of sunlight on skin; the second speeds the renewal of the extra-cellular matrix – a dual brake/accelerator strategy.

The approach likewise consists of two delivery systems, including a topical cream to apply actives which can easily enter the skin; and an oral form which delivers the water-soluble actives.

There are a number of links in the chain of events from sunlight to skin damage, and as many of these as possible must be blocked to achieve maximum inhibition of the catabolic processes. The anti-catabolic (anti-breakdown) formulation should, therefore, include a UV filter, lipid-soluble anti-oxidants to protect cell membranes; water-soluble anti-oxidants including Vitamin C to support the lipid-soluble anti-oxidants; MMP-blockers and other anti-inflammatory agents.

The pro-anabolic (pro-repair) formulation should include zinc, copper and Vitamins C and B6 to accelerate collagen and elastin synthesis; and glucosamine, manganese and betaine to boost the amino-sugar polymers which form the other main constituents of the matrix.

Your Vitamin E regime – is Vitamin C included?

Most anti-oxidant nutrients work in tandem. An approach which singles out only one or two anti-oxidants is simplistic, and may be counter-productive[13].

Taking Vitamin E to protect the skin without taking Vitamin C could cause more damage than taking no vitamins at all.

Complete sun protection and anti-ageing formula

Anti-catabolic = UV filter, Vitamin E, Vitamin C, mixed carotenoids, OPC flavonoids

Pro-anabolic = Vitamins C and B6, copper, zinc, glucosamine, manganese and betaine.

A nutraceutical formulation based on this approach is on trial at a major UK clinical research centre. The results will be available by February 2002, and spin-off skin rejuvenating products should be available later that year.

CO-ENZYME Q10

Co-enzyme Q10 is another prime anti-ageing candidate. Like melanin, Q10 is a dual purpose compound. It is a potent anti-oxidant which supports Vitamin E, and it also boosts the function of the mitochondria, improving the energy balance of the cells and acting as a general stimulant. Like Vitamin E, Q10 is fat soluble, so it can also be applied topically.

Water soluble micro-nutrients, on the other hand, including Vitamin C, glucosamine, the B group of vitamins and the anti-oxidant minerals, are more logically taken orally.

This forms the basis of a thorough anti-ageing skin care strategy. It's effectively an inside/outside strategy. The outside half of the skin care strategy comprises lipid-soluble anti-oxidants and matrix stabilisers delivered through the skin. The inside half consists of water-soluble micro-nutrients arriving at the skin via the bloodstream after oral ingestion. This micro-nutrient pincer movement significantly reduces photic ageing[14-17].

Plants to block ageing

Blackcurrant (Ribes Nigrum), the perennial herb, Lady's Mantle (Alchemilla Vulgaris) and elderberry contain flavonoids which block most of the destructive MMP enzymes [4-6].

Bilberry, ginkgo, pycnogenol and red wine or green tea extract contain flavonoids with similar MMP blocking properties[7-11].

Some citrus flavonoids (ie tangeritin) may be equally effective[29].

MMP blockade

Two garden plants are rich sources of flavonoids which block MMPs. These are blackcurrant (Ribes Nigrum L), and the perennial herb Lady's Mantle (Alchemilla Vulgaris L). Both contain flavonoids which are potent inhibitors of just about all of the metallo-protease enzymes, including the elastases, hyaluronidases and collagenases[4-6, 21]. Of the two, I would recommend blackcurrants, manifestly safe and delicious. Elderberries and bilberries are excellent alternatives.

Commercially available alternatives include ginkgo, pycnogenol, and red wine or grapeseed extract. These preparations are not identical to blackcurrant and Lady's Mantle, but contain related flavonoids which are very good at stabilising collagen and elastin fibres in the extra-cellular matrix, and protecting them from enzymic attack[7-11].

Matrix protection is best combined with enhanced matrix regeneration, see previous page for details.

CROSS-LINKS

There is one more key aspect of skin ageing which can be blocked; namely, the cross-linking of collagen and elastin. When these micro-fibres are cross-linked together, usually by sugar molecules (a process called glycosylation), they lose their strength and elasticity[18].

The flavonoids in blackcurrant and the other plants mentioned inhibit cross-link formation[19]. This is another way in which they protect the micro-fibres, and another crucial anti-ageing property. High doses of Vitamins C and E have a similar effect[20] as does turmeric[2], or half an aspirin per day.

Looking for skin savers

There are a number of pharmaceutical approaches to the problem of skin ageing.

Dr Young, a photobiologist at the Dermatology Centre at St Thomas's Hospital in London, has been working with compounds found in the bergamot orange (used to flavour Earl Grey tea). This stimulates the tanning process, and offers fair-skinned people the same protection against the sun that dark-skinned people have. In other words, it increases your natural SPF rating, and may double it or even better.

Other scientists are looking at agents that enhance the rate of skin regeneration. Among these are the retinoids (Vitamin A and its close relatives), which have well-known growth promoting effects. The first of these was RetinA.

Unfortunately RetinA often irritates the skin before improving it, and leaves it extremely sensitive to sunlight. Currently awaiting FDA approval is Renova, the same drug in a more soothing base. Perhaps more excitingly, a licence application has also been made by Hoffman LaRoche for topical isotretinoin, a close chemical cousin to RetinA.

Isotretinoin is well known as an oral treatment for acne, and it's now being screened in clinical trials for topical use for repairing sun-damaged skin. Experimenters say that it improves skin colour and texture, with less reddening and scaling than RetinA.

But the best member of the Vitamin A group so far appears to be retinyl palmitate, a compound initially dismissed because it could not penetrate the skin. Researchers have now succeeded in making a formulation of retinyl palmitate which does penetrate.

Initial studies show that this compound can promote skin cell renewal, help wound healing, reverse sun-induced damage, increase skin elasticity and thicken age-thinned skin, without the side effects associated with the other retinoids.

Coral relief

Researchers at the Scripps Institute in La Jolla, California, have found that certain soft corals produce compounds which, like the flavonoids in blackcurrant and the other plants, inhibit the skin-damaging enzymes elastase and collagenase.

These are probably defence compounds. Corals need to defend themselves against predators just as plants do and it's not

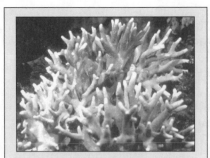

A new and unexpected area of research which may pay big dividends in skin care is soft coral.

surprising that some defence substances in coral are very similar to those which occur in plants. Others, however, are found nowhere else in the plant or animal kingdom.

This latter group includes cell division inhibitors, which may find a role in anti-cancer treatments, neuromuscular toxins and anti-inflammatory agents.

The Scripps scientists have identified a whole host of novel compounds in soft corals, including some which are interesting because they have the ability to remove excess iron from the tissues. They also bind to a wide range of enzyme active sites. Two of these, the cembrenes and the pseudopterosins, are powerful anti-inflammatory agents[2], which is why Estée Lauder is currently investigating their suitability for inclusion in their skin care range for sensitive, easily inflamed skin.

The anti-inflammatory properties of the coral compounds, if they help to stabilise the micro-fibres in the skin, should exert a marked anti-ageing effect.

Silicon and skin

Skin cells called fibroblasts are important in building the extra-cellular matrix. They may often be below par, slowed down by aluminium intoxication[25, 26].

Silicic acid removes the aluminium 'brake' and can boost fibroblast activity[23, 24].

CAROTENOIDS

Carotenoids have much to offer. Drs Kune and Bannerman at the University of Melbourne recently showed that a high intake of fish and vegetables, plus foods containing beta carotene and Vitamin A, offered a degree of protection against basal cell carcinoma and squamous cell carcinoma[1]. These are two skin cancers caused by over-exposure to sunlight.

Carotenoids on their own reduce inflammation of the skin (sunburn) after exposure to UV, but are unlikely to help much if you seriously overdo the sunbathing[9, 12], or are depleted in Vitamin C.

Beauty sleep

From the deep to deep sleep, otherwise known as core sleep or more technically sleep stages 3 and 4.

Core sleep triggers the release, from the pituitary gland located just below the brain, of Growth Hormone. Growth Hormone (GH) is one of the great restoratives. It increases the amount of nutrients taken up by the cells, encourages the growth and repair of muscle and bone, and stimulates the immune system.

Unfortunately, as we age, the pituitary's ability to synthesis GH falters. The resulting fall in GH levels is associated with loss of lean tissue, and an increased risk of heart disease. (GH therapy is increasingly being used to reverse some of the symptoms of ageing.)

The rate of tissue growth and repair is greatest at night because, under the influence of GH, this is the time when our body cells are most active, and when they are most actively dividing (which they must do in order to multiply). This is why lack of sleep shows in the skin, and why the old idea that lack of sleep stunts growth may have something in it.

The skin cells are constantly being replaced, which keeps the skin clean and healthy. A large part of the renewal takes place at night, during core sleep. If we don't get enough of this restorative sleep the pituitary gland produces less GH, the rate of skin cell replacement slows down, and our skin loses its clarity and bloom.

When the need for growth is greatest (such as during pregnancy, adolescence, or recovery from anorexia), the duration of core sleep, and the amount of GH released, increase.

A similar response occurs when daily energy expenditure increases, either through exercise, or in some medical conditions such as hyperthyroidism. But when we use less energy, the amount of core sleep, and GH release, is reduced.

This is why a rewarding and stimulating day, especially when exercise takes place, leads to improved sleep and more GH. This means that a happy and well-balanced lifestyle will improve your looks, your physique and your immune system – another example of modern science rediscovering the classical idea of a healthy mind in a healthy body.

Finally, sex causes a burst of GH release. This is not only good for the skin (unless it keeps you up all night) but could also explain why a good sex life is associated with slower ageing.

Beauty sleep

The notion of 'beauty sleep' is not just an old wives' tale.

Growth hormone released while we sleep repairs tissues. This is why a string of late nights resulting in reduced growth hormone synthesis shows in the skin.

... and Arginine

Why do fit people look healthier? Exercise triggers deeper, longer sleep, which produces more Growth Hormone, which repairs the body better. Sex does the same.

If you can't change your lifestyle to incorporate more sleep, sex or exercise, try an arginine supplement.

This amino acid stimulates the synthesis and release of Growth Hormone, and has a place in serious skin rejuvenation programmes.

Many athletes and bodybuilders use GH boosters. Most of these are based on the amino acids arginine and ornithine.

Preventing ageing skin

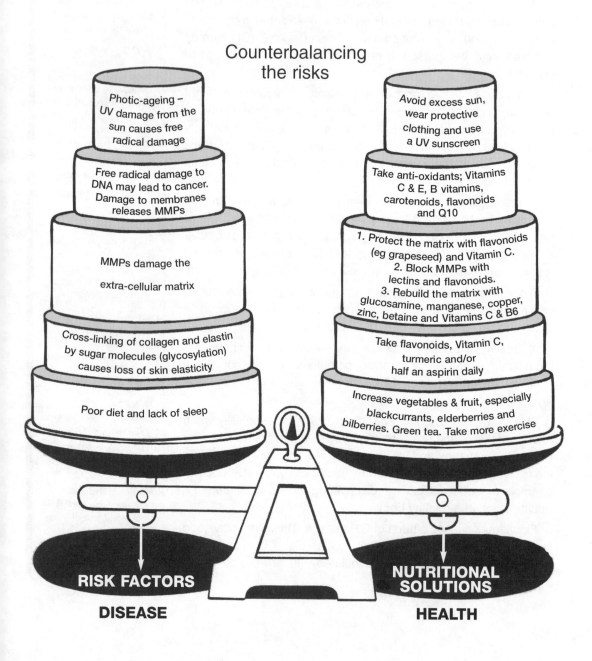

Counterbalancing
the risks

Photic-ageing –
UV damage from the
sun causes free
radical damage

Free radical damage to
DNA may lead to cancer.
Damage to membranes
releases MMPs

MMPs damage the

extra-cellular matrix

Cross-linking of collagen and elastin
by sugar molecules (glycosylation)
causes loss of skin elasticity

Poor diet and lack of sleep

Avoid excess sun,
wear protective
clothing and use
a UV sunscreen

Take anti-oxidants; Vitamins
C & E, B vitamins,
carotenoids, flavonoids
and Q10

1. Protect the matrix with flavonoids
(eg grapeseed) and Vitamin C.
2. Block MMPs with
lectins and flavonoids.
3. Rebuild the matrix with
glucosamine, manganese, copper,
zinc, betaine and Vitamins C & B6

Take flavonoids, Vitamin C,
turmeric and/or
half an aspirin daily

Increase vegetables & fruit, especially
blackcurrants, elderberries and
bilberries. Green tea. Take more exercise

RISK FACTORS

DISEASE

**NUTRITIONAL
SOLUTIONS**

HEALTH

SUMMARY

Keep young and beautiful ...

Avoiding UV

▶ Even in temperate countries such as the UK, there are many cases of skin cancer in people who have never been abroad.

So during the summer months:

▶ Keep children out of the sun between 11 am and 3 pm (this also applies, to a lesser extent, to adults, especially those with fair skin).

▶ Stay in the shade.

▶ Wear loose, cool clothing which doesn't leave vulnerable areas like the shoulders exposed.

▶ Wear a hat with a broad brim to protect the face.

▶ Use a sunscreen, minimum SPF 15, with UVA and UVB filters.

▶ Sunglasses (or contacts) with UV filters should be used.

▶ Don't forget UV protection for your hair.

Skin savers

▶ Stop smoking.

▶ Stock up on anti-oxidants C, E, Q10, mixed carotenoids and flavonoids.

▶ Eat lots of blackcurrants and/or blueberries and/or elderberries, which contain matrix stabilising flavonoids. Combine with glucosamine, manganese and betaine.

▶ If you don't like fruit products, take half an aspirin daily. The salicylate it contains slows the cross-linking in collagen, as well as reducing the risk of heart attacks.

▶ Take more exercise, and ...

▶ Get a good night's sleep.

▶ Look for skin care products that contain a well-balanced range of anti-oxidants and matrix stabilisers in liposome or phytosome form to ensure penetration into the skin. The best include a good sun block.

▶ Drink plenty of water.

▶ Take a tablespoonful of silicic acid (sold in Europe as Silicol) daily. Found in foods such as watercress, it is claimed to reduce fine lines in ageing skin.

It may work by protecting the fibroblasts that help to build the extra-cellular matrix from aluminium poisoning .

Part 4

DIETS WHICH PROMOTE HEALTH

*T*he direct link between nutrition and health or illness is increasingly clear. The respective roles of diet and supplements are emerging too.

For many reasons – our reduced calorie requirements, the depleted soil our crops are grown in, the prolonged storage of fruit and vegetables, food-processing methods, increased pollution – the diet we eat today does not provide all the nutrients we need to stay really healthy.

Supplements fill the gaps. And as we have seen, supplements taken strategically, whether to ward off the flu or heart disease, are among the most potent medicines.

But there's little point in dosing yourself up every morning if your diet consists of burgers and chips. The everyday foods which make up our diet are vitally important – a crucial and basic link in the supplement-lifestyle-diet circle which can give us longer, healthier lives.

This section provides a guide to all the elements explored in Health Defence. Which nutrients, at what levels, and in what forms should you be getting?

Chapter 19

Health care through Functional Foods

The wars against cancer, Alzheimer's, coronary artery disease, osteoporosis and the other major killers will not be won in the pharmaceutical labs. Indeed the industry's singular lack of success in these areas reinforces the conviction that drugs cannot be an adequate answer to problems caused largely by multiple micro-nutrient depletion.

Nor will popular victory come from molecular biology – because although genetically engineered agents will undoubtedly make a difference to some, they will be proprietary, expensive and unavailable for mass use.

If we want to ensure healthier (and longer) lives for all: if we want to have the same impact on coronary artery disease, for example, as the sanitation engineers had on cholera, turning it from an epidemic to a medical curiosity; the way forward is through the improvement of the public diet.

Functional foods

A definition

Foods which either naturally contain ingredients with health benefits; or, increasingly, foods to which such ingredients have been added.

Pills or foods?

Supplements are invaluable and the first choice for many people, but there are many others who don't like taking tablets and capsules.

Unfortunately, many of the so-called one-a-day supplements are inadequate in terms of the number, type and level of micro-nutrients used. Products that feature 100% of all the RDAs usually do not contain enough of the classical micro-nutrients to give optimal protection. And they usually do not contain any of the newly discovered micro-nutrients such as isoflavones, carotenoids, flavonoids, etc.

This is where so-called 'functional foods' should come to the fore. These are basically food products, in a variety of forms, with enhanced levels of the key micro-nutrients, sometimes accompanied by reduced levels of ingredients judged to be less beneficial such as refined sugar or animal fat.

Whilst the current way forward is through supplements, I strongly believe that the true medicine of the 21st century will eventually be food – a 'superfood' containing all the ingredients in the right form and at optimum levels that provide the highest chance of a long and healthy life.

But what would the superfood contain?

The reader who has got this far will have understood the importance of a wide range of micro-nutrients in reducing the impact of the ageing process.

Anti-oxidants have received most of the publicity; but there is a great deal more to comprehensive anti-ageing nutrition. Apart from the anti-oxidants, there are at least eight other categories of micro-nutrients which must be available in adequate amounts if the body is to receive optimal nutritional support, and the best chance of realising its true biological potential.

Initially you may have to buy these nutrients in traditional capsule/tablet form, but I hope that some manufacturer will eventually develop a 'functional' food that includes all the key ingredients. Such a functional or superfood might take the form of a chew, a non-bake biscuit, or even a yoghurt-type dessert.

On a more limited scale some functional foods are beginning to appear – because as the connections between our diet and our health become clearer, and are supported by more studies, industry is beginning to catch on.

We've been through the low-fat, low-calorie, low-taste, low-salt phase. Instead of taking things out, the new wave of foods *adds* value by adding new nutrients to old recipes in order to actively promote health.

Food manufacturers have, of course, been putting vitamins in our breakfast cereals and iodine in our table salt for years. Now they're adding phyto-nutrients, minerals, fibres and other kinds of nutrients to our milk, biscuits, chocolate bars, quiches and soft drinks.

**Functional foods
A national example**

Hypertension is an important cause of heart failure and stroke, and requires distinct nutritional care and prevention.

In Finland, country-wide trials have shown conclusively that replacing sodium in the diet with potassium and magnesium is the most cost-effective way of lowering blood pressure safely.

Between 1986 and 1996, the national diastolic blood pressure fell an average of 10mm mercury; and the numbers of heart attacks and strokes fell by a massive 50%.

No drugs were involved; when the food industry switched from common salt to the salt substitute PanSalt, they did more good than the entire Finnish health care budget. (PanSalt is made by the Finnish company Raiso.)

The doses are generally smaller than in supplements, because food manufacturers are committed to preventing even the remotest possibility of accidental overdose – and must take a conservative position, based on consensus science. But the main difference is in the presentation.

Whereas tablets and capsules only reach a proportion of consumers, the same ingredients added to yoghurts or breads, for example, can reach the mass market and change public health statistics. This has happened in Finland, where the extensive use of PanSalt – which substitutes a potassium/magnesium formula for common salt (sodium chloride) – has lowered blood pressure safely and reduced the incidence of stroke on a national scale.

You won't find a functional food section in your local supermarket yet, but you will find an increasing number of foods with added Omega 3s, 'friendly' bacteria (eg live yoghurts and other fermented milk products), and anti-oxidants.

Can functional foods improve public health?

Some commentators[11] regard functional foods as just an attempt by food manufacturers to increase their profit margins at the expense of the consumer. In some cases they may be right but the evidence suggests that genuinely functional foods will be of real benefit. Many studies have found widespread malnutrition among the public at large. It is increasingly accepted that this malnutrition is a risk factor for conditions ranging from spina bifida to coronary artery disease to cancer; and conversely that enhanced nutrition is the best way to reduce risk.

Breakfast cereals were the first foods to be routinely fortified and can be considered as early functional foods. Breakfast eaters have a higher intake of fibre, B vitamins, calcium, iron and Vitamins A, C and E than non-breakfast eaters, thanks largely to breakfast cereal consumption[1]. Even this slight dietary improvement has been linked to a reduced risk of cerebral palsy in new-born babies[3].

There is much research to be done, but I have no doubt that functional foods can greatly improve public health.

But isn't all food functional?

The more conservative scientists don't like the term 'functional foods', and they have a point.

It's hard to think of a food which isn't functional, even if that function is only to provide taste, or bulk, or calories. And foods like soy, red wine, blueberries, dark chocolate, green tea, cranberry juice, oatmeal and herring – to give just a few examples – are undoubtedly and intrinsically functional.

Uphill climb

It won't happen overnight. Exaggerated health claims by the media will inevitably cause disappointment, as will sub-standard products, which make implicit claims they cannot fulfil.

In the UK, for example, the sale of nutritional supplements is relatively unregulated, except in terms of the claims that can be made. Apart from that fig-leaf (and it's actually counter-productive in that it prevents the consumer from finding out what a given supplement will do) consumers have insufficient protection.

They have no way of knowing whether the tablet, capsule, or bar has been so badly formulated that its contents cannot be absorbed – or whether the amount of each nutrient will actually do any good.

Some supplement manufacturers only put a token amount of some of the most expensive nutrients in their product, so the list on the pack looks impressive. That's why I have listed (on pages 338-340) the levels I believe are genuinely therapeutic.

The regulatory authorities, who are over-influenced by the drug companies, continue to adopt a defensive position.

They maintain that any product which makes a medical claim or alludes to a medical condition is a medicine, must therefore have a licence (costing anything between £100,000 – £100 million), and may even require a prescription.

This is entirely appropriate when dealing with a novel molecule, but is not a suitable way of handling extracts of food crops we have co-evolved with and which are widely eaten without known toxicity.

Another problem with the regulatory authorities is that they dislike compound formulations. 'Polypharmacy', as they call it, is considered inferior. The pharmaceutical companies are always looking for a better 'magic bullet', designed to hit one single link in the disease chain so hard that it kills the disease, an approach almost guaranteed to produce side effects.

The nutritionist, on the other hand, tries to modify as many of the links as possible, subtly, gently, effectively and hopefully without side effects.

Setting standards

Reputable trade associations such as the Health Food Manufacturers' Association (in Britain) are particularly concerned with maintaining and raising production standards: but there are still too many companies operating outside the HFMA's limits.

Food as preventative medicine

An ageing population, rising health-care costs, a growing awareness of the limitations of traditional 'crisis management' health care, and a public which is generally more health-conscious, all mean that foods which can help sustain health are increasingly seen as the way forward.

Wedded as they are to the single agent approach, the regulatory authorities find it hard to understand the more complex relationships between multiple food ingredients and health.

To give just one example, fish oil has been shown to reduce the risk of coronary artery disease, as have Vitamins E and C. From the herbal community we learn that hawthorn has very significant benefits on heart health, and recent investigations have shown that some of its active ingredients work in a way which complements the C, E and fish oil.

Then there's work from the USA and Finland showing the role of the B vitamins and betaine in reducing plasma levels of homocysteine, an amino acid which raises the risk of clot formation.

When you know how each of these actives works, it is logical to combine all of them – and illogical of the medical regulatory authorities to refuse to deal with nutraceutical combinations like this.

Whilst the public needs to be protected against fraud, it's also true that reputable manufacturers are prevented from getting information to the general public that could save many millions of lives. Indeed that has been a major motive in writing this book.

FOSHU to you

In Japan, which has the most highly developed market in these products, they are termed 'Foods for Specified Health Use' (FOSHU or TOKUHO).

These terms, although accurate, are unlikely to become popular in the West!

In Japan

Q: Why does the Japanese Ministry for Health actively promote functional foods?

A: The ageing Japanese population creates increasing health-care costs. Functional foods are seen to be not only the most effective way of improving public health – but also the most cost-effective.

THE FUNCTIONAL FOOD RACE

Japan was first in the race, and remains in front. Japanese manufacturers of functional foods work to exacting standards. Labelling is easily understood, and the customer has a clear idea of the health benefits of the food he or she is buying.

As a result, the Japanese market in functional foods has expanded to $11 billion – approximately eight percent of the processed food market.

Functional foods include drinks, wafers, candies, bars and even noodles.

The European approach is quite different. Current law forbids medicinal claims; and statements like 'cardio-protective nutrition', although justifiable on the basis of scientific evidence, have been disallowed.

In this rather hostile climate, food manufacturers in the West are understandably reluctant to invest in new functional foods. However, policy recommendations such as the Joint Health Claims Initiative (UK) and the Health Canada Initiative will help to grow the market.

Through the red tape

In the USA the FDA have grudgingly admitted health claims for only a few items, including dietary fibre and whole grains in reducing the risk of colon cancer and heart disease; lipids in affecting the risk of cancer and heart disease; calcium and osteoporosis; and sodium and hypertension. These are not particularly good claims. Calcium by itself is not a good treatment for osteoporosis, nor is sodium reduction on its own very important except in a sub-set of hypertensive patients.

There are many other stronger health claims which could and should be made, but cannot because of administrative stonewalling.

In contrast, the Japanese government has recognised 12 broad classes of food ingredients as promoting health[1] including:

- Dietary fibres, eg inulin: which reduce the risk of colo-rectal cancer and heart disease, and modify sugar absorption in diabetics.

- Oligosaccharides: which modify gut flora, reduce the risk of food poisoning, diarrhoea, and probably colo-rectal cancer. There is also evidence for some immuno-enhancement.

- Lactic acid bacteria (in live yoghurts): which have functions similar to the oligosaccharides.

- Poly-unsaturated fatty acids: beneficial effects on coronary artery disease, arthritis, eczema, asthma, cancers, diabetes, weight control and osteoporosis.

- Phytochemicals (plant extracts like flavonoids and isoflavones) and anti-oxidants: which reduce free radical related and inflammatory diseases.

The future now

We have instinctively known for many generations that we are what we eat. Increasingly, old wisdom and new science show how true that is – and the way forward. If we take note of the new science – and put more emphasis on prevention rather than cure, – we can achieve a dramatic effect on the public health statistics.

STOP PRESS!

The Food and Drug Administration in America has just accepted a well-substantiated claim that soy protein lowers cholesterol, and may reduce the risk of heart disease.

Goldrush

The multi-nationals are investing large amounts of money and time in phytochemicals[4]. Nestlé, for example, have taken a special interest in carnosol and carnosic acid, derived from the herb rosemary.

These compounds are powerful anti-oxidants, bind destructive free iron, and have anti-cancer properties[5, 6]. You can expect to see rosemary or rosemary extract listed as an ingredient in functional foods in the future as well as catechins, strong anti-oxidants that survive cooking well[7-11].

A functional food that included all the nutritional categories we reviewed in the early sections of this book and the specific nutrients and levels detailed in the next chapter would, I believe, make a dramatic impact on our health.

If each of us ensured that our diet included these nutrients and foods, we would see a rise in healthy longevity and a very significant fall in the amount of money being spent on the National Health Service.

21st Century Health Care?

Until recently, few people knew more about their bodies than their weight, or their blood group. New health monitoring devices mean we'll all be better informed.

The current generation of breathalysers can already detect diabetes, colon cancer, kidney failure, liver failure, lactose intolerance, Helicobacter pylori infection and other problems. The devices will be miniaturised and sold like personal stereos before long.

Laser acoustics can already measure blood glucose via a probe placed on the skin which gives a read-out, Star Trek style in seconds.

The next generation of probes will use tunable laser diodes. One touch on the wrist will provide a comprehensive read-out of your biochemistry. The data can either be fed down a phone line to a clinical centre for diagnosis or into your own personal computer.

Add diagnostic software and you have a home diagnostic centre, capable of detecting potential illness long before symptoms appear, long before a doctor might pick it up.

Your genetic make-up will become a factor. (Some people are salt-sensitive, some do not respond to fish oil, others cannot utilise folic acid, etc.) This will create a new science of nutrigenomics.

The next phase will link your health and your genetic data to your shopping habits, so your virtual on-line supermarket can flag potential hazards or recommend beneficial foods according to your body's personal requirements.

Ultimately we will no longer have to worry about nutrition and health because optimum nutrition will become embedded in the consumer environment.

EXISTING SUPERFOODS

Foods you should include frequently in your diet:

- Fruit, especially bilberries, elderberries, tomatoes, blackcurrants, prunes, raisins, strawberries, bananas

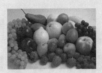

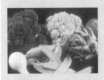

- Vegetables, especially soy and other beans, broccoli, Brussels sprouts, cabbage, Jerusalem artichokes, kale, lentils, peas, chick peas, peppers, sweet potato and onions

- Oily fish, eg salmon, mackerel, herring, sardines
- Herbs, including rosemary, oregano, and thyme

- Juices, especially orange, grapefruit, cranberry, blackcurrant and black grape

- Red wine
- Spices, especially turmeric, ginger and garlic
- Eggs
- Seeds, eg sunflower, linseed
- Soya products
- Tea, especially green
- Wholegrains, including oatmeal and wheat
- Dark chocolate

SUMMARY

Health care through functional foods and supplements

- Categories of nutrients that offer a comprehensive positive health-care strategy include
  * anti-oxidants
  * vitamins and minerals
  * isoflavones (eg genistein)
  * Pre-biotics
  * Omega 3 oils

  * carotenoids (mixed)
  * flavonoids (grapeseed, elderberry, bilberry)
  * betaine
  * co-enzyme Q10
  * adaptogens (Withania Somnifera)

- Start with a better diet. This is now widely agreed to contain more fruits, vegetables, wholegrains and fish; less animal products, sugars, and salt; alcohol in moderation (not spirits), and no tobacco.

- Emphasise foods which are naturally good sources of micro-nutrients (see above).

- Look for functional processed foods, and/or top up with supplements.

Chapter 20

Countering the ageing process

Nobody dies of old age. At this stage of the book we can finally begin to answer the questions posed in the first paragraphs of the first chapter.

- Are we really old at 70?

- Why do we sicken and die in our seventies and eighties when our biological potential lifespan is so much longer?

- Shouldn't we really regard the seventh and eighth decades as middle age?

- And if so, why do the vast majority of us age so prematurely?

The answers to these riddles are all linked. They are also relatively easy to apply.

1 As we age, our diet and life style ensures that we develop increasingly severe multiple micro-nutrient depletion; causing progressive metabolic and physiological imbalances.

2 These imbalances shackle the body's power of repair and allow the process of decay to predominate. This is the ultimate cause of most of the diseases that cripple our later years and eventually kill us, long before our full biological potential.

3 Comprehensive micro-nutrient support is the only way to rectify multiple micro-nutrient depletion, and to reduce the risk of the diseases of ageing. And when we delay the diseases of ageing, we are slowing the process of ageing itself.

Putting it all together

This chapter summarises **fourteen** support or defence strategies that together make up a comprehensive nutritional programme.

The programme will greatly reduce the risk of most of the chronic degenerative diseases, and lower the incidence of many infectious illnesses.

The way ahead

Until today, anti-ageing strategies have been largely unsuccessful. This is because we did not know what the nature of the ageing process was.

I believe that we can now, for the first time, decode the process of ageing: break it down into its sub-routines, and propose rational strategies designed to modify each and perhaps all of the major components of mortality.

Clearly, a wide range of micro-nutrients have a role to play in reducing the impact of ageing.

Anti-oxidants have received most of the publicity; but there is a great deal more to anti-ageing nutrition. Apart from the anti-oxidants, there are at least eight other categories of micro-nutrients which must be available in adequate amounts if the body is to receive optimal nutritional support, and the best chance of realising its true biological potential.

This chapter describes how these nine categories of micro-nutrients modify all fourteen of the sub-routines of ageing being described in the following pages. It presents a composite nutritional anti-ageing strategy, which reflects current leading edge research. It will greatly reduce the risk of most chronic degenerative diseases, lower the incidence of many infectious illnesses, and extend your healthy life.

I have included an optional hormone replacement module. Growth Hormone, testosterone, DHEA, melatonin and other hormones may play a significant role in anti-ageing programmes, but are outside the remit of this nutritional guide. I suspect that an optimal nutritional programme as described below will reduce age-related damage to the hormone-producing tissues, and slow the decline of the endocrine system, thereby making hormone replacement programmes partially or totally redundant.

The following programmes should ideally be added on to a basically healthy lifestyle (ie no smoking, moderate exercise and moderate drinking). But if you are not yet ready to live the good life, the programme acts as a partial antidote, and should still confer considerable health and life-extending benefits.

Healthy lifestyle

The following 14 programmes should ideally be added on to a basically healthy lifestyle (ie moderate exercise, no smoking, moderate drinking).

But if you are not yet ready to live the good life, the programme is designed to act as an antidote, and should still confer considerable health and life-extending benefits.

Nutraceuticals

Nutraceuticals are extracts from foods, presented as capsules or tablets, which have health benefits.

THE FOOD SUPPLEMENTS BALANCE: Ageing

Ageing Mechanisms	Nutritional Counters
1 Excessive free radicals **Aim:** To reduce free radical damage to DNA, proteins, cell membranes and other lipid components such as LDL cholesterol.	a) The trace minerals needed for optimal anti-oxidant enzyme activity include zinc, copper, manganese and selenium. Iron is also required, but should probably not be used unless iron deficiency symptoms have been diagnosed. The enzymes can be up-regulated by moderate exercise. b) Vitamins C and E are well documented. To these can be added the flavonoids, the carotenoids, alpha lipoic acid, Co-enzyme Q10, and possibly melatonin.
2 Excessive cross-links **Aim:** To protect proteins and other types of molecule in the body from cross-linking and loss of function (glycosylation). This form of tissue damage plays an important role in many of the end-effects of diabetes, including kidney damage, cataract, and lesions of the blood vessels; and in the ageing of the connective tissues such as occurs in skin.	a) Many flavonoids have the ability to block abnormal glycosylation of proteins and this property, together with their anti-oxidant effects, makes them invaluable therapeutic and anti-ageing compounds. Green tea, red wine, pycnogenol, ginkgo, turmeric and other sources are all suitable. b) Aspirin is also a good anti-glycosylant, and a widely available alternative to flavonoids in this respect. Gastric irritation is an occasional side effect.
3 Methyl group depletion **Aim:** To supply the body with sufficient methyl groups to achieve adequate DNA methylation, optimise the immune system, the hypothalamic-adrenal axis, liver and kidney function, phospholipid, and lipid metabolism and neurotransmitter synthesis; and prevent the toxic accumulation of homocysteine—thereby reducing the risk of heart disease and Alzheimer's.	a) Betaine. b) Vitamin B complex is an alternative, but is not universally effective. c) Choline is less effective than either of the above.

Ageing Mechanism	Nutritional Counters
4 Pre-biotic depletion **Aim:** To normalise bowel microbiology and function, and reduce the risk of food poisoning, constipation, colitis, colon and colorectal cancer, liver cancer and possibly breast cancer.	Mixed short- and long-chain non-digestible oligosaccharide fibres (NDOs). Short-chain NDOs such as FOS or beta glucans from oats provide cover for the proxmal colon. Longer chain NDOs such as inulin are likely to be more helpful for the distal colon and rectum.
5 Membrane breakdown **Aim:** To prevent the loss of cell membrane components and function which develop when the rate of breakdown of phospholipid structures outstrips the rate at which the body can replace them.	a) Appropriate anti-oxidants to slow phospholipid oxidation. b) Betaine to increase endogenous phospholipid synthesis in the liver. c) Phosphatidyl Serine (PS)
6 Mitochondrial damage **Aim:** To prevent the run-down in cellular energy caused by progressive oxidative damage to the mitochondria.	Co-enzyme Q10 and beta carotene to enhance the rate of energy production in the mitochondria and protect the mitochondrial structure. Acetyl carnitine can also improve mitochondrial stability.
7 Cardiovascular damage **Aim:** To prevent coronary artery disease, or to reduce pre-existing atheroma.	a) Anti-oxidants to stabilise both the lipids (fats) and the structural elements in the arteries (ie Vitamins E, C, mixed carotenoids and flavonoids). b) Betaine to reduce homocysteine and increase HDL. Lecithin (or another source of mixed phospholipids) can be used to increase HDL levels. c) Omega 3 PUFAs to reduce inflammatory microlesions in the blood vessels, platelet stickiness and cardiac electrical instability.

Ageing Mechanism	Nutritional Counters
8 a) **Elevated blood pressure** **Aim:** To reduce blood pressure. b) **Thromboembolic stroke** (when a blood vessel in the brain is blocked by atheroma and/or platelets) **Aim:** To reduce the risk of thrombus (blockage)	a) Hypertension is an important cause of heart failure and stroke. Switch from sodium salt to a potassium/magnesium substitute. b) Flavonoids and Omega 3 PUFAs to reduce inflammation in the blood vessels, platelet stickiness and cardiac electrical instability.
9 **Nervous system deterioration** **Aim:** To prevent oxidative damage in the central and peripheral nervous systems.	a) Phosphatidyl Serine (PS) combined with appropriate anti-oxidants, ie Vitamins C and E, to support peripheral nerves b) Thyme oil as additional anti-oxidant. Betaine to increase phospholipid synthesis and to reduce homocysteine levels; with B complex for additional support.
10 **Immune system run-down** **Aim:** To maintain near-optimal immune cover.	a) Broad spectrum vitamins and minerals, including Vitamin E and carotenoids. b) Betaine to supply essential methyl groups. c) Glutamine to prevent exercise-induced immuno-suppression. d) An adaptogen such as Eleutherococcus or Withania to prevent stress-related immuno-suppression. e) Q10 to increase cellular capacity. f) Prebiotics to enhance resistance to gastro-intestinal infections. g) Anti-adhesins: cranberry juice to reduce severity and risk of urinary tract infection; carrot soup to reduce severity and risk of upper bowel infections.

Ageing Mechanisms	Nutritional Counters
11 Connective tissue deterioration **Aim:** To maintain the extra-cellular matrix. Also to prevent the loss of connective tissue in joints, ligaments, bone, the extra-cellular matrix and skin which occurs when the rate of tissue renewal is outstripped by tissue erosion.	a) Glucosamine hydrochloride plus manganese and betaine boosts synthesis of the amino sugar polymers in cartilage and synovial fluid. b) The combination of Vitamin C and zinc increases collagen synthesis, with silicic acid as an optional extra[1-3]. c) The above micro-nutrients are all essential for the formation of osteoid, the precursor of new bone; but for optimal bone regeneration, they must be combined with copper, and Vitamins B6, K1 and D3. d) If significant inflammation is involved, an anti-inflammatory ingredient like turmeric (curcumin), ginger, and/or ginkgo is essential. For skin protection, add carotenoids and flavonoids.
12 Cancer #1 **Aim:** To prevent genetic damage to your cells.	a) Don't smoke, and avoid excessive exposure to the sun. b) Eat plenty of fruit and vegetables, reduce pickles, fried and smoked foods. c) Anti-oxidant and flavonoid supplements. d) Betaine.
13 Cancer #2 **Aim:** To prevent the uncontrolled growth and spread of cancer cells.	a) Carotenoids (lycopene and alpha carotene) and soy isoflavones to force cancer cells to redifferentiate/commit suicide. b) In the case of colorectal cancer, pre-biotics to increase levels of butyrate (another redifferentiator) in the colon should also be considered.

Ageing Mechanism	Nutritional Counters
Cancer #2 cont.	c) Protease inhibitors (soy beans) and MMP inhibitors (blackcurrant and other flavonoids) to prevent blood vessel growth and metastatic spread. d) Baseline (broad spectrum) vitamins and minerals to support immune function. e) Q10 should also be considered as an immuno-potentiator, especially in the elderly. f) Selenium at 150-200mcg a day.
14 Hormone imbalance Aim: To maintain levels of key anabolic and parent hormones at optimal levels.	a) DHEA (in some countries) OR Yam extract containing standardised amounts of diosgenin boosts levels of DHEA, the parent steroid hormone. b) Growth Hormone levels may be increased by physical exercise, better sleep patterns and the amino acid arginine.

If you look at the above list, you will see that a truly comprehensive nutrition (or nutraceutical) plan would include:

1 Anti-oxidants
2 Vitamins and minerals
3 Carotenoids (like lutein lycopene and beta carotene)
4 Flavonoids (like grapeseed extract)
5 Isoflavones (like genistein)
6 Betaine
7 Omega 3 oils
8 NDO (non-digestible pre-biotic oligosaccharides)
9 Co-enzyme Q10, and glucosamine
10 Adaptogens

Apart from the last nutrient (ie adaptogens), which has a slightly specialist function, all these nutrients are involved in the nutritional jigsaw we referred to in *The Big Picture* at the beginning of the book.

Specialist cases (like brain function in the elderly) might call for extra nutrients like phosphatidyl serine and thyme oil; but in the majority of cases the nutritional jigsaw approach provides comprehensive cover against all the major components of ageing.

ANTI-OXIDANT SCORES

The average Western diet provides about 1400 ORAC (anti-oxidants) units per day (see *The Big Picture*).

The USDA Home Nutrition Research Centre on Ageing recommend we double or treble this level of intake for better health.

The supplement programme recommended on page 338 would provide approximately 3,500 ORAC units a day.

Chapter 21

Selecting the right supplements –

Suggested Optimum Daily Amounts

For anyone who wishes to use nutraceuticals or functional foods to protect their health or to treat a medical condition, this book aims to provide a guide to the best micro-nutrients and phyto-chemicals currently available.

Identifying the appropriate ingredients, however, is only half the battle; it is equally important to take them in the form that the body can most effectively absorb. **And** at the optimum levels. **And** to combine them rationally.

The list on page 338 is my best estimate, based on the literature, of the dose levels of the key micro-nutrients for prophylactic use; ie for the healthy who wish to stay healthy.

It is outside the scope of this book to offer precise nutritional recipes for existing illness, although it is generally true that in nutraceutical medicine, the levels of micro-nutrients required to cure a problem are often higher dose versions of levels for preventative health care.

Individual nutritional needs may differ depending on levels of activity, smoking habits, diet, sex, age and other factors. For that reason, the doses given represent a mid-point, suitable for the great majority of people. The list will be updated as further information becomes available.

In the appendices I have recommended a specific form for certain micro-nutrients, where there is evidence that this form is more bio-available, ie better absorbed by the body. For example, some minerals may be better absorbed as chelates (ie bound with

---

Caveat emptor!

Over 40 per cent of British adults now take supplements. Sadly, the great majority are *not* receiving the health benefits they are hoping for – as the simple ORAC test quoted on page 335 makes clear.

a protein). Some vitamins are more efficiently absorbed when pre-dissolved in edible oil. Others (generally the water-soluble vitamins) are better given as sustained release preparations. If these are not available, divided doses taken morning and night are an alternative. Isoflavones are better absorbed as aglycones (ie stripped of sugar molecules), and so on.

Beware of the quality of some supplements

Sadly, too many vitamin and mineral supplements still contain the wrong micro-nutrients, in the wrong doses and in the wrong combinations. Until national quality standards can be set in place to protect the consumer, you will have to check the ingredients in your supplement very carefully before you can be sure whether or not it can deliver on its promises.

Plenty of multi-vitamin/mineral tablets contain iron in the form of iron oxide (otherwise known as rust). Iron in this form is not recommended. It is not well absorbed into the body, and by generating free radicals in the gut, may actually harm the gastrointestinal tract. In fact, many of the cheaper mineral salts used by manufacturers to cut costs are so poorly absorbed that they simply pass right through you.

Other micro-nutrient formulations are nearly as bad. Check, for example, the percentage of Omega 3 or 6 essential fatty acids in your fish oil or evening primrose oil capsules. This can be surprisingly low. (Thus a 1000mg fish oil capsule may have as little as 200mg of Omega 3 as EPA/DHA.) To make matters worse, if they are the cheaper esters, or free acids rather than triglycerides, these will be less well absorbed – so you will need more of them.

High-dose poly-unsaturate formulations without an accompanying hefty dose of an appropriate anti-oxidant mix will increase your free radical load, and can eventually cause serious health problems – yet there are still plenty of these on sale.

Q10 tablets are cheaper than Q10 pre-dissolved in edible oil in capsules, and may look a better buy; but pre-dissolved Q10 is so much better absorbed that the capsules generally provide better value for money.

WARNING

Check the label of any supplement against the recommended amounts provided on page 338.

Too often manufacturers include too few of the important nutrients, at too low levels, and in cheap, poorly absorbed forms.

For example, I submitted three of the leading UK multi-vitamin and mineral supplement brands to ORAC testing, which measures their capacity to absorb free radicals.

They scored 111, 117 and 137 on the ORAC scale respectively. In contrast five servings of fruit or vegetables a day should produce an average of 1,400 ORAC units.

Finally, extracts can be confusing. Thus 20mg of soy extract sounds impressive on the pack, but, even if the percentage of isoflavones is as high as 40 per cent, you will only be getting 8mg of the actual soy isoflavones themselves – against the 40mg level I think you may need.

Unless you know about micro-nutrients, it is probably better to stick with the brands used by professional nutritionists. These may be more expensive, but it is often worth paying a little more to ensure quality, and value for money.

Amino Acids

The essential amino acids are not included in my recommended daily supplement, as amino acid depletion is uncommon in anyone eating a diet containing reasonable amounts of animal or soy protein, micro-algae or a balanced intake of vegetables.

Many amino acids can, however, be used as therapeutic tools, and a section on amino acid therapy may be included in the next edition.

Inadequate Amounts

My biggest complaint about many supplement brands is that they use phrases like 'Mega Dose', or 'High Strength' misleadingly.

Look at the pack and you will see a long and impressive list of ingredients. Check more carefully, however, and you find that levels of many of the more expensive ingredients (which are often among the most important nutrients) are token amounts designed to impress by merely being listed on the pack.

Claiming "100% of all the RDAs" is also misleading. Some nutrients, like Vitamins C and E, need much higher levels to be effective; and many micro-nutrients do not yet have an RDA!

One well-known 'Ultra' formula includes just 0.6mg of beta carotene – whereas the minimum level that will make a difference to your health is probably 20 times that dose. And it includes none of the other carotenoids like lycopene or lutein (probably because they are expensive).

Another 'Super' formula did include the other carotenoids but at levels of about 20mcg (sometimes written µg). I would want to see a supplement containing at least 15mg of carotenoids. Since a milligram is 1000 micrograms, this 'Super' formula contains about 1000 times less of the other carotenoids than research indicates is really effective. (It also contained about 10mg of Vitamin E as opposed to the 266mg (or 400IU) that evidence shows to be cardio-protective.)

I am aware that the shelves of the typical health food store and the pack declarations on the typical supplement can be very confusing.

A major motivation in writing this book has been to simplify your task in choosing a diet and in selecting supplements that really will improve your health.

The anti-ageing supplement

Research indicates that the ideal diet designed to protect against cancer, stroke, heart disease, Alzheimer's and ageing is fundamentally the same. This is the basis of my recommended supplement.

The list of nutrients overleaf includes a column headed 'recommended supplement level', plus a comparison with the current RDAs, the average person's daily intake and the upper safe levels for supplements. The recommended levels should help protect against most of the degenerative diseases, as you will see from page 339. Do not exceed them without professional advice.

> **Important**
>
> The recommended doses should not be exceeded without individual nutritional advice.
>
> Pregnant women and patients on medication should consult their physicians before self-treating.

VARYING REQUIREMENTS

Higher risk groups such as smokers, drinkers, athletes, diabetics and sun-worshippers should opt for upper range doses of the anti-oxidants, as their requirements are increased.

Sunbathers should also choose higher doses of the B vitamins, as many of these are degraded by the action of sunlight on skin, and higher doses of carotenoids and flavonoids to protect their skins from UV damage.

My recommended doses of nutrients can be taken by adults of all ages. The only exception is iron. Teenagers and pre-menopausal women are frequently in need of an iron supplement and I recommend 10mg a day.

Men and post-menopausal women don't usually need an iron supplement, so it is not recommended unless iron deficiency anaemia has been diagnosed.

Additional supplements are not needed and are not recommended, unless suggested elsewhere in this book for a particular therapeutic purpose.

As a general rule supplements should be taken with meals, to facilitate absorption and minimise the risk of gastric irritation.

Recommended supplement levels, RDAs and average current daily intakes

	Av. daily intake from a typical Western diet*	My recommended supplement level	Upper safe limit to supplement†	RDA
Vitamin A	1012mcg(3370IU)	800mcg(2664IU)	2300mcg	800mcg
Vitamin C	58mg	500mg	2000mg	60mg
Vitamin D	2.9mcg	15mcg	20mcg	5mcg
Vitamin E	9.3 mg (14IU)	265mg (400IU)	800mg	10mg
Vitamin K	25mcg	50mcg	1000mcg	Not established
Beta carotene ⎫	1.9mg	10mg	20mg	Not established
Lutein	0.5-2.0mg	6mg	Not established	Not established
Lycopene Carotenoids	1-4mg	5mg	Not established	Not established
Zeaxanthin ⎭	0.05-0.1mg	100mcg	Not established	Not established
Vitamin B1	1.7mg	7.5mg	100mg	1.4mg
Vitamin B2	2.0mg	7.5mg	200mg	1.6mg
Niacin	39mg	15mg	450mg	18mg
Pantothenic acid	5mg	15mg	500mg	6mg
Vitamin B6	2.4mg	7.5mg	200mg	2.0mg
Folic acid	252mcg	200mcg	400mcg	200mcg
Vitamin B12	7.2mcg	6.75mcg	500mcg	1mcg
Selenium	35mcg	150mcg	200mcg	75mcg
Zinc	11.1mg	10mg	15mg	15mg
Calcium	917mg	100mg	1500mg	800mg
Magnesium	308mg	50mg	300mg	300mg
Chromium	30mcg	120mcg	200mcg	125mcg
Copper	1.5mg	2mg	5mg	2.5mg
Manganese	4.6mg	4mg	15mg	5mg
Iodine	180mcg	100mcg	1000mcg	200mcg
Molybdenum	50mcg	100mcg	300mcg	Not established
Biotin	30mcg	200mcg	Not established	150mcg
Betaine	5-25mg	450mg	Not established	Not established
Oligoproantho-cyanidins (OPC) ⎫	25mg	100mg	Not established	Not established
Polyphenol complex Flavonoids	95mg	150mg	Not established	Not established
Isoflavones ⎭	2-5mg	40mg	100mg	Not established
Omega 3	100-200mg	600mg	Not established	Not established
Oligo-saccharides (FOS)	1-3g	4g	Not established	Not established
Co-Q10	10mg	30-60mg	Not established	Not established
Glucosamine	N.A.	500mg	Not established	Not established

*Sources: Council For Responsible Nutrition and trade sources   †Source: Council for Responsible Nutrition

The protective roles of the main nutrient groups

	Anti-oxidants (vitamins and minerals)	Vitamin E	Carotenoids (lycopene, beta and alpha carotene, lutein, zeaxanthin)	Flavonoids (grapeseed, OPCs, green tea, red wine)	Isoflavones (genistein, daidzein)	Omega 3	Betaine	Q10	Magnesium/calcium Vitamin D	Glucosamine	Pre-biotics
Heart disease	✔	✔	✔	✔	✓	✔	✔	✔	✔		✓
Stroke	✔	✔		✔	✓	✓	✔	✓	✔	✓	✓
Cancer	✔	✔	✔	✔	✔	✔	✔	✓	✓		✔
Alzheimer's / Mental decline	✔	✔	?	✓	✔	✔	✔	?			?
Ageing	✔	✔	✔	✔	?	✓	✓	✔		✔	✓
Diabetes	✔	✔	?	✔		?					✓
Arthritis	✓	✓	?	✔		✔				✔	
Osteoporosis	?		✓	✔	✔			✔	✔	?	
Asthma	?	?	?	✓		✔	?	?	✔		
Age-related eye disease (macular degeneration)	✔	?	✔	✔				?			
Skin ageing	✔	✔	✔	✔	✓	?	?	?		✔	

Key: ✔ = strong protective effect ✓ = a degree of protection ? = possible protective effect

Note: The strength of effectiveness of protection will vary between nutrient groups and individuals. There is also often a synergy between the different nutrient groups which affects overall protection levels.

Risk Reduction

At the beginning of the book I explained that I believe you can reduce your risk of almost all the degenerative diseases through healthy eating, supplemented by a particular combination of nutrients. I then likened those groups of nutrients to nine pieces of a jigsaw, which all have to be in place to offer comprehensive protection.

The previous two pages specify which nutrients and at what levels. In the appendix on page 343 I have suggested the best **form** of each nutrient. This information is the basis for creating all nine pieces in the nutritional big picture:

- Vitamins and minerals – at levels that are optimum rather than simply RDAs to support the metabolic and immune systems.

- Anti-oxidants – including Vitamins C and E. plus the anti-oxidant minerals to cut the risk of heart disease, cancer and Alzheimer's.

- Carotenoids – beta carotene, lycopene and lutein to cut the risk of many cancers and heart disease, and protect the eyes, skin, etc.

- Flavonoids – as grapeseed/bilberry extract and green tea which act as additional anti-oxidants and protect not only against heart disease and cancer but also against asthma and arthritis.

- Omega 3 fish oil – for added cardio-protective function and for its role in defending against arthritis and asthma.

- Soy isoflavones – genistein and daidzein to cut cancer risks.

- Betaine – which helps protect the heart, liver, nervous and immune systems.

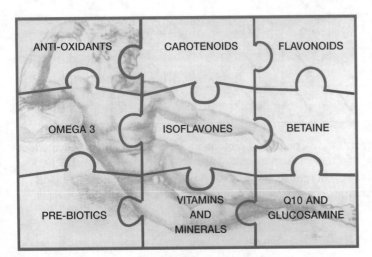

ANTI-OXIDANTS	CAROTENOIDS	FLAVONOIDS
OMEGA 3	ISOFLAVONES	BETAINE
PRE-BIOTICS	VITAMINS AND MINERALS	Q10 AND GLUCOSAMINE

- CoQ10 and Glucosamine – which support the mitochondria and connective tissue (skin and joints) respectively.

- Pre-biotics – which help protect against bowel, liver and, possibly, breast cancers.

Tangible benefits

Such a combination of nutrients is not the cheapest option*– but in health, prevention is definitely better (and cheaper!) than cure. To wait until a health problem manifests itself is to wait too long.

I am very aware that taking supplements can seem like an act of faith. This is why I have not hesitated to give you the research on which I base my conclusions, even though the knowledge base is large and complex.

However for at least one benefit – the anti-oxidant strength of nutritional supplements – science now offers an accurate measurement. The anti-oxidant capacity of my recommended combination of supplements was measured by the ORAC method (as described on page 335), and produced an ORAC score of over 3,000!

To put that into context, five servings of fruit and vegetables deliver an average ORAC score of 1,400, while, as you have seen, the average leading multi-vitamin and mineral formulae at 100% of the RDAs, deliver an average ORAC score of only 122!

It's true that a truly comprehensive nutritional supplement will cost more than most people are used to paying for their vitamins and minerals. However, it is the best form of 'health insurance' I know.

As we get older we begin to plan more for our future – for example taking out a pension. But it doesn't make sense to pay into a pension plan without also taking the 'nutritional insurance' to live out a maximum healthy life span.

Longevity by itself is an over-simple objective. It is the twin objectives of longevity with a high quality of life that most of us seek. I trust this will be a significant contribution to 'quality longevity' for you.

Keep up to date through the Internet

The internet allows instant and inexpensive communication. I shall always be pleased to hear from any reader who has comments, criticisms or new information to offer.

Moreover should later research indicate any modifications in my recommended amounts, I will post them on

www.healthdefence.com

*W*hat are the best nutrient forms?

*D*rug/nutrient reactions

WHAT ARE THE BEST NUTRIENT FORMS?

In some cases the **form** of the nutrient matters a great deal. So if you follow the optimum supplement programme proposed on page 338, you should check to ensure that the following nutrients are in the form recommended.

Vitamins

Vitamin E	natural (dA tocopherol succinate)
Vitamin A	retinol (oil filled capsules)
Vitamin B1	thiamin hydrochloride
Vitamin B3	nicotinamide
Vitamin C	without sodium

Carotenoids

Mixed	oil-filled, light-opaque capsules

Minerals

Iodine	potassium iodide
Molybdenum	sodium molybdate
Iron	ferrous fumarate

Flavonoids

Polyphenols	Green tea powder or leaves
Oligo-proanthocyanidin (OPCs)	Grapeseed or bilberry extract
Isoflavone complex	Soy extract containing genistein, daidzein and other isoflavones in aglycone form

Other nutrients

Omega 3	gel capsules with Vitamin E. Look for the highly concentrated fish oils containing 60% Omega 3 oils, delivering approx 330mg EPA and 220mg DHA (both are Omega 3 oils)
Q10	oil-filled, light-opaque capsules
Glucosamine	hydrochloride, not sulphate

Notes: FOS: Doses of Oligofructose should not exceed 5g unless laxative effects are desired. Start with a low dose and build up in stages; some people are very sensitive to these compounds. It can be stirred into fruit juice or yoghurt or sprinkled on cereal.

Iron: Iron-deficiency anaemia is common amongst teenagers and women of child-bearing age. This group should supplement with iron at 10mg a day, if indicated.

DRUG/NUTRIENT INTERACTIONS

A final note of caution to all self-supplementers. The micro-nutrients listed in this book have many positive effects, and can bring about striking improvements in function and well-being. But this very activity may, in some circumstances, amplify or reduce the effects of certain medications. This is one of the reasons why we urge you to check with your doctor before embarking on any intensive nutraceutical programme.

The better known drug/nutrient interactions are listed below. The list is not comprehensive, and I will be grateful to hear from any practitioners or clinical scientists who know of any other interactions.

A Nutrients which may amplify the effects of certain drugs. Here, taking a supplement may permit the dose of a drug to be reduced; or it may necessitate reducing the dose of the drug(s) to prevent overdose.

Bromelian	Anti-coagulant, thrombolytic and anti-hypertensive drugs
Betaine	Anti-depressants
Carnitine (high dose)	Anti-angina, anti-arrhythmic and lipid-lowering drugs
Cayenne	Anti-coagulants
Chromium	Oral hypoglycaemic drugs
Co-enzyme Q10	Anti-hypertensive, anti-angina and anti-arrhythmic drugs
Garlic (high dose)	Anti-coagulant drugs
Ginkgo	See proanthocyanidins
Ginseng (Korean)	Diuretics
Hawthorn	Anti-hypertensive, anti-arrhythmic and anti-angina drugs, also tranquillisers
Magnesium	Anti-hypertensive, anti-angina, anti-arrhythmic and anti-coagulant drugs
Niacin (high dose)	Cholesterol-lowering drugs
Non-digestible oligo-saccarides (pre-biotics)	Cholesterol-lowering drugs
Omega 3 fish oils (low dose)	Anti-arrhythmic drugs
Omega 3 fish oils (high dose)	Anti-coagulant, lipid-lowering and anti-inflammatory drugs

Potassium	Anti-hypertensive, anti-angina and anti-arrhythmic drugs
Proanthocyanidins (and most flavonoids)	Anti-coagulant, anti-hypertensive and anti-inflammatory drugs, and in some cases anti-histamines also
Soy isoflavones	HRT, Tamoxifen
Taurine	Anti-hypertensive, anti-angina, anti-arrhythmic and lipid-lowering drugs
Vitamin E (high dose)	Anti-coagulant and anti-arrhythmic drugs
5-HTP	Prozac and similar serotonin-specific anti-depressants

B Nutrients which may reduce the efficacy of certain drugs. Here, taking a supplement may contribute to treatment failure.

Fibre (ie brans)	May reduce absorption of minerals including iron and calcium
Fibre (insoluble, ie pectins)	May reduce absorption of the cholesterol-lowering drug lovastatin
Folic acid	Anti-folate drugs such as methotrexate, trimethoprim
Iron	May reduce absorption of carbidopa (anti-convulsant), thyroxine (thyroid hormone), captopril (anti-hypertensive)
Vitamin B6	Anti-Parkinsonism drug levodopa
Vitamin K	Anti-K anti-coagulant drugs such as warfarin

GLOSSARY

adaptogen
Compound which damps the body's response to stress, making it less damaging to our health.

amino acid
Basic building block from which proteins are assembled.

amino sugar
A molecule which combines a sugar with an amino acid, eg glucosamine. These are the basic building blocks from which hyaluronic acid and other micro-fibres in the extra-cellular matrix are assembled.

angiogenesis
The growth of new blood vessels, an important step in the development of diseases including cancer and arthritis.

angiostat
Compound which prevents the formation of new blood vessels (eg shark cartilage, genistein, certain flavonoids, troponin 1 blockers, thalidomide, etc).

anti-adhesin
A molecule which prevents bacteria and other pathogens from binding to docking sites on cells in the body. Can be either a sugar or a flavonoid.

anti-oxidant
A substance or an enzyme capable of neutralising free radicals, which could otherwise cause tissue damage in the body.

apoptosis
Cellular 'suicide'.

arteriosclerosis
Literally, hardening of the arteries. Generally includes atheroma, thickening and/or stiffening of the arterial walls, and some degree of calcification.

astaxanthin
A red carotenoid (responsible for the red in lobster shell and flamingoes' legs) which has relatively unexplored anti-oxidant and anti-cancer properties.

atheroma
The fatty material which deposits inside the lining of the arteries (if you eat the wrong diet and/or smoke) – which can culminate in a heart attack.

betaine/trimethyl glycine
The most efficient dietary source of vital methyl groups.

bifido-bacteria
Health-promoting bacteria, occur in throat, lower bowel and vagina where they form an important defence against infections.

bioavailability
The degree to which a compound can be absorbed into the body.

breakers
New drugs which 'break' cross-links. These are caused by excess sugar linking to protein molecules in the body, 'sticking' them together and impairing their function. This is an important part of the ageing process, so 'breakers' are as critical in anti-ageing as anti-oxidants. Many flavonoids are natural 'breakers'.

carcinogen	A substance which can cause cancer.
carotenoids	A group of compounds derived from foods which have anti-oxidant, immuno-stimulating, anti-cancer and other health-promoting properties. Typically coloured, varying from red (lycopene, astaxanthin) to yellow (lutein) and orange (alpha and beta carotene).
catechins	A group of flavonoids found in various plants, including green tea.
chelation	A process whereby trace minerals are bonded to other molecules (amino acids or sugars) which makes them more bioavailable.
cholesterol	A waxy fat which is a vital constituent of cell membranes. It is also present in the blood, and is the precursor for steroid hormones and bile acids; some of which are carcinogenic.
cholesterol oxidation products (COPs)	When cholesterol in the blood or in cell membranes is oxidised, it breaks down into cholesterol oxidation products. These are highly toxic, and are implicated in various diseases including coronary artery disease.
choline	A methyl group donor. Less effective than betaine.
co-enzyme/co-factor	An atom or molecule which is an essential aid to enzyme function.
collagen	A protein micro-fibre, one of the key components of the extra-cellular matrix. Gives tensile strength.
colloid/colloidal system	A solution in which very fine particles of a substance are suspended in a liquid, eg minerals in water. It is claimed these are better absorbed: there is little data to support this.
cosmaceutical	Cosmetic containing molecules which modify skin chemistry and physiology to produce genuine structural improvements (eg anti-ageing).
cross-linkage	See **breakers** and **glycosylation**.
cytokines	Messenger substances formed by cells for local (ie cell to cell) interactions. Involved in speeding or slowing inflammation.
deficiency	A serious state of malnutrition, where intake of a micro-nutrient is so low that characteristic symptoms of disease appear, typically within weeks or months.
deficiency disease	An illness with a consistent pattern of symptoms that appear soon after the intake of a micro-nutrient, such as Vitamin C, falls below critical levels.
depletion	A type of malnutrition where intakes of several micro-nutrients are sub-optimal; causing metabolic imbalances that, if left untended, surface many years later as a chronic degenerative disease.
DHA/docosahexaenoic acid	One of the Omega 3 acids found in oily fish. It is cardio-protective and essential for the growing brain.
DHEA	A steroid hormone, made in the body from cholesterol. DHEA is linked to sustained health, and is used in various anti-ageing regimes.

GLOSSARY

electrolyte
Sodium, potassium and magnesium are examples of electrolytes, ie charged atoms which contribute to the density and pH of body fluids, the efficiency of enzyme function and the maintenance of electrical voltages over cell membranes.

elastin
A protein micro-fibre, one of the key components of the extra-cellular matrix. Gives elasticity.

enzyme
A protein molecule, made in the body, which catalyses specific chemical reactions.

enzyme inducers
Substances in the diet which stimulate the body to produce increased amounts of various (generally detoxifying) enzymes.

EPA/eicosapentaenoic acid
One of the Omega 3 fatty acids found in oily fish. It is cardio-protective.

extra-cellular matrix
The matrix of micro-fibres (collagen, elastin and amino-sugar polymers) that makes up our 'soft skeleton', and provides structure to all our soft tissues.

flavonoids
A group of compounds derived from foods which have anti-oxidant, anti-glycosylant, anti-inflammatory, anti-bacterial and anti-viral properties. Formerly known as Vitamin P, these are vital ingredients in our diet. Often coloured, they range from curcumin (yellow) to anthocyanins (typically red, blue and purple).

folate/folic acid
Folate is a B vitamin found in foods; folic acid is the synthetic form.

free radical
A highly reactive atom or molecule which, if unchecked, can damage cells in the body. This is thought to be a major cause of illnesses such as coronary artery disease, cancer, cataract and many other chronic degenerative diseases.

fructo-oligosaccharide
A non-digestible oligosaccharide found in onions, leeks and garlic – a good prebiotic.

functional foods
Foods which either naturally contain ingredients with health benefits; or, increasingly, foods to which such ingredients have been added.

GAGs/glycosaminoglycans
Important structural molecules which form (among other things) part of the extra-cellular matrix. Built partly from amino sugars.

genistein
An isoflavone found in soy with many therapeutic indications, including heart disease, cancer, osteoporosis, menopause, etc.

GLA/gamma linoleic acid
Omega 6 fatty acid found in plant oils such as borage oil.

glucosamine
An amino sugar that is the basic building block for hyaluronic acid, and the amino sugar polymers in the extra-cellular matrix. Bypasses the rate-limiting enzyme, glucosamine synthetase.

glutathione
A critical anti-oxidant compound inside your cells which is made in the body. Also involved in detoxification reactions and may be substituted by alpha lipoic acid.

glutathione peroxidase

A key anti-oxidant enzyme. It requires selenium to function.

glycaemic index (GI)

The extent to which the carbohydrate elements in food increase blood sugar levels. Refined, and easily digested, carbohydrates have a high GI, while unrefined carbohydrates have, in general, a low GI. A high GI diet is linked to an increased risk of Type 2 diabetes.

glycosylation

The addition of sugar to other molecules in the body. May cause considerable tissue damage via cross-linking; or increase the risk of infection by providing more docking sites for bacteria. A major cause of ageing, but one which can be blocked by certain flavonoids.

HDL (high density lipoprotein) cholesterol

Cardio-protective form of blood cholesterol. Removes cholesterol from the tissues and deposits it in the liver, and takes phospholipids from the liver and distributes them in the tissues.

homocysteine

An amino acid formed in the body, toxic if there are insufficient methyl groups in the diet. Linked to coronary artery disease and Alzheimer's.

hormone

Messenger substances made in our glands for remote (ie organ to organ) interaction. Hormones include insulin, growth hormone, oestrogen, adrenalin, etc.

hyaluronic acid

A polymer of glucosamine found in the synovial fluid in joints. Provides some cushioning and lubrication.

hypertension

Excessive blood pressure. Risk factor for heart attacks and strokes.

immune system

Complex system of cells and cell messengers which defend us against infection and cancers. May deteriorate with age, and does deteriorate in multiple micro-nutrient depletion.

insulin

A hormone made by the pancreas, needed to transport glucose into cells.

inulin

A non-digestible oligosaccharide found in Jerusalem artichokes and other plants – a pre-biotic.

isoflavones

Flavonoids with hormonal properties found in soy beans and other plants – see **genistein**.

LDL (low density lipoprotein) cholesterol

In excess, and if unprotected by anti-oxidants, a risk factor for coronary artery disease. Essential for taking fat-soluble micro-nutrients such as Vitamin E and Q10 from the liver to the tissues.

lectin

A glycoprotein with a tightly packed structure, generally found in plant foods. Many lectins are resistant to digestion, and are biologically active, ie they block protease, or trigger cell division. Some are toxic; others are potentially important nutraceuticals.

lipid oxidation products (LOPs)

When lipids in the blood or in cell membranes are oxidised, they form lipid oxidation products. These are highly toxic, and implicated in various diseases including coronary artery disease. See **cholesterol oxidation products**.

GLOSSARY

lipofucsin
The brown pigment in age or 'liver spots', formed when lipids in the body are oxidised. Large numbers of age spots indicate that your anti-oxidant defences are inadequate, and your cells are ageing.

lipoic acid
Like Q10, this is a co-factor in oxidative phosphorylation and an anti-oxidant. Interacts very positively with Vitamin E.

lutein
Carotenoid derived commercially from marigold and chrysanthemum petals. Occurs also in kale and spinach. Protects against macular degeneration of the eye, and probably cardio-protective also.

lycopene
A carotenoid derived from tomatoes. Anti-cancer agent, and powerful cardio-protectant.

matrix metallo-proteases
A group of up to 20 enzymes which between them dissolve all the elements in the extra-cellular matrix. Produced by cancer cells, so-called 'flesh-eating' bacteria, and cells whose membranes have been damaged by oxidation.

metabolism
The complex chemistry, consisting of many thousands of reactions, that is the basis of life – and all our bodily functions.

methyl group
A simple group of atoms (1 carbon and 3 hydrogen atoms) which cannot be synthesised in the body, and must be obtained from the diet. Essential for DNA replication, detoxification mechanisms, stress responses and many other metabolic functions.

micro-nutrient
Compounds derived from the diet, typically in milligram or microgram amounts, which are essential for normal growth and for maintaining health. Classically, only vitamins and trace minerals fall into this group; but flavonoids, carotenoids and certain other groups of molecules also qualify.

mineral
A chemical element such as calcium or magnesium. If you need less than 100mg/day, it is termed a trace element; such as iron, copper, zinc and selenium.

mitochondria
Tiny bean-shaped structures in the cells where energy from the food you eat is transferred to the cell by a process called oxidative phosphorylation. This is a slow form of burning; carbon is burned in oxygen to produce carbon dioxide, water and heat.

mono-unsaturates
Mono-unsaturated fatty acids (MUFAs) contain a single double bond, and are liquid at room temperatures (eg olive, peanut oils)

multiple micro-nutrient depletion
A form of malnutrition prevalent in the West, where the diet is low in many or most micro-nutrients. Increases the risk of many diseases.

neurotransmitter
Chemicals made in the body which transfer information between nerve cells. These include acetyl choline, serotonin, dopamine and noradrenaline.

non-digestible oligosaccharide	A type of carbohydrate which is not digested in the small bowel, so passes intact into the large bowel where it stimulates the growth of healthy bacteria. A pre-biotic.
nutraceutical	Extracts from foods, presented as pills or tablets, which have health benefits.
nutrient	Compounds derived from the diet, typically expressed in gram amounts, which are essential for normal growth and health. Proteins, fats and carbohydrates fall into this group; more recent work indicates that certain fibre types also qualify.
oestrogen	A female sex hormone made in the ovaries and uterus.
OPs/organo-phosphates	New pesticides which have replaced the organo-chlorine poisons such as DDT. Implicated in many disease states.
OPCs/oligomeric proanthocyanidins	Flavonoids, found in red wine, grapeseed, pine bark and other plant sources, with many therapeutic indications.
osteoporosis	Thinning of the bones leading to increased risk of fracture. Nutritional factors are very important.
oxidation	The biological equivalent of rusting, which occurs when free radicals attack the body.
PCBs/poly-chlorinated biphenyls	Industrial chemicals used, among other things, as coolants. Implicated in various disease states.
PGs/proteoglycans	Important structural molecules which form (among other things) part of the extra-cellular matrix. Built partly from amino sugars.
phosphatidyl choline	A phospholipid which forms the bulk of cell membranes, and is fairly unreactive. Some is broken down to form the neurotransmitter acetyl choline.
phosphatidyl serine	A phospholipid which anchors proteins such as ion pumps into cell membranes. Some may be transformed into phosphatidyl choline.
phospholipids	Molecules which contain fatty acids, and are the building blocks of cell membranes and HDL cholesterol particles. Derived from food or made in the liver.
phytochemical	Compounds derived from plants.
phytoestrogen	Substance derived from plants that mimics oestrogen. One example is genistein, from soy.
phytonutrient	Compounds derived from plants, generally food plants, which have been shown to be important for health, such as the carotenoids and flavonoids.
poly-unsaturate	Poly-unsaturated fatty acids (PUFAs) contain more than one double bond, and are liquid at room temperature (eg sunflower, safflower oils).

GLOSSARY

pre-biotic   A dietary substance which stimulates the growth of bifidobacteria and other healthy bacteria in the gut. Non-digestible oligosaccharides and resistant starches do this. More effective than ...

pro-biotic   Healthy bacteria, consumed either in fermented milk products or as supplements. Not very effective.

progesterone   Female sex hormone, made in the ovaries by the corpora lutea.

prostaglandins   Messenger substances made in the body from fatty acids. May be pro- or anti-inflammatory, depending on the type of fats and oils in the diet.

protease   Enzyme produced by damaged cells, and cancer cells. Activates the destructive matrix metallo-protease enzymes.

Q10   The rate-limiting co-factor in oxidative phosphorylation, an anti-oxidant, and a mitochondrial protector.

quercitin   A flavonoid found in onions and apples. Probably the quantitatively most important flavonoid in the Western diet.

resistant starch   When starches have been cooked and cooled several times (ie in food processing), they become resistant to digestion and may function as pre-biotics.

saturated fatty acids   Saturated fatty acids (SAFAs) contain no double bonds. They are solid at room temperature, and are mostly derived from meat and dairy foods.

SOD/super oxide dismutase   One of the key antioxidant enzymes. Requires zinc and copper to function.

tocopherols   A group of important fat-soluble anti-oxidants, derived from plant foods. One of these is D-alpha tocopherol, or natural Vitamin E.

trans fats   Generally plant oils which have been modified for food processing. The process alters the molecular structure, producing a fat which is considered to be cardiotoxic.

vitamin   One of the classically defined types of micro-nutrient. Essential for normal growth and the maintenance of health.

zeaxanthin   A carotenoid involved in protecting the eyes from oxidative damage. Found in green, leafy vegetables.

REFERENCES

INTRODUCTION: The Big Picture

1   Vitamin and Mineral Nutrition Lab, *National Dietary Survey*, Beltsville Human Nut Res Centre, US Dept Agric, Beltsville MD, 1993
2   Prior RL, Cao G, *J Am Nutraceutical Assn* 2:46-56, 1999
3   Prior RL et al, *Free Radical Biol Med* 27:173-1181, 1999
4   Johnston CS, Thompson LL, *J Am Col Nut* 17:336-370, 1996
5   Wadsworth M et al, *Public Health Nutrition*, Dec. 1999
6   Schweitzer C et al, *CSFII: 1994-1999, A National Survey*, 12th Intl. Carotenoids Symposium, Cairns, July 1999
7   Hallfrisch J et al, *Am J Clin Nut* 60(2):176-182, 1994
8   Shaw GM et al, *Epidemiology* 6(3):205-207, 1995
9   Stiles NJ, Boosalis MG, *Clin Lab Science* 8(1):39-42, 1995
10 Naurath HJ et al, *Lancet* 346:85-89, 1995
11 Finch S et al, *National Diet & Nutrition Survey*, Vol 1, HMSO, London, 1998
12 Volkert D et al, *Menschen Ern Umschau* 35:348-351, 1988
13 Schümann K, *Intl J Vitamin Nut Res* 69:173-178, 1999
14 Krall E et al, *J Am Den Assn* 129(9):1261-1269, 1998
15 McCance & Widdowson, *Composition of Foods*, 1st and 5th Editions, Royal Soc of Chemistry and Min of Agriculture, Fisheries & Food
16 Lichtenstein P et al. *New Eng J Med, 13 July, 2000*

WHY DISEASE STRIKES
Chapter 2: Malnutrition

1   Mariotti S et al, *Lancet* 339:1506-1508, 1992
2   Chandra R, *Lancet* 340:1124-1127, 1992
3   Sahyoun NR et al, *Am J Epidemiol* 144(5):501-511, 1996
4   Jeandel C et al, *Annales Med de Nancy et de l'Est* 33(6):433-436, 1994
5   De Pee S et al, *Lancet* 346:75-81, 1995
6   Hume EM, Krebs HA, *MRC Special Report 264*, HMSO, London, 1949
7   Carlier C et al, *Br J Nutrition* 68:529-540, 1992
8   Allen LH, *Advances Experim Med Biol* 34:173-186, 1994
9   Morrison H et al, *JAMA* 275:189-196, 1996
10 Shaw GM et al, *Epidemiology* 6(3):205-207, 1995
11 De-Kun Li et al, *Epidemiology* 6(3):212-218, 1995
12 Girodon F et al, *Ann Nut & Metab* 41:90-107, 1997
13 Guidozzi F et al, *S Africa Med J* 85(3):170-173, 1995
14 Beaufrere B et al, *Archives de Pediatrie* 2(4):373-376, 1995
15 Hallfrisch J et al, *Am J Clin Nut* 60(2):176-182, 1994
16 Ji LL, *Free Rad Biol & Med* 18(6):1079-1086, 1995
17 Hartmann A et al, *Mutation Res Letters* 346(4):195-202, 1995
18 Jacob RA et al, *J Nutrition* 124(7):1072-1080, 1994
19 Yao Y et al, *Archives Family Med* 3(10):918-922, 1994
20 Lindenbaum J et al, *Am J Clin Nut* 60(1):2-14, 1994
21 Nichols HK, Basu TK, *J Am College Nut* 13(1):57-61, 1994
22 van der Wielen RPJ et al, *Lancet* 346:207-210, 1995
23 Favier M, Faure P, *Review Fr Gynecol Obstet* 89(4):210-215, 1994
24 Kiremidjian-Schumacher L et al, *Biol Trace Element Res* 41:115-127, 1994
25 Thurnham DI, *Proc Nutrition Society* 53:77-87, 1994
26 Chopra M & Thurnham D I, *Food and Cancer Prevention; Chemical & Biological Aspects*, Eds. Waldron, Johnson, Fenwick, Royal Soc Chem, Cambridge, 1993; pp125-129
27 Van der Wielen RPJ et al, *Eur J Clin Nut* 49:665-674, 1995
28 Van Wouwe JP, *Biol Trace Element Res* 49:211-225, 1995
29 Uden S et al, *Aliment Pharmacol Thr* 6:229-240 1992
30 Braganza J et al, *Pancreas* 2:489-494, 1987
31 Sandilands D et al, *Gastroenterology* 98:766-772, 1990
32 Kluklinski B, Zimmerman R, *Med Clin* 90 (Suppl 1), 36-41, 1995
33 Gregory JF, *Folate in Health and Disease*; Ed. Bailey LB, Marcel Dekker, New York, 1995; pp195-235
34 Naurath HJ et al, *Lancet* 346:85-89, 1995
35 O'Keefe CA et al, *J Nutrition* 125:2717-2725, 1995
36 Paoliso G et al, *J Am Geriat Soc* 46:833-838, 1998
37 Cuskelly, GJ et al, *Lancet* 347:657-659, 1996
38 Keane GM et al, *Br J Clin Prac* 49: 301-303, 1995
39 Gloth FM et al, *J Am Geriat Soc* 43:1269-1271, 1995
40 Rudman D et al, *J Am Col Nut* 14:604-613, 1995
41 Torronen R et al, *Nut Res* 16:565-575, 1996
42 Amorim Cruz, JA, et al, *Eur J Clin Nut* 50:s77-85, 1996
43 Vitamin and Mineral Nutrition Lab, *National Dietary Survey*, Human Nut Res Centre, US Dept Agric, Beltsville MD, 1993
44 Rimm, EG, et al, *New Eng J Med* 283:1450-1457, 1993
45 Crawford M, Doyle W, personal communication
46 Crawford M, Doyle W, *Eur J Clin Nut* 46:S51-S62, 1992
47 Hiemstra SJ, *Food Consumption, Prices and Expenditures*, US Dept Agriculture, Econ Rep 138, Washington DC, 1968
48 Putnam JJ, *Food Consumption, Prices and Expenditure, 1966-1987* US Dept. Agriculture Stat Bull 773, Washington DC 1989
49 Putnam JJ, *Food Consumption, Prices and Expenditure, 1966-1987* US Dept. Agriculture Stat Bull 804, Washington DC 1989
50 Grunfeld J, personal communication
51 Cairella M et al, *Lecithin Consumption in the Western European Diet* in *Lecithin and Healthcare*, Eds. Paltauf F, Lekim D, Semmelweis Verlag, Austria, 1988
52 MacPherson A et al, *Trace Elements in Man and Animals*, Proc 8th Intl Symposium, Dresden, May 1993
53 Bowen HJM, Peggs J, *J Science Food Agric* 35:1225-1229, 1984
55 Key TJ et al, *BMJ* 313:775-779, 1996
56 Pandey DK, et al, *Am J Epidemiol* 142(12):1269-1278, 1995

Chapter 3: Immune System

1   Waldron KW, Selvendran RR, *Food & Cancer Prevention: Chemical & Biological Aspects* Eds. Waldron, Johnson, Fenwick, Royal Soc Chem, Cambridge, 1993; pp307-326
2   Kiecolt-Glaser J et al, *Lancet* 346:1194-1196, 1995
3   Pocock S et al, *Lancet* 303:197-201, 1987
4   Breeze E et al, *OPCS Series GHS No 20*, HMSO, London, 1991
5   McCormick A, Rosenbaum M,*OPCS Series MS5 No 2*, HMSO, London, 1990
6   *OPCS Series DS No 8*, HMSO, London, 1988
7   *OPCS Series DH3 No 24*, HMSO, London, 1992
8   *OPCS Series DS No 6*, HMSO, London, 1986
9   Murphy SP et al, *Am J Clin Nut* 52:361-367, 1990
10 Bolton-Smith PT et al, *Br J Nutrition* 65:321-335, 1991
11 Morgan M et al, *J Epidemiol Commun Health* 42:162-167, 1989
12 Marmot MG, *Lancet* 337:1387-1393, 1991
13 Krantz DS et al, *Psychological Bulletin* 96:435-464, 1984
14 Marmot MG, *New Horizons in the Pathogenesis of Coronary Heart Disease*, Conference Report, June 1992
15 Marmot MG et al, *Lancet* (1):1003-1006, 1984
16 Shaper AG et al, *J Epidemiol Commun Health* 39:199-209, 1985
17 Marmot MG, *Proc Natl Acad Science* 123, No 4, 1994

REFERENCES

18   Wilkinson, R G, *Unhealthy Societies, the Applications of Inequality* Routledge, PA 1996
19   Meydani SM et al, *Ann NY Acad Science* 570:283-290, 1989
20   Bendich A et al, *J Nutrition* 116:675-681, 1986
21   Meydani SM et al, *Am J Clin Nut* 52:557-563, 1990
22   Penn ND et al, *Age & Ageing* 20:169-174, 1991
23   Meydani SM et al, *Antioxidants, Vitamins & Beta Carotene in Disease Prevention* 2nd Intl Conf, Berlin 1994; Abs p34
24   Meydani SM, Hayek MG, *Clin Geriat Med* 11:567-576, 1995
25   Ripa S, Ripa A, *Minerva Medica* 86:315-318, 1995
26   Bogden JD, *Am J Clin Nut* 60:437-447, 1994

Chapter 4: Free radicals

1   Tribble DL et al, *Am J Clin Nut* 58:886-890, 1993
2   Hallfrisch J et al, *Am J Clin Nut* 60(2):176-182, 1994
3   Orr WC, Sohal RS, *Science* 263:1128-1130, 1994
4   Sohal RS et al, *J Biol Chem* 270:20224-20229, 1995
5   Sohal RS et al, *Proc Natl Acad Sci USA* 90:7255-7259, 1995
6   Agarwal S et al, *Proc Natl Acad Sci USA* 91:12332-12335, 1994
7   Ku HH et al, *Free Rad Biol Med* 15:621-6227, 1993
8   Wartanowicz M et al, *Am Nut Metab* 28:186-191, 1984
9   Tolonen M et al, *Bio Trace Element Res* 17:221-228, 1988
10   Lund E K et al, *Am J Clin Nut* 69:250-5, 1999
11   James P, Rowett Institute, UK, personal communication
12   Nandy K, Bourne GH, *Nature* 210:313-314, 1966
13   Nandy K, *Mech of Ageing & Dev* 8:131-138, 1978
14   Hochschild R, *Experim Gerontology* 8:177-183, 1973
15   Mercer D, Hopkins SM, *Age & Ageing* 6:123-131, 1977
16   Horrobin D, personal communication and work in progress
17   Deans SG et al, *Role of Free Radicals in Biological Systems* , Eds. Feher, Blazovics, Matkovics and Mezes, Akademiai Kiado, Budapest, 1993; pp159-165
18   Evans DJ et al, *Lancet* 346:545-546, 1995
19   Harding AE et al, *Ann Neurol* 12:419-424, 1982
20   Raynor R et al, *Archives Dis Child* 69:602-603, 1993
21   Addis P, personal communication and work in progress
22   Drevon CA et al, *Can J Cardiol* 11 Suppl G:47G-54G, 1995
23   Ronsen O, personal communication
24   Peters EM et al, *Am J Clin Nut* 57:170-174, 1993
25   Hartmann A et al, *Mutation Res* 346:195-202, 1995
26   Davies KJA et al, *Biophys Res Commun* 107:1198-1205, 1982
27   Apple FS, Rhodes M, *J Applied Physiol* 65:2598-2600, 1988
28   Sumida S et al, *Intl J Biochem* 21:835-838, 1989
29   Cannon JG et al, *Am J Physiol* 259:R1214-R1219, 1990
30   Novelli GP et al, *Free Rad Biol Med* 8:9-13, 1990
31   Rokitzi L et al, *Acta Physiologica Scanda* 151:149-158, 1994
32   My own personal experience.
33   De Ritter MB et al, *Antioxidants, Vitamins & Beta Carotene in Disease Prevention* 2nd Intl Conf, Berlin 1994; Abs p45
34   Miyajima T et al, *Ibid*, Abs p46
35   Soussi B et al, *Antioxidants & Disease Prevention: Biochem, Nut & Pharmacol Aspects* ILSI Intl Sympsm Stockholm June/July 1993; p110
36   Rokitzki L et al, *Acta Physiol Scanda* 151:149-158, 1994
37   Dekkers JC et al, *Sports Med* 21:213-238, 1996
38   Rokitzki L et al, *Intl J Sport Nut* 4:253-264, 1994
39   Keaney JF et al, *J Clin Investig* 93:844-851, 1994
40   Itoh H et al, *Bulltn Phys Fitness Res Inst* 91:36-44, 1996
41   Arthur JR et al, *Am J Clin Nut* 57:2365-2395, 1993

42   Stiles NJ, Boosalis MG, *Clin Lab Science* 8(1):39-42, 1995
43   Klevay LM, *Am J Clin Nut* 28:764-774, 1975
44   Robins A, Rowatt Inst, personal communication
45   Thorn J et al, *Br J Nutrition* 39:391-396, 1978
46   MacPherson A et al, *Trace Elements in Man & Animals*, Eds. Anke, Meissner & Mills, TEMA 8, Verlag Media Touristik, 1993
47   Allen LH, *Advances Experim Med Biol* 34:173-186, 1994
48   Naurath HJ et al, *Lancet* 346:85-89, 1995
49   Shaw GM et al, *Epidemiology* 6(3):205-207, 1995
50   De-Kun Li et al, *Epidemiology* 6(3):212-218, 1995
51   Jeandel C et al, *Annales Med de Nancy et de l'Est* 33(6):433-436, 1994
52   Guidozzi F et al, *S Africa Med J* 85(3A):170-173, 1995
53   Beaufrere B et al, *Archives de Pediatrie* 2(4):373-376, 1995
54   Hallfrisch J et al, *Am J Clin Nut* 60(2):176-182, 1994
55   Ji LL, *Free Rad Biol & Med* 18(6):1079-1086, 1995
56   Nichols HK, Basu TK, *J Am College Nut* 13(1):57-61, 1994
57   Jacob RA et al, *J Nutrition* 124(7):1072-1080, 1994
58   Yao Y et al, *Archives Family Med* 3(10):918-922, 1994
59   Lindenbaum J et al, *Am J Clin Nut* 60(1):2-14, 1994
60   Favier M, Faure P, *Review Fr Gynecol Obstet* 89(4):210-215, 1994
61   Van der Wielen RPJ et al, *Lancet* 346:207-210, 1995
62   Iavier M, Faure P, *Review Fr Gynecol Obstet* 89(4):210-215, 1994
63   Kiremidjian-Schumacher L et al, *Biol Trace Element Res* 41:115-127, 1994
64   Birlouez-Aragon I et al, *Intl J Vit Nut Res* 65:261-266, 1995
65   Jialal I et al, *Arteriosclerosis, Thromb & Vasc Biol* 15(2):190-198, 1995
66   Aus J Science & Med in Sport, 25:94-99, 1994
67   Salonen JT, *Iron Nutrition in Health & Disease*, Swedish Nutrition Foundation, 20th Intl Symposium, Stockholm August 1995; p46
68   Jacob RA et al, *J Nutrition* 124(7):1072-1080, 1994
69   Prior RL et al, *Free Redical Biol Med* 27:173-1181, 1999
70   Kent S, *Geriatrics* 31:128-137, 1976
71   Hanssen M, personal communication
72   Richard MJ, Roussel AM, *Proc Nut Soc* 58(3):573-578, 1999
73   Reidel WJ, Jorissen BL, *Current Opinion Clin Nut Care* 1(6):579-585, 1998
74   Shephard RJ et al, *Exercise Immunol Rev* 4:22-48, 1998
75   Kanter M, *Proc Nutrition Society* 57(1):9-13, 1998

Eleutherococcus (Siberian ginseng)

80   Barenboim GM et al, *Khim Farm Zh* 28:914-917, 1986
81   Wagner H et al, *Arzneimittelforschung*, 34:659-661, 1984
82   Farnsworth NR et al, *Proc 2nd Intl symp on Eleutherococcus*, Far East Science Centre, USSR Acad Sci, Vladivostock 1986; pp63-69
83   German Pharmacopeia, *Monograph on Eleutherococcus senticosus*, 1991
84   Shandrin V et al, *Proc 2nd Intl symp on Eleutherococcus*, Far East Science Centre, USSR Acad Sci Vladivostock 1986; p289
85   Galanova LK, *Ibid*, pp126-127
86   Krylov AV, *Acta Virol* 16:75-76, Prague 1972
87   Barkan AI et al, *Pediatrya* 4:65-66, Moscow 1980
88   Vershchagin IA et al, *Antibiotiki* 27:65-69, 1983
89   Bohn B et al, *Arzneimittelforschung* 37:1193-1196, 1987
90   Bohn B et al, *Drug Research* 7: (11) No.10, 1987
91   Wagner H et al, *Economical & Medicinal Plant Res* 1: 206-207 Academic Press, Orlando, 1985
92   Kupin VJ et al, *Proc 2nd Intl symp on Eleutherococcus*, Far East Science Centre, USSR Acad Sci, Vladivostock 1986
93   Wagner H et al, *Zeitshift für Phytostempie* 13:42-54,1992

Echinacea

95 Helbig G, *Med Klin* 56:1512, 1961

96 Kleinschmidt H, *Ther der Gegen* 12:58, 1965

97 Wacker A, Hilbig W, *Planta Med* 33(1):89-102, 1978

98 Amman M & Suter K, *Deutsche Apoth-Zeit* 127: 853, 1987

99 Bauer R et al, *Arzneimittelforschung* 38: 276, 1988

100 Bauer R, *Zeit Phytotherapie* 10: 43, 1989

101 Lohman-Matthes ML & Wagner H, *Zeit Phytotherapie* 10: 52, 1989

102 Lasch HG, *Die Med Welt* 34:1463, 1983

103 Wagner H & Proksch A, *Economical & Medicinal Plant Res* 1:113, Academic Press, Orlando, 1985

104 Enbergs H & Woestmann A, *Tierarztliche Umschau* 11: 878, 1986

105 Wagner H et al, *Phytotherapie,* Hippokrates Verlag, Stuttgart, 1988; pp127-135

106 Jurcic K et al, *Zeit Phytotherapie* 10(2):67-70, 1989

107 Coeugniet E & Kuhnast R, *Therapiewoche* 36: 3352, 1986

108 Chone B & Manidakis G, *Deutsche Med Woch* 27:1406, 1969

109 Bauer R, Remiger P, *Phytochem* 27:2339-2342, 1988

110 Mose JR, *Die Med Welt* 34:1463, 1983

112 Stotzem CD et al, *Med Science Res* 20:719-720, 1992

113 Bauer R, Wagner H, *Econ & Med Plant Res* 5:253-321, 1991

114 Tubaro A, Tragni E, *J Pharmacol* 39:567-569, 1987

115 Tubaro A, Galli P, *Pharmacol Res Comm* 20(S5):87-90, 1988

116 Wagner H, Breu W, *Planta Med* 55:566-567, 1989

117 Luettig B, Steinmuller C, *J Natl Cancer Inst* 81(9):669-675, 1989

118 Orinda D, Diederich J, *Arzneimittelforschung* 23(8):1119-1120, 1973

THE DEFENCE BOOSTERS

Chapter 5: Anti-oxidants

1 Genot C et al, *Antioxidants in Food,* Royal Soc Chem Symposium, London, December 1994

2 Yamamoto Y, *Ibid*

3 Howarth JM et al, *Am Review Respir Dis* 123:496-499, 1981

4 Scheider JF et al, *Stable Isotopes,* Proc 3rd Intl Con, Eds. Klein, Klein, Academic Press, NY 1974; pp507-516

5 Jackson MJ et al, *Proc Nutrition Society* 53:53-57, 1994

6 Turnlund JR, *Trace Elements in Man & Animals ,* Ed. Momcilovic, IMI, Zagreb, 1991; pp56-61

7 Underwood EJ, *Trace Elements in Human & Animal Nutrition,* Academic Press, London 1977; p321

8 Scott R et al, *Br J Urol* 82(1):76-90, 1998

9 Luck MR et al, *Biol Reprod* 52(2):262-266, 1995

10 Davies S, Harley St, London, personal communication

11 Willekens H et al, *Antioxidants & Disease Prevention: Biochem, Nut & Pharmacol Aspects,* ILSI Intl Symposium, Stockholm June/July 1993; p115

12 Gollnick H et al, *Proc Intl Life Sci Inst,* Europe, 1993; pp88-89

13 Kapitanov AB, Pimenov AM, *Antioxidants & Disease Prevention: Biochem Nut & Pharmacol Aspects,* ILSI Intl Symposium, Stockholm June/July 1993; p99

14 Sarma L, Kesavan PC, *Intl J Radia Biol* 63:759-764, 1993

15 Dworschak E et al, *Antioxidants & Disease Prevention: Biochem, Nut & Pharmacol Aspects,* ILSI Intl Symposium, Stockholm June/July 1993; p95

16 Meydani S et al, *Antioxidants, Vitamins & Beta Carotene in Disease Prevention,* 2nd Intl Conf, Berlin 1994, Abs p26

17 Levine M et al, *Ibid,* Abs p15

18 Oettinger AP et al, *Antioxidants & Disease Prevention: Biochem, Nut & Pharmacol Aspects,* ILSI Intl Symposium, Stockholm June/July 1993; p105

19 Rabl H et al, *Kidney International* 43:912-917, 1993

20 Nourooz-Zadeh J et al, *Annals Biochem* 220:403-409, 1994

21 Abbey M et al, *Am J Clin Nut* 58:525-532, 1993

22 Prasad K, Kalra J, *Am Heart J* 125:958-973, 1993

23 Lemoyne M et al, *Am J Clin Nut* 46:267-272, 1987

24 Nourooz-Zadeh J et al, *Antiox, Atherosclerosis & Diabetes,* William Harvey Research Conference, London, October 1994

25 Morrow et al, *Proc Natl Acad Sci USA* 87:9383, 1990

26 Takahashi K et al, *J Clin Investig* 90:136, 1993

27 Collins A et al, *Proc Nutrition Society* 53:67-75, 1994

28 Suzukawa M et al, *J Am College Nut* 14(1):46-52, 1995

29 Gaziano JM et al, *Atherosclerosis* 112(2):187-195, 1995

30 Jacques PF et al, *Ann Epidemiology* 5(1):52-59, 1995

31 Gaziano JM et al, *Circulation* 82:Suppl 3:201,1990

32 Chopra M et al, *Proc Intl Life Science Inst,* Europe, p92, 1993

33 Esterbauer H et al, *Am J Clin Nut* 53:314S-321S, 1991

34 Taylor A, *J Am College Nut* 12:138-146, 1993

35 West S et al, *Archives Opthalmol* 112:222-227, 1994

36 Taylor A, *Antioxidants, Vitamins & Beta Carotene in Disease Prevention,* 2nd Intl Conf, Berlin 1994; Abs p32

37 Snodderly DM, *Ibid,* Abs p33

38 Seddon JM et al, *JAMA* 272:1413-1420, 1994

39 Handelman GJ et al, *Investig Opthalmol and Visual Science* 29:850-855, 1998

40 Ritter LL, Shoff SM, *Am J Epidemiology* 141(4):322-334, 1995

41 Fahn S, *Ann Neurol* 32:S128-S132, 1992

42 Arthur JR et al, *Am J Clin Nut* 57:236S-239S, 1993

43 Bower B, *Science News* 141(21):351, 1992

44 Adler LA et al, *Am J Psychiatry,* 150(9):1405-1407, 1993

45 Peet M et al, *Intl Clin Psychopharmacol* 8:151-153, 1993

46 Wartanowicz M et al, *Ann Nut Metab* 28:186-191, 1984

47 Tolonen M et al, *Biol Trace Element Res* 17:221-228, 1988

48 Tolonen M et al, *Biol Trace Element Res* 7:161-168, 1985

49 Meydani SM et al, *Nut Res* 5:1227-1236, 1985

50 Ingold KU et al, *Lipids* 22:163-172, 1987

51 Burton GW et al, *Accounts of Chem Res* 19:194-201, 1986

52 Britton J et al, *Lancet* 344:357-361, 1994

53 Rolla G et al, *Allergy* 42:186-188, 1987

54 Heliovaara M et al, *Ann Rheum Dis* 53:51-53, 1994

55 Bachmann H et al, *Antioxidants, Vitamins & Beta Carotene in Disease Prevention,* 2nd Intl Conf, Berlin 1994; Abs p83

56 Srivastava KC, *Prostaglandins, Leukotrienes and Medicine* 13:227-235, 1984

57 Barja G et al, *Antioxidants, Vitamins & Beta Carotene in Disease Prevention,* 2nd Intl Conf, Berlin 1994; Abs p45

58 Bartoli G-M et al, *Ibid,* Abs p14

59 Clark RM et al, *Ibid,* Abs p52

60 Palozza P, Krinsky NI, *Archives Biochem Biophys* 297(1):184-187, 1992

61 Knekt P et al, *BMJ* 305:1392-1394, 1992

62 Niki E, *Antioxidants, Vitamins & Beta Carotene in Disease Prevention,* 2nd Intl Conf, Berlin 1994; Abs p12

63 Hennekens CH, *Am J Med* 97 (Suppl 3A):26, 1994

64 Wandzilac TR et al, *J Urol* 151:834-837, 1994

65 McLarty J, *Antioxidants, Vitamins & Beta Carotene in Disease Prevention,* 2nd Intl Conf, Berlin 1994; Abs p31

REFERENCES

66 Antonenkov VD, Sies H, *Ibid*, Abs p44

67 Omara FO, Blakely BR, *J Nutrition* 123:1649-1655, 1993

68 Sies H, *Oxidative Stress*, Academic Press, NY 1985

69 O'Donnell VB, Azzi A, *Biochem Soc Trans* 239S, 1995

70 Engman L et al, *Antioxidants & Disease Prevention: Biochem, Nut & Pharmacol Aspects*, ILSI Intl Symposium, Stockholm, June/July 1993; p71

71 Gers-Barlag H et al, *Antioxidants, Vitamins & Beta Carotene in Disease Prevention*, 2nd Intl Conf, Berlin 1994; Abs p69

72 Aeschbach R et al, *Food & Chem Toxicol* 32:3136, 1994

73 Scherat T et al, *Antioxidants, Vitamins & Beta Carotene in Disease Prevention*, 2nd Intl Conf, Berlin 1994; Abs p49

74 Amit K, *Ibid*, Abs p96

75 Julius M et al, *J Clin Epidemiology* 4:1021-1026, 1994

76 Lang CA et al, *J Lab Clin Med* 120:720-725, 1992

77 Shklar G et al, *Nut Cancer* 20:145-151, 1993

78 Cantilena LR et al, *Am J Clin Nut* 55:659-663, 1992

79 Hodges S, Eastman Hospital, London, personal communication

80 Bruckdorfer KR, Ettelaie C, *Biochem Soc Trans* 23:243S, 1995

81 Morris DL et al, JAMA 272(18):1439-1441, 1994

82 Schwartz J, Weiss ST, *Am J Clin Nut* 59(1):110-114, 1994

83 Wu D et al, *J Nutrition* 124(5):655-663, 1994

84 Riemersma R, personal communication

85 Koller LD, Exon JH, *Can J Vet Res* 50:297-306, 1986

86 Salonen JT et al, *Am J Epidemiology* 120:342-349, 1984

87 Salonen JT et al, *Intl J Epidemiology* 16:323-328, 1987

88 Westermark, *Acta Pharmacol Toxicol* 41:121-128, 1977

89 Tarp U et al, *J Trace Elem Electrolytes Health Dis* 3:93-95, 1989

90 Barclay MNI, MacPherson A, *J Sci Food Agric* 37:1133-1138, 1986

91 MacPherson A et al, *Trace Elements in Man & Animals*, Proc 8th Intl Sympsm, Dresden, May 1993

92 Clemens MR, *Ther Umsch* 51(7):483-488, 1994

93 Symons MCR, *Proc Royal Soc Biochem Annual Gen Meeting*, Brighton, Dec 1994; Abs 111

94 Reaven PD et al, *Arteriosclerosis Thromb* 14(7):1162-1169, 1994

95 Nyssonsen K et al, *Eur J Clin Nut* 48(9):633-642, 1994

96 Gey KF et al, *Ther Umsch* 51(7):475-482, 1994

97 Oels C, Elmadfa J, *Aktuel Ernahr Med Klin Prax* 19(3):155-259, 1994

98 Britton RS, Bacon BR, *Hepato-Gastroenterology* 41(4):343-348, 1994

99 Comoglio A et al, *Free Rad Res Comms* 11:109-124, 1990

100 Everette SA et al, *Proc Royal Soc Biochem Annual Gen Meeting*, Brighton Dec 1994; Abs 85

101 Truscott TG et al, *Ibid*, Abs 238

102 Shenberg C et al, *J Trace Elem Electrolytes Health Dis* 3(2):71-75, 1989

103 Schrauzer GN, White DA, *Bio-inorganic Chem* 8:303-318, 1978

104 Eiserich JP et al, *Proc Royal Soc Biochem Annual Gen Meeting*, Brighton, Dec 1994; Abs 103

105 Garcia-de-la-Asuncion JG et al, *Ibid*, Abs 59

106 Cynthia Leaf, Free Radical Sciences Inc, Cambridge, USA, presented at William Harvey Conference, London 1995

107 Steinberg D et al, *New Eng J Med* 320:915-924, 1989

108 Bolton CH et al, *Biochem Soc Trans* 23:245S, 1995

109 Stampfer M et al, *New Eng J Med* 328:1444-1450; 1993

110 Rimm EB et al, *New Eng J Med* 283, 1450-1457; 1993

111 Stocker R, *Antioxidants & Disease Prevention: Biochem, Nut & Pharmacol Aspects*, ILSI Intl Symposium, Stockholm June/July 1993; pp45-46

112 Cadenas E, *Ibid*, pp20-21

113 Ordoñez ID, Cadenas E, *Biochem J* 286:481, 1992

114 Camejo G, *Antioxidants & Disease Prevention: Biochem, Nut & Pharmacol Aspects*, ILSI Intl Symposium, Stockholm June/July 1993; pp66-67

115 Bruchelt G et al, *Ibid*, p90

116 Roberfroid MB et al, *Ibid*, pp72-73

117 Taper H, Roberfroid M, *Anticancer Res* 12:1651-1654, 1992

118 Biesalski HK et al, *Antioxidants & Disease Prevention: Biochem, Nut & Pharmacol Aspects*, ILSI Intl Symposium, Stockholm, June/July 1993; p88

119 Gollnick H et al, *Ibid*, p89

120 Krinsky NI, *Ibid*, pp27-29

121 Hodis HN et al, *JAMA* 273(23):1849-1854, 1995

122 Khaw K-T et al, *BMJ* 310:1548-1549 & 1559-1563, 1995

123 Stahl W et al, *Antioxidants & Disease Prevention: Biochem, Nut & Pharmacol Aspects*, ILSI Intl Symposium, Stockholm June/July 1993; pp23-24

124 Hertog MGL et al, *Lancet* 342:1007-1011, 1993

125 Clayton RM, Edinburgh University, personal communication

126 Jorge, PAR , et al, *Atheroscler* 140:333-339, 1998

127 Fitzpatrick, DF et al, *J Cardiovasc Pharmacol* 32:509-515, 1998

128 Hennekens CH et al, *New Eng J Med* 334:1145-1149, 1996

129 Kohlmeier L et al, *Am J Epidemiology* 146:618-626, 1997

130 Hills, BA, *Thorax* 51:1-4. 1996

131 Hills, BA, *Med Hypoth* 46:33-41, 1996

132 Hills, BA, *Med Sci Res* 20:543-55-, 1992

133 Kune JF et al, *Nut & Cancer* 18/(3):237-44, 1992

134 Hills BA, Masters ITS, *Arch Dis Child Fetal Neonatal* Ed 79: F221-F222, 1998

135 Hills, BA, *J Applied Physiol* 73:1034-1039, 1992

136 Maini RM et al, *Arthr Rheuma* 41:1552-1563, 1998

137 Maini RM et al, *Lancet* 354:1932-1939, 1999

138 Mikhail MS et al, *Am J Obs & Gyne* 171:150-158, 1994

139 Jain SK, *Mol Cell Biochem* 151:33-38, 1995

140 Shaaraway M, *Intl J Gyne & Obs* 60:123-128, 1998

141 Gratacos E et al, *Am J Obs & Gyne* 178:1072-1076, 1998

142 Yanik FF et al, *Intl J Gyne & Obs* 64:27-33, 1999

143 Klesges LM et al, *Am J Epidemiol* 147:127-135, 1998

144 Paston L et al, *Lancet* 354:810-819, 1999

145 Apple FS, Rhodes M, *J Applied Physiol* 65:2598-2600, 1988

146 Dekkers JC et al, *Sports Med* 21:213-238, 1996

147 Peters EM et al, *Am J Clin Nut* 57:170-174, 1993

148 Sumida S et al, *Intl J Biochem* 21:835-838, 1989

149 Cannon JG et al, *Am J Physiol* 259:R1214-R1219, 1990

150 Novelli GP et al, *Free Rad Biol Med* 8:9-13, 1990

151 Rokitzi L et al, *Acta Physiologica Scanda* 151:149-158, 1994

152 My own personal experience

153 Soussi B et al, *Antioxidants & Disease Prevention: Biochem, Nut & Pharmacol Aspects*, ILSI Intl Symposium; p110

154 De Ritter MB et al, *Antioxidants, Vitamins & Beta Carotene in Disease Prevention*, 2nd Intl Conf, Berlin 1994; Abs p45

155 Miyajima T et al, *Ibid*, Abs p46

156 Devaraj S et al, *Arteriosclerosis Throm* 13:601-608, 1993

157 Brown KM et al, *Am J Clin Nut* 65:496-502, 1997

158 Upston JM et al, *J Biol Chem* 272:30067-30074, 1997

159 Hammond BR et al, *Optometry & Vision Science* 74:499-504, 1997

160 Hammond BR et al, *Investig Opthalmol & Visual Science* 38:1795-1801, 1997

161 Landman JT et al, *Experim Eye Res* 65:57-62, 1997

162 Bone RA et al, *Experim Eye Res* 64: 211-218, 1997

163 Martynenko LD, *Antioxidants, Vitamins & Beta Carotene in Disease Prevention*, 2nd Intl Conf, Berlin 1994; Abs p97

164 Krinsky NI, *Antioxidants & Disease Prevention: Biochem, Nut & Pharmacol Aspects*, ILSI Intl Sympsm, Stockholm June/July 1993; pp27-29

165 Upstone JM et al, *FASEB J* 13:977-994, 1999

166 Tribble DL et al, *Am J Clin Nut* 58:886-890, 1993

168 Gaziano JM, *Am J Med* 97 (Suppl 3A):25, 1994

169 Stiles NJ, Boosalis MG, *Clin Lab Science* 8(1):39-42, 1995

170 Klevay LM, *Am J Clin Nut* 28:764-774, 1975

171 Robins A, Rowatt Inst, personal communication

172 Thorn J et al, *Br J Nutrition* 39:391-396, 1978

173 MacPherson A et al, *Trace Elements in Man & Animals*, Eds. Anke, Meissner & Mills, TEMA 8, Verlag Media Touristik, 1993

174 Parkinson Study Group, *Ann Neurol* 39:29-36, 1996

175 Parkinson Study Group, *Ibid 37-45, 1996*

176 Chopra M, Thurnham D I, *Food and Cancer Prevention: Chemical & Biological Aspects*, Royal Soc Chem, Cambridge 1993; pp125-129

177 Davies KJA et al, *Biophys Res Comm* 107:1198-1205, 1982

178 Parkinsonism Study Group, *New Eng J Med* 325:176-183, 1993

179 Herbaczynska-Cedro K et al, *Eur Heart J* 16:1044-1049, 1995

180 Bellisola G et al, *Clinica Chimida Acta* 205:75-85, 1992

181 Folmer M, *Cand scient opgave i ernaeringsphysiologie*, Institutt for Ernaeringsforskning, Universitet i Oslo, 1993

182 Ringstad J et al, *J Trace Elem Electrolytes Health Dis* 1:27-31, 1987

183 Ringstad J et al, *J Epidemiology Comm Health* 41:329-332, 1987

184 Lane HW et al, *Nutrition Research* 3:805-817, 1983

185 Zachara BA et al, *Archives Env Health* 42:223-229, 1987

186 Yang G et al, *J Trace Elem Electrolytes Health Dis* 3:77-87, 1989

187 Yang G et al, *Ibid* 3:123-130, 1989

188 Yang G et al, *Am J Clin Nut* 37:872-881, 1993

189 Natl Cancer Inst, *Techn Rep Ser 194*, NIH, Bethesda, USA, 1980

190 Anundi I et al, *Chem Biol Interactions* 50:277-288, 1984

191 Bunce GE, Hess JL, *Experim Eye Res* 33:505-514, 1981

192 Maitra I et al, *Free Rad Biol Med* 18:823-829, 1995

193 Princen HMG et al, *Arteriosclerosis Thromb Vasc Biol* 15:325-333, 1995

194 Goode HF et al, *Hepatology* 19:354-359, 1994

195 Rothman KJ et al, *New Eng J Med* 333:1369-1373, 1995

196 Nenseter MS et al, *Scand J Clin & Lab Investig* 55:477-485, 1995

197 Jialal I, Fuller CJ, *Can J Cardiol* 11/suppl G:97G-103G, 1995

198 Reiter RJ, *Frontiers in Neuroendocrinology* 16:383-415, 1995

199 Kadrabova J et al, *Biol Trace Elem Res* 50:13-24, 1995

200 Mavor J, *A Book of the Farm, Being Practical Letters and Hints for Improving Farmers in Modern Times*, Vol. 2, London 1781; p309

201 Stephens NG et al, *Lancet* 347:781-786, 1996

202 Hodges NG, Beer WE, *Lancet* 347:966, 1995

203 Pieri C et al, *Life Science* 55:271-276, 1994

204 Grune T et al, *Phytomedicine* 2:205-207, 1996

205 Vijayalazmi, Reiter R, Meltz M, *Mutation Research* 346:23-31, 1995

206 Fotouhi N et al, *Am J Clin Nut* 63:553-558, 1996

207 Torronen R et al, *Nutrition Research* 16:565-575, 1994

208 Mian I, personal communication

209 Grievink L et al, *Am J Epidemiol* 149:306-314, 1999

210 Parkinson-Mercado JD et al, *J Am College Nut* 14:614-620, 1995

211 Fontham ETH et al, *Cancer Epidemiol, Biomarkers & Prevn* 4:801-803, 1995

212 Beal FM, *Biomed & Clin Aspects of Coenzyme Q*, 9th Intl Symposium, Ancona, May 1996; Abs pp30-32

213 Horstink MWIM, Strijks E, *Ibid*, Abs p58

214 Parkinson Study Group, *Ann Neurol* 39:29-45, 1996

215 Brigham, *Eur Respir J* 3:482S-484S, 1990

216 Bernard et al, *Am J Respir & Crit Med* 149:A24, 1994

217 Kalayjian et al, *J Acquired Immune Def Syndromes* 7:369-374, 1994

218 Salim AS, *Scot Med J* 36:019-121, 1991

219 Salim AS, *J Lab Clin Med* 119:710-717, 1992

220 Salim AS, *World J Surgery* 15:264-269, 1991

221 Salim AS, *Surgery, Gynecol & Obstet* 176:484-490, 1993

222 Faucheux B et al, *Proc Natl Acad Sci* 92:9603-9607, 1995

223 Faucheaux B et al, *Acta Neuropath* 91:566-577, 1996

224 Soares KVS, McGrath JJ, *Schizophrenia Module of Cochrane*, Eds. Adams C, Anderson J, De Jesus Mari J, Database of Systematic Reviews, BMJ Publishing Group, London 1996

225 Kost J, Eliaz R, *Cytokine* 8:482-487, 1996

226 Reilly M, *Circulation* 94(1):19-25, 1996

227 Curran-Celento J, Henkel Symposium, Pine Mountain, Georgia, June 1996

228 International Study of Asthma & Allergy in Children (ISAAC), preliminary results, 1996

229 Street DA et al, *Circulation* 90:1154-1161, 1994

230 Chen H, Tappel AL, *Free Rad Biol & Med* 16:437-444, 1994

231 Wahlqvist ML et al, *Am J Clin Nut* 60:936-943, 1994

232 Curhan GC et al, *J Urology* 155:1847-1851, 1996

233 Dexter DT et al, *Neuroreport* 5:1773-1776, 1994

234 Hartmann A et al, *Mutation Research* 346:195-202, 1995

235 Handelman GJ et al, *Am J Clin Nut* 59:1025-1032, 1994

236 Keaney JF et al, *J Clin Investig* 93:844-851, 1994

237 Vezina D et al, *Biol Trace Element Res* 53:65-83, 1996

238 Malm C et al, *Acta Physiol Scandinavica* 157:511-512, 1996

239 Ben-Amotz A, Levy Y, *Am J Clin Nut* 63:729-734, 1996

240 Awasthi S et al, *Am J Clin Nut* 64:761-766, 1997

241 Eberlein-Konig B et al, *J Am Acad Derm* 38:45-48, 1998

242 Lopez-Torres M et al, *Br J Derm* 138:207-215, 1998

243 Mangles AR et al, *JADA* 93:284-296, 1993

244 Micozzi MS et al, *J Natl Cancer Inst* 82:282-285, 1990

245 Parker RS, *FASEB J* 10:542-551, 1996

246 Weber P et al, *Nutrition* 13:450-460, 1997

247 La Chance P, *Clin Nut* 7:118-122, 1988

248 Truscott TG, *J Am Chem Soc* 119:621-622, 1997

249 Bendich A, Machlin LJ, *Am J Clin Nut* 48:612-619, 1988

250 Kuklinski B, Schweder R, *J Nut Env Med* 6:393-394, 1996

251 Ward Burton G, *Am J Clin Nut* 67:669-684, 1998

252 Lykkesfeldt J et al, *FASEB J* 12:1183-1189, 1998

253 Chan AC, *J Nutrition* 128:1593-1596, 1998

254 Plotwick GD et al, *JAMA* 278:1682-1686, 1997

255 Deans SG et al, *Role of Free Radicals in Biological Systems*, Eds. Feher, Blazovics, Matkovics and Mezes, Akademiai Kiado, Budapest 1993; pp159-165

256 Leske MC et al, *Opthalmol* 105:831-836, 1998

257 Brown K et al, *Biol Psychiat* 43:863-867, 1998

258 Edmonds SE et al, *Ann Rheum Dis* 56:649-655, 1997

259 Bierenbaum ML et al, *Nut Reports Intl* 31:1171-1180, 1985

260 Sano M et al, *New Eng J Med* 336:1216-1222, 1997

261 Reaven PD, Wiztrim JL, *Atherosclerosis Thromb* 13:601-608, 1993

262 Meydani SN et al, *Ann NY Acad Science* 570:283-290, 1989

263 Penn ND et al, *Age and Ageing* 20:169-174, 1991

264 Meydani SN et al, *JAMA* 277:1380-1386, 1997

265 Allen LH, *Advances Experim Med Biol* 24:173-186, 1994

REFERENCES

266 Naurath HJ et al, *Lancet* 346:85-89, 1995
267 Shaw GM et al, *Epidemiology* 6(3):205-207,1995
268 De-Kun Li et al, *Epidemiology* 6(3):212-218, 1995
269 Jeandel C et al, *Annales Med de Nancy et de l'Est* 33(6):433-436, 1994
270 Guidozzi F et al, *S Africa Med J* 85(3A):170-173, 1995
271 Beaufrere B et al, *Archives de Pediatrie* 2(4):373-376, 1995
272 Birlouez-Aragon I et al, *Intl J Vit Nut Res* 65:261-266, 1995
273 James P, Rowett Institute, UK, personal communication
274 Jialal I et al, *Arteriosclerosis, Thromb & Vasc Biol* 15(2):190-198, 1995
275 Rokitzki L et al, *Acta Physiol Scanda* 151:149-158, 1994
276 Molis TM et al, *J Pineal Res* 18:930103, 1995
277 Lissoni P et al, *Br J Cancer* 69:196-199, 1994
278 Lissoni P et al, *Support Care Cancer* 3:194-197, 1995
279 Arendt J et al, *Ergonomics* 30:1379-1393, 1987
280 Claustrat B et al, *Biol Psychiat* 32:705-711, 1992
281 Lino A et al, *Biol Psychiat* 34:587, 1993
282 Petrie K et al, *Biol Psychiat* 33: 526-530, 1993
283 Schmid L, *Sport Med Phys Fitness* 32(4):432-434, 1992
284 Wilson BR, *Res Q Exercise Sport* 61(1):1-6, 1990

Chapter 6: Flavonoids and isoflavones

1   Harborne JB, *Plant Flavonoids in Biology & Medicine 2: Biochemical, Cellular & Medicinal Properties*, Eds. Cody, Middleton, Harborne, Beretz, Alan R Liss Inc., NY 1988; pp17-27
2   Brown, JP, *Mutation Research* 75:243-277, 1980
3   Hertog MGL et al, *Lancet* 342:1007-1011, 1993
4   Birt DF & Bresnick E, *Human Nutrition* 7:221-260 1991
5   Stich HF, Rosin MP, *Nutritional and Toxicological Aspects of Food Safety*, Ed. M Friedman, Plenum Press, NY 1984; pp1-29
6   Intern Agency for Research on Cancer, *Monograph on Evaluation of Carcinogenic Risks to Humans, Some Food Additives, Feed Additives and Naturally Occurring Substances*, Lyon, 31:213-229, 1983
7   Pierpoint WS, *Flavonoids in Medicine & Biology 3: Current Issues in Flavonoid Research*, Ed. Das NP, Natl Univ Singapore 1990; pp 497-514
8   Herrman K, *J Food Technology* 11:433-448, 1976
9   Havsten B, *Biochem Pharmacol* 32:1141, 1983
10 Middleton E, *Trends Pharmacol Science* 5:335, 1984
11 Alcaraz MJ, Jimenez MJ, *Fitoterapia* 59:25-38, 1988
12 Moroney MA et al, *J Pharmacol* 40:787, 1988
13 Cazenave JP et al, *Flavonoids & Bioflavonoids*, Eds Farkas, Gabor, Kallay, Elsevier 1986; pp373-380
14 Ferriola PC et al, *Biochem Pharmacol* 38:1617, 1989
15 Kuppusamy VR et al, *Biochem Pharmacol* 40:397, 1990
16 Ono K et al, *Eur J Biochem* 190:469, 1990
17 Vlietink DA et al, *Plant Flavonoids in Biology & Medicine 2: Biochemical, Cellular & Medicinal Properties*, Eds. Cody, Middleton, Harborne, Beretz, Alan R Liss Inc., NY 198; pp283-299
18 Hodnick WF et al, *Biochem Pharmacol* 36:2873, 1987
19 Tauber AI et al, *Biochem Pharmacol* 33:1367, 1984
20 Elliott AJ et al, *Biochem Pharmacol* 44:1603, 1992
21 Appleby PN, et al, *Am J Clin Nut* 70(3Suppl):525S-531S,1999
22 Bors W et al, *Methods in Enzymology* 186:343, 1990
23 Comoglio A et al, *Free Rad Res Comm* 11:109-124, 1990
24 Thompson EB et al, *J Pharmaceutical Sciences* 63:1936-1937, 1974
25 Rewerski W et al, *Arzneimittelforschung* 21:886-888, 1971
26 Rodale JI, *The Hawthorn Berry for the Heart*; Rodale Books, Emmaus PA, 1971
27 Robert AM et al, *Path Biol* 38:601, 1990

28 Morazzoni P et al, *Eur J Drug Metab Pharmacokinet* 17:39, 1992
29 Groult N et al, *Path Biol* 39:277, 1991
30 Mennicke WH et al, *Hepatology, Rapid Literature Review* V, 411, 1979
31 Rice-Evans C, Free Radical Group, Guy's Hospital, personal comm.
32 Bauman J et al, *Archives Pharmacol* (Weinheim) 313:330, 1980
33 Robak J, Gryglewski RJ, *Biochem Pharmacol* 37:837, 1988
34 Blasig IE et al, *Biomed Biochim Acta* 47:S252, 1988
35 Pincemail J et al, *Experientia* 45:708, 1989
36 Sichel G et al, *Free Radical Biol Med* 11:1, 1991
37 Husain RS et al, *Phytochemistry* 26:2489, 1987
38 Cilard J et al, *Flavonoids in Medicine & Biology 3: Current Issues in Flavonoid Research*, Ed. Das NP, Natl Univ Singapore 1990; pp143-160
39 Deby C et al, *Experientia* 39:1113, 1983
40 Sorata Y et al, *Biochem Biophys Acta* 799:313, 1984
41 Afanaslev IB et al, *Biochem Pharmacol* 38:1763, 1989
42 Erben Russ M et al, *Intl J Radiat Biol* 52:393, 1987
43 Torel J et al, *Phytochemistry* 25:383, 1986
44 Thompson M et al, *Anal Chim Acta* 85:375, 1976
45 Takahama U, *Phytochemistry* 24:1443-1446, 1985
46 Harper KA et al, *J Food Technol* 4:255, 1969
47 Clegg KM, Morton AD, *J Food Technol* 3:277, 1968
48 De Whalley CV et al, *Biochem Pharmacol* 39:1743-1749, 1990
49 Laughton MJ et al, *Biochem Pharmacol* 42:1673-1681, 1991
50 Hollman PCH et al, *Antioxidants & Disease Prevention: Biochem, Nut & Pharmacol Aspects*, ILSI Intl Sympsm, Stockholm June/July 1993
51 Miller N, Free Radical Group, Guy's Hospital; personal communication
52 Laparra, J et al, *Plantes Medicinales et Phytotherapie* XI:133, 1977
53 Laparra J et al, *Acta Therapeutica* 4:233, 1978
54 Masquelier J et al, *Bulltn Soc Pharmacol Bordeaux* 118:95, 1979
55 Masquelier J, *Parfums, Cosmetiques, Aromas* 95: 1990
56 Masquelier J et al, *Intl J Vit Nut Res* 49:307, 1979
57 Pincemail J et al, *Flavonoids & Bioflavonoids*, Eds Farkas, Gabor, Kallay, Elsevier 1986; pp423-436
58 Hagerman AE, Butler LG, *J Biol Chem* 256:4494, 1981
59 Tixier JM et al, *Biochem Pharmacol* 33:3933-3939, 1984
60 Frankel EN et al, *Lancet* 341:454-457, 1993
61 Werbach MR & Murray MT, *Botanical Influences in Illness: A Sourcebook of Clinical Research*, Third Line Press, Tarzana, CA 1994
62 Rice-Evans C, Bruckdorfer KR, *Molec Aspects of Med* 13:1-111, 1992
63 Green ESR et al, *Biochem Pharmacol* 45:357-366, 1993
64 Rice-Evans C, *Antioxidants & Disease Prevention: Biochem, Nut & Pharmacol Aspects*, ILSI Intl Sympsm, Stockholm, June/July 1993
65 Uchida S et al, *Plant Flavonoids in Biology & Medicine 2: Biochemical, Cellular & Medicinal Properties*, Eds. Cody, Middleton, Harborne, Beretz, Alan R Liss Inc., NY 1988; pp135-138
66 Ozaki M et al, *Flavonoids in Medicine & Biology 3: Current Issues in Flavonoid Research*, Ed. Das NP, Natl Univ Singapore 1990; pp 259-265
67 Elstner EF et al, *Ibid*, pp227-235
68 Salvayre R et al, *Flavonoids & Bioflavonoids*, Eds. Farkas, Gabor, Kallay, pp437-442, Elsevier 1986
69 Maridonneau I et al. *Ibid*, pp427-436
70 Pincemail J et al, *Experientia* 43:181, 1987
71 Zhao J et al, *Carcinogenesis* 20:9: 1737-1745, 1999
72 Horrobin D, Scotia Pharmaceuticals; personal communication
73 Kapitanov AB et al, *Antioxidants & Disease Prevention: Biochem Nut & Pharmacol Aspects*, ILSI Intl Symposium Stockholm, 1993
74 Kuttan R et al, *Experientia* 37:221-223, 1981
75 Masquelier J et al, *Acta Therapeutica* 7:101-105, 1981

76   Kakegawa H et al, *Chem Pharmacol Bulltn* 33:5079 1985

77   White D, Intl Sympsm on Pycnogenol, Bordeaux, France, Oct 1990

78   Feine-Haake G, *Zeitschrift für Allgemeinemedizin* 51:839, 1975

79   Blaszo G, Gabor M, *Acta Phys Scient Hungaricae* 56(2):235-240, 1980

80   Schmidke I, Schoop W, *Schweizerische Gesellschaft für Phebologie*, January 1984

81   Leydhecker HCW, *Report on Efficacy of Pycnogenol in Diabetic Retinopathy*, University Eye Clinic, Wurzburg

82   Passwater R, *The New Super-Antioxidant*, Keats Publishing, New Canaan, CT 1992

83   Masquelier J, *Reports from Centre d'Experimentation Pharmaceutiques*, Bordeaux, France

84   Steinmetz KA, Potter JD, *Cancer Causes Control* 2:325-357, 1991

85   Block G et al, *Nutrition & Cancer*, 18(1):1-26, 1992

86   Mitscher LA, Gollapudi SR, *Flavonoids in Medicine & Biology 3: Current Issues in Flavonoid Research*, Ed. Das NP, Natl Univ Singapore 1990; pp447-456

87   Wood AW et al, *Proc Natl Acad Sci USA* 79:5513-5517, 1924

88   Mukhtar H et al, *Carcinogenesis* 5:1565-1571, 1984

89   Teel RW, *Cancer Letters* 30:329-336, 1986

90   Wheeler EL, Berry DL, *Carcinogenesis* 7:33-36, 1986

91   Nishino H et al, *Gann* 75:113-116, 1984

92   Wang ZY et al, *Carcinogenesis* 10:411-415, 1989

93   Wei H et al, *Cancer Research* 50:499-502, 1990

94   Nagabhushan M, *The Toxicologist* 10:166, 1990

95   Wiltrout RH, Hornung RL, *J Natl Cancer* 80:220-222, 1988

96   Yu CL, Swaminthan B, *Food Chem Toxicol* 25(2):135-139, 1987

97   Volkner W, Muller E, Cytotest Cell Research GmbH, Projects 143010, 143021, 1989

98   International Bio-Research Inc, Acute & chronic toxicity tests, Hanover, Germany

99   Hiemstra SJ, *Food Consumption, Prices and Expenditures*, US Dept Agriculture, Econ Res Serv, Agric Econ Rep 138, Wash. DC, 1968

100 Putnam JJ, *Food Consumption, Prices and Expenditures 1966-1987* Stat Bulltn 773, US Dept Agriculture, Econ Res Serv, Wash. DC 1989

101 Putnam JJ, *Food Consumption, Prices and Expenditures 1966-1987* Stat Bulltn 804 US Dept Agric Econ Res Serv, Wash. DC 1989

102 Mitscher LA, Gollapudi SR, *Flavonoids in Medicine & Biology 3: Current Issues in Flavonoid Research*, Ed. Das NP, Natl Univ Singapore, 1990; pp447-456

103 Middleton E, Drzwieki G, *Biochem Pharmacol* 33:333-338, 1984

104 Middleton E, Drzwieki G, *Intl Archives Allergy Applied Immunol* 77:155-157, 1985

105 Amella M et al, *Planta Medica* 51:16-20, 1985

106 Pearce F et al, *J Allergy Clin Immunol* 73:819-823, 1984

107 Renaud S, de Lorgeril M, *Lancet* 339:1523-1526, 1992

108 Renaud S et al, *Am J Clin Nut* 55:1012-1017, 1992

109 Steinberg G et al, *New Eng J Med* 320:915-924, 1989

110 Frankel EN et al, *Lancet* 341:454-571, 1993

111 Werbach M & Murray MT, *Botanical Influences in Illness: A Sourcebook*, Third Line Press, Tarzana, CA 1995

112 Werbach M & Murray MT, *Nutritional Influences in Illness: A Sourcebook of Clinical Research*, 2nd edition,Third Line Press, Tarzana, CA1993

113 Maffei Facino R et al, *Antioxidants, Vitamins & Beta Carotene in Disease Prevention*, 2nd Intl Conf, Berlin 1994; Abs p60

114 Maxwell S et al, *Lancet* 344:193-194, 1994

115 De Whalley CV et al, *Biochem Pharmacol* 39:1743-1750, 1990

116 Peng H et al, *Artery* 20:122-134, 1993

117 Mitchinson MJ, *Br J Clin Prac* 48:147-151, 1994

118 Rice-Evans C, Bruckdorfer KR, *Molec Aspects of Medicine* 13:1-111, 1992

119 Duthie GG et al, *Antioxidants, Vitamins & Beta Carotene in Disease Prevention*, 2nd Intl Conf, Berlin 1994; Abs p44

120 Serafini M et al, *Lancet* 344:626, 1994

121 Sakai A et al, *Teratogen, Carcinogen, Mutagen* 10:333-340 1990

122 Natl Res Council, *Diet, Nutrition & Cancer*, chap 13, Natl Academic Press, Wash DC 1982

123 Ueno I et al, *Jpn J Experim Med* 53:41-50, 1983

124 Birt DF & Bresnick E, *Human Nutrition* 7:221-260 1991

125 Troll W, Yavelow J, *Diet, Nutrition & Cancer: From Basic Research to Policy Implication*, Ed. Roe DA, Alan R Liss, NY 1983; pp167-176

126 Nagabhushan M et al, *Food Chem Toxicol* 25(7):545-547, 1987

127 Huang MT et al, *J Cell Biochem Suppl* 27:26-34, 1997

128 Nagabhusan M et al, *J Am College Nut* 11(2):192-198, 1992

129 Maurya AK, *Cancer Letters* 57(2):121-129, 1991

130 Nagabhushan M et al, *Antioxidants, Vitamins & Beta Carotene in Disease Prevention*, 2nd Intl Conf, Berlin 1994; Abs p73

131 Birkedal-Hansen H et al, *Crit Reviews in Oral Biol & Med* 4:197-250, 1993

132 Liotta LA et al, *Cell* 64:327-336, 1991

133 Matrisian LM et al, *Am J Med Science* 302:157-162, 1991

134 Mignatti P, Rifkin DB, *Physiol Review* 73:161-195, 1993

135 Ray JM, Stetler-Stevenson WG, *Eur Respir J* 7(11):2062-2072, 1994

136 Stetler-Stevenson WG et al, *Ann Review Cell Biol* 9:541-573, 1993

137 Stetler-Stevenson et al, *FASEB J* 7:1434-1441, 1993

138 Bonfil RD et al, *J Natl Cancer Inst* 81:587-594, 1989

139 Powell WC et al, *Cancer Research* 53:417-422, 1993

140 Streenath T et al, *Cancer Research* 52: 4942-4947, 1992

141 Levy AT et al, *Cancer Research* 51:439-444, 1991

142 Lyons JG et al, *Biochem* 30:1449-1456, 1991

143 Sato H et al, *Oncogene* 7:77-83, 1992

144 Weidner N et al, *New Eng J Med* 324:1-8, 1991

145 Albini A et al, *AIDS* 1994

146 Murphy AN et al, *J Cell Physiol* 157:351-358, 1993

147 Mignatti P et al, *Cell* 47:487-498, 1986

148 Moses MA, Langer R, *Biotech* 9:630-634, 1991

149 Moses MA et al, *Science* 248:1408-1410, 1990

150 Takigawa M et al, *Biochem Biophys Res Comm* 171:1264-1271, 1990

151 Alvarez OA et al, *J Natl Cancer Inst* 82:589-595, 1990

152 Schultz RM et al, *Cancer Research* 48:5539-5545, 1988

153 Giavazzi R, Taraboletti G: personal communication

154 Tierney GM et al, *Eur J Cancer* 35(4):563-568, 1999

155 Beattie G et al, *Clin Cancer Res* 4(2):1899-1902, 1998

156 Folkman J, *J Natl Cancer Inst* 82:4-6, 1990

157 Folkman J, *Nature Medicine* 1:27-31, 1995

158 Horak ER et al, *Lancet* 340:1120-1124, 1992

159 Weidner et al, *J Natl Cancer Inst* 84:1875-1887, 1992

160 Bosari S et al, *Human Pathology* 23:755-761, 1992

161 Gasparini G et al, *Clin Oncol* 12:454-466, 1994

162 Machiarani P et al, *Lancet* 340:145-146, 1992

163 Craft PS, Harris AL, *Ann Oncology* 5:305-311, 1994

164 Hayes DF, *Hematol Oncol Clin North Am* 8:51-71, 1994

165 Pincemail J et al, *Flavonoids in Medicine & Biology 3: Current Issues in Flavonoid Research*, Ed. Das NP, Natl Univ Singapore 1990; pp161-179

166 O'Brien T et al, *Cancer Research* 55(3):510-513, 1995

REFERENCES

167 Moghaddam A et al, *Proc Natl Acad Sci USA*, 1995

168 Zhang HT, Rees G, Bicknell R, unpublished observations

169 Bouskela et al, *Intl J Microcirc* 14:S1:79, 1994

170 Friesenecker B et al, *Intl J Microcirc* 14:50-55, 1994

171 Jaeger A et al, *Plant Flavonoids in Biology & Medicine 2: Biochemical, Cellular & Medicinal Properties*, Alan R Liss Inc, 1988; pp379-394

172 Stich HF et al, *Mutation Research* 95:119-128, 1985

173 Matrka & Marhold, *Proc 3rd Sympsm on Tox Testing for Safety of New Drugs*, Prague 1976; pp307-310

174 *BMJ* editorial, pp235-237, 25th Jan 1969

175 Vertommen J et al, *Phytotherapy Research* 8:430-432, 1994

176 Grønbæk M et al, *BMJ* 310:1165-1169, 1995

177 Klatsky AL, Armstrong M, *Am J Cardiology* 71:467-469, 1993

178 St Leger AS et al, *Lancet* 2:1017-1020, 1979

179 Gerdes L, *Ugeskr Lager* 154:3580-3586, 1992

180 Sælan H et al, *Alcohol & Drug Abuse 1992*, 21st edition, Copenhagen, Natl Board of Health 1993

181 Handa K et al, *Am J Cardiology* 65:287-289, 1990

182 Frankel EN et al, *Lancet* 341:1103-1104, 1993

183 Pace-Asciak CR et al, *Clin Chimica Acta* 235(2):207-219, 1995

184 Lamuela-Raventós RM et al, *J Agric Food Chem* 42:281-283, 1995

185 Demrow HS et al, *Circulation* 91(4):1182-1188, 1995

186 Ruf JC et al, *Arteriosclerosis Thromb Vasc Biol* 15(1):140-144, 1995

187 Lavy A et al, *Ann Nut Metab* 38/5:287-294, 1994

188 Baum RM, *Chem Eng News* , p20-26, 9 Apr 1984

189 Gonzales R et al, *Cancer Research* 44:4137-4139, 1984

190 Norback IH et al, *Ann Surg* 214:671-678, 1991

191 Cedarbaum AI, *Free Rad Biol Med* 7:537-539, 1989

192 Teli MR et al, *Lancet* 346:987-990, 1995

193 Axelson M, Setchell KDR, *FEBS Letters* 122:49-53, 1980

194 Setchell KDR et al, *Nature* 287:740-742, 1980

195 Stitch SR et al, *Nature* 287:738-740, 1980

196 Axelson M et al, *Biochem J* 201:353-357, 1982

197 Bannwart C et al, *Clin Chim Acta* 136:165-172, 1984

198 Bannwart C et al, *Fin Chem Letters* 4-5:120-125, 1984

199 Adlercreutz H et al, *Am J Clin Nut* 54:10931100, 1991

200 Setchell KDR et al, *Role of Gut Flora in Toxicity & Cancer*, Ed. Rowland IR, Academic Press, London 1988; pp315-345

201 Schultz TD et al, *Nutrition Research* 11:1089-1011, 1991

202 Lampe JW et al, *Am J Clin Nut* 60:122-128, 1994

203 Thompson LU et al, *Nut Cancer* 16:45-52, 1991

204 Kelly GE et al, *Clin Chim Acta* 223:9-22, 1993

205 Hollman PCH et al, *Am J Clin Nut* 62:1276-1282, 1995

206 Deihm C et al, *Lancet* 347:292-294, 1996

207 Deihm C et al, *VASA* 21:188-192, 1992

208 Rudofsky G et al, *Phlebol Proktol* 15:47-54, 1986

209 Steiner M, Hillmanns HG, *Munch Med Wochenschr* 31:551-552, 86

210 Thompson WG, *Lancet* 347:5-6, 1995

211 Siemann EH, Creasy LL, *Am J Enol Vitic* 43:49-52, 1992

212 Bell GD et al, *Atherosclerosis* 36:47-54, 1980

213 Renaud S, de Lorgeril M, *Lancet* 339:1523-1526, 1992

214 Klatsky AL et al, *Ann Epidemiology* 3:375-381, 1993

215 Key TJ et al, *BMJ* 313775-779, 1996

216 Poston RN, Johnson-Tidey R, *Am J Path* 149: 1996

217 Springer TA, *Cell* 76:301-304, 1994

218 Cybulski ML, Gimbrona MA. *Science* 251:788-791, 1991

219 Poston RN et al, *Am J Path* 140:665-673, 1992

220 Van der Wal AC et al, *Am J Path* 141:1427-1430, 1992

221 Wood KM et al, *Histopathol* 22:437-444, 1993

222 Johnson-Tidey RR et al, *Am J Path* 144:952-961, 1994

223 Hollman PC et al, *Am J Clin Nut* 62:1276-1282, 1996

224 Negre-Salvayre A, Salvayre R, *Free Rad Biol Med* 12:101-106, 1992

225 Knekt P et al, *BMJ* 312:478-481, 1996

226 Hertog MG et al, *Archives Intern Med* 155:381-386, 1995

227 Rimm EB et al, *Ann Intern Med* 125:384-389, 1996

228 Loew D et al, *2nd Intl Congress on Phytomedicine*, SL-70, Sept 11-14, Munich 1996

229 Loew D, *Ibid*, PL-4, Sept 11-14, Munich 1996

230 Franck U et al, *Ibid*, SL-71, Sept 11-14, Munich 1996

231 Serafini M et al, *Eur J Clin Nut* 50:28-32, 1996

232 Li D et al, *J Lipid Res* 37:1978-1986, 1996

233 Jang M et al, *Science* 275:218-220, 1997

234 Clifford AJ et al, *Am J Clin Nut* 64:748-756, 1996

235 Bravo L et al, *Br J Nutrition* 71:933-946, 1994

236 Osawa T, *Phenolic Antioxidants in Plants as Mutagens: Phenolic compounds in Food & their Effect on Health*, Eds. Huang HT, Ho CT, Lee CY, Am Chem Soc, Washington DC 1992; pp269-283

237 Ito N et al, *Ibid*, pp269-283

238 Yoshizawa S et al, *Ibid*, pp316-325

239 Kellof GJ et al, *J Cell Biochem* 20S:1-24, 1994

240 Stavric B, *Clin Biochem* 27:245-248, 1994

241 Wang H et al, *J Agric Food Chem* 44:701-705, 1996

242 Bonser H et al, *Planta Medica* 62:212-216, 1996

243 Hodges S, personal communication

244 Anonymous, *Diet, Nutrition & Cancer*, Natl Academic Press, Washington DC 1982; p358

245 Cao G et al, *Am J Clin Nut* 68:1081-1087, 1998

246 Cao G et al, *Clin Chem* 45:574-576, 1999

247 Thompson WG, *Lancet* 347:5-6, 1995

248 Fontham ET, *Intl J Epidemiology* 19 Suppl 1:S32-S42, 1990

249 Miller HE et al, *Cereal World* 45:59-63, 2000

250 Holmes-McNary M et al, *Cancer Res* July 2000

Soy

251 *Protein Quality Evaluation*, Report of a Joint FAO/WHO Expert Consultation, UN FAO, Rome and WHO, Geneva 1990

252 Young VR, *JADA* 91:828-835, 1991

253 Raper NR et al, *J Am College Nut* 11:304-308, 1992

254 Troll W, Kennedy A, Workshop Report, Division of Cancer Aetiology, National Cancer Institute, *Cancer Research* 49:499-503, 1989

255 Abou-Issa H et al, *Eur J Cancer* 28A:784-788, 1992

256 Troll W et al, *Carcinogenesis* 1:469-472, 1980

257 St Clair WH et al, *Cancer Research* 50:580-586, 1990

258 Witschi H et al, *Carcinogenesis* 10:2275-2277, 1989

259 Takahashi M et al, *Chemically Induced Cell Proliferation*, Wiley Liss Inc, New York 1991; pp145-154

260 Messadi DV et al, *JNCI* 76:447-452, 1986

261 Von Hofe E et al, *Carcinogenesis* 12:2147-2150, 1991

262 Weed HG et al, *Carcinogenesis* 6:1239-1241, 1985

263 Shamsuddin AM et al, *Carcinogenesis* 9:577-580, 1988

264 Raicht RF et al, *Cancer Research* 40:403-405, 1980

265 Tanizama H et al, *Proc Sympsm Wakan-Yaku*, 15:119-123, 1982

266 Elias R et al, *Mutagenesis* 5:327-331, 1990

267 Newmark HL, *Can J Physiol Pharmacol* 65:461-466, 1987

268 Adlercreutz H et al, *Scand J Clin Investig* 48:190, 1988

269 Barnes S et al, *Mutagens & Carcinogens in the Diet*, Ed. Pariza MW, Wiley-Liss, New York 1990; pp239-253

270 Barnes S, Univ Alabama, personal communication, Jan 1993

271 Akiyama T, Ogawara H, *Meth Enzymol* 201:362-370, 1991

272 Akiyama T et al, *J Biol Chem* 262:5592-5595, 1987

273 Watanabe T et al, *Experim Cell Res* 183:335-342, 1989

274 Fotsis T et al, *Proc Natl Acad Sci USA* 90:2690-2694, 1993

275 Chen A et al, *BMJ* 303:276-282, 1991

276 Brown MS, Goldstein JL, *Science* 232:34-47, 1986

277 D'Adamo PJ, *Re: Lectins*, posted 10 March 1997 @ http:www.dadamo.com

278 Ornish D et al, *Lancet* 336:129-133, 1990

279 Carroll KK, *JADA* 91:820-827, 1981

280 Van Raaij JMA et al, *Am J Clin Nut* 35:925-934, 1982

281 Potter SM et al, *Am J Clin Nut* 58(4):501-506, 1993

282 Sirtori CR et al, *Ann NY Acad Science* 676:188-201, 1993

283 Jackson RL et al, *Med Res Review* 13:161-182, 1993

284 Kuller L, Lilienfeld A, *Circulation* 34:1056-1058, 1966

285 Turnbull WH et al, *Am J Clin Nut* 55:415-419, 1992

286 Burley VJ et al, *Eur J Clin Nut* 47:409-418, 1993

287 Kennedy AR, *J Nutrition* 125/3:733S-743S, 1995

288 Young VR et al, *Am J Clin Nut* 39:16-24, 1984

289 Torun B et al, *Protein Quality in Humans: Assessment and in vitro Estimation*, Eds. Bodwell CE, Adkins JS, Hopkins DT, AVI Publishing Co Inc, 1991; pp347-389

290 Wayler A et al, *J Nutrition* 113:2485-2491, 1983

291 Anderson JW et al, *New Eng J Med* 333:276-282, 1995

292 Sugano M et al, *Ann Nut Metab* 28:192-199, 1984

293 Carroll KK, *Fed Proc* 41:2792, 1982

294 Kritchevsky D, *Atherosclerosis* 41:429, 1982

295 Ikeda I et al, *Lipid Research* 29:1573-1582, 1988

296 Oakenfull D, Sidhu GS, *Eur J Clin Nut* 44:79-88, 1990

297 Mattson FH et al, *Am J Clin Nut* 35:697-700, 1982

298 Walker A, personal communication

299 Mattson FH et al, *Am J Clin Nut* 35:697-700, 1982

300 Ikeda et al, *Lipid Research* 29:1573-1582, 1988

301 Dakenfull D, Sidhin GS, *Eur J Clin Nut* 44:79-88, 1990

302 Freed DLJ, *Dietary Lectins and Disease* in *Food Allergy & Intolerances*, Eds. Brostoff J, Challacombe SJE, Bailliese Tindall, 1987; pp395-400

303 Wattenberg LW, *Food & Cancer Prevention: Chem & Biolog Aspects*, Eds. Waldron, Johnson, Fenwick, Royal Soc Chem, 1993; pp12-23

304 D'Adamo PJ, *Many lectins not inactivated by digestion*, posted 2 Sep. 1997 @ http:www.dadamo.com

Tea

311 Huang MT. Ferraro T, *Phenolic Compounds in Foods and their Effects on Health 2*, Eds. Huang MT, Ho C and Lee CY, ACS Symposium Series 507, New York 1992; p834

312 Ziegler RG et al, *Cancer Research* 52: 2060s-2066s, 1992

313 Lunder TL, *Phenolic Compounds in Foods and their Effects on Health 2*, Eds. Huang MT, Ho C and Lee CY, ACS Symposium Series 507, New York 1992; pp114-120

314 Soc Prod Nestlé, *Green tea catechins to solubilise tea cream*, Eur Pt 0.201.000, 1986

315 Soc Prod Nestlé, *Green tea rich in catechins*, patent applied for 1992

316 Klaunig JE, *Preventive Medicine* 21:510-519, 1992

317 Rosen FB et al, *Preventive Medicine* 21:520-525 1992

318 Stich K et al, *Mutation Research* 95:119-128 1985

319 Akinyanja & Yudkin, *Nature* 214:426-427 1967

320 Green & Jucha, *J Epidemiology Commun* 40:324-329 1986

321 Jenkins GN, *Proc Finn Dent Soc* 87:571-579 199

322 Yamaga et al, *J Dental Research* 66:919 1987

323 Nakahara K et al, *Intl Sympsm on Tea Science*, New York, August 1991

324 Fusi F et al, *Antioxidants & Disease Prevention: Biochem Nut & Pharmacol Aspects*, ILSI Intl Sympsm Stockholm, June/ July, 1993

325 Wakai K et al, *Jap Cancer Research* 84(12):1223-1229, 1993

Chocolate

331 Kris-Ethertom P, *Effects of whole food diets high in stearic acid on serum lipids of free-living subjects*, American Cocoa Institute, McLean, VA, 1994

332 Grundy, S, *Effects of diets high in stearic acid on serum lipids in metabolic studies*, American Cocoa Institute, McLean, VA,1994

333 Committee on Medical Aspects of Food Policy, *Report on Health & Social Subjects 46: Nut Aspects of Cardiovascular Disease*, Report, Cardiovascular Review Group, HMSO Nov 1994; pp138, 143

334 Waterhouse AL et al, *Lancet* 348:834, 1996

335 Donovan JL, *J Nutrition* 129:1662-1668,1999

336 Lee IM, Paffenbarger RS Jr., *BMJ* 317:1683-1684, 1998

Chapter 7: Pre-biotic fibre

1 Rutherford PP, Whittle R, *J Horticul Science* 57:349-356, 1982

2 Darbyshire B, *J Horticul Science* 53:195-201, 1978

3 Van Loo, J et al, *Inulin and Oligofructose in food, Critical Reviews in Food Science & Nutrition*, Tiense Suikkerraffinaderij Services, Tienen, Belgium, 1995.

4 Delamare JM, Levebvre C, Mémoire de fin d'études à l'Institut Supérieur d'Agriculture à Lille, 1971

5 Van Der Linden R, *Cikorei Kon Bond der Oostvlaamse Volkskundingen*, Gent 1973

6 Roberfroid M, *J Nutrition* 129 (7 Suppl):1398S-1401S, 1999

7 Delzenne N, poster presented at 10th Meeting at Nutrition Centre, Univ Limburg, 1992

8 De Laether M, Thesis at UCL Faculty of Medicine, Belgium 1992

9 Gibson G et al, *Gastroenterology* 104:19, 1993

10 Wang X, Gibson G, *J Applied Bacteriol* 75:373-380, 1993

11 Wang X, PhD Thesis at Dunn Institute, Cambridge Univ, 1993

12 Whitton PD et al, *FEBS Letters* 98:85-87, 1979

13 Remesy C et al, *Dietary Fiber – a Component of Food*, Eds. Schweizer TF & Edwards CA, Springer Verlag, 1992; pp137-150

14 Anderson JW, Bridges SR, *Diabetes* 30:133A, 1981

15 Hidaka H et al, *Bifidobacteria Microflora* 5:37-50, 1986

16 Okada J et al, *Proc 2nd Neosugar Research Conference*, Meija-Seika Publications, Tokyo 1984; pp69-85

17 Mitsuoka T et al, *Die Nabrung* 31:426-436, 1987

18 McKellar RC, Modler HW, *Applied Microbiol & Biotech* 31:537-541, 1989

19 Roberfroid M, *Critical Reviews in Food Sci & Nut* 33:103-148, 1993

20 Roberfroid M et al, *Nutrition Reviews* 51:137-146, 1993

21 Levrat MA et al, *J Nutrition* 121:1730-1737, 1991

22 Ohta A et al, *Nippon Eiyo Shokuryo Gakkaishi* 46:123-129, 1993

23 Harmuth-Hoene AE, Schelling R, *J Nutrition* 10:1774-1784, 1980

24 De Schrijver R, Conrad S, *J Ag Food Chem* 40:1166-1171, 1992

25 Wright PS et al, *Proc Soc Experim Biol Med* 195:26-29, 1990

REFERENCES

26 Hata N et al, *Proc 1st Neosugar Research Conference*, Meija-Seika Publications, Tokyo 1982; pp63-72

27 Takeda U, Niizato T, *Ibid*, pp88-99

28 Tokunaga T et al, *J Nut Science & Vitamins* 32:11-121, 1986

29 Coussement P, personal communication

30 Gibson GR, Wang X, *J Applied Bacteriol* 77(4):412-420, 1994

31 Wang X, Gibson GR; *J Applied Bacteriol* 75:373-380, 1993

32 Gibson GR et al, *Gastroenterology* 108(4):975-982, 1995

33 Reddy BS, Rivenson A, *Cancer Research* 53:3914-3918, 1993

34 Koo M, Rao AV, *Nut Review* 51:137-146, 1991

35 Kohwi Y et al, *Gann* 69:613-618, 1978

36 Sekine K et al, *Cancer Research* 45:1300-1307, 1985

37 Delzenne N et al, *Am J Clin Nut* 57:820S, 1993

38 Chun W et al, *Digestion* 42:22, 1989

39 Dowling RH, *Scand J Gastroenterol* 17:(Suppl 74) 53, 1982

40 Todesco et al, *Am J Clin Nut* 54(5):860-865, 1991

41 Schweizer TF et al, *Eur J Clin Nut* 44:567, 1990

42 Yamashita K et al, *Nutrition Research* 4:961, 1984

43 Davidson MH et al, *Proc.1st Orafti Research Conference*, Université Catholique de Louvain, Jan 17 1995; pp83-94

44 Takahashi Y, *Topic 1-3, Proc 3rd Neosugar Research Conference*, Tokyo 1986

45 Kritchevsky D, *Ann Review Nut* 8:301, 1988

46 Miller TL, Wolin MJ, *Am J Clin Nut* 32:164, 1979

47 Lee SC, Prosky L, *Intl Survey on Dietary Fibre Reference Materials* (Abstr) 6th Intl Sympsm Biol Environ Ref Materials, 1994

48 Balows A et al, *Manual of Clin Microbiol*, 5th edition, ASM Press, Washington 1991

49 Leder A, Leder P, *Cell* 5:319-322, 1975

50 Kim YS et al, *Falk Symposium* 31:317-323, 1982

51 Gibson GR, Wang X, *J Applied Bacteriology* 77:412-420, 1994

52 Wiggins HS, Cummings JH, *Gut* 17:1007-1011, 1976

53 Byrne BM, Dankert J, *Infection & Immunity* 23:559-563, 1979

54 Dodd HM, Gasson MJ, *Genetics & Biotech of Lactic Acid Bacteria* , Eds. Gasson MJ, de Vos WM, Chapman & Hill, London 1994; pp211-251

55 Hurst A, *Advances in Applied Microbiol* 27:85-123, 1981

56 Fowler GG, Gasson MJ, *Antibiotics In Food Preservatives*, Eds. Russel NJ, Goulds GW, Blackie & Sons, Glasgow 1990; pp135-152

57 Gibson GR, Wang X, *FEBS Microbiology Letters* 118:121-128, 1994

58 Drasar BS, Roberts AK, *Control of Large Bowel Microflora in Human Microbiol Ecology*, Eds. Hill MJ, Marsh PD, CRC Press, Boca Raton 1990; pp87-110

59 Yoshioka M et al, *Bifidobacteria Microflora* 10:11-17, 1991

60 Bullen CL, Willis AT, *BMJ* 3:338-343, 1971

61 Bezkorovainy A, *Biochem & Physiology of Bifidobacteria*, Eds. Bezkorovainy A, Miller-Catchpole R, CRC Press, Boca Raton 1989; pp29-72

62 Wells CL et al, *Eur J Clin Microbiol Infect Dis* 7:107-113, 1988

63 Yamazaki S et al, *Bifidobacteria Microflora* 1:55-60, 1982

64 Yamazaki S et al, *Immunology* 56:43-50, 1985

65 Bouhnik Y et al, *Gastroenterology* 102:875-878, 1992

66 Orafti internal note, *Impact of Oligofructose on Gut Function*, 1994

67 Orafti internal note, *Bifidous Effect of Inulin & Oligofructose*, 1994

68 Demigne N et al, *J Nutrition* 116:77-86, 1986

69 Delzenne N et al, Internal report, Orafti 1994

70 Roediger WEW, *Gut* 21:793-798, 1980

71 Venter CS et al, *Am J Gastroenterol* 85:549, 1990

72 Venter CS et al, *J Nutrition* 120:1046, 1990

73 McBurney MI, Thompson LU, *Nut Cancer* 13:271, 1990

74 Leischer SZ, *Kinderheik*, 85:265-276, 1961

75 Goldin BR, Gorbach SL, *Probiotics: The Scientific Basis*, Ed. Fuller R, Chapman & Hall, London 1992; pp355-376

76 Fiordaliso MF et al, *Lipids* 30(2):163-167, 1995

77 Delzenne N, *Proc 1st Orafti Research Conference*, Université Catholique de Louvain, Jan 17th 1995; pp75-82

78 Bell LP et al, *JAMA* 261:3419-4323, 1989

79 Cummings JH, *Proc 1st Orafti Research Conference*, Université Catholique de Louvain, Jan 17th 1995; pp95-108

80 Delzenne N et al, *Ibid*, pp275-278

81 Shannon JA, Smith HW, *J Clin Investig* 14:393-401, 1935

82 Hata Y et al, *Geriat Med* 21:156-167, 1983

83 Mitsuoka T et al, *Topic 1-4, Proc 3rd Neosugar Research Conference*, Tokyo 1986

84 Touhami M et al, *Ann Pediat* 39(2):79-86, 1992

85 Siitonen S et al, *Ann Med* 22(1):57-59, 1990

86 Faulds CB, Williamson G, *Microbiol* 140:779-787, 1994

87 Borneman WS et al, *Applied Environ Microbiol* 58:3762-3766, 1992

88 Faulds CB, Williamson G, *Biochem Soc Trans* 23:253S, 1995

89 Graf E, *Free Rad Biol Med* 13:435-448, 1992

90 Scott BC et al, *Free Rad Res Comm* 19:241-253, 1993

91 Moller ME et al, *Food Chem Toxic* 26:841-845, 1988

92 Nersessian AK, *Food & Cancer Prevention: Chem & Biolog Aspects*, Eds. Waldron, Johnson, Fenwick, Royal Soc Chem, 1993; pp62-63

93 Isolauri E et al, *Pediatrics* 88:90-97, 1991

94 Oksanen P et al, *Ann Medicine* 22:53-56, 1990

95 Wells CL et al, *Eur J Clin Microbiol Infect Dis* 7:107-113, 1988

96 Yamazaki S et al, *Immunology* 56:43-50, 1985

97 Yoshioka M et al, *Bifidobacteria Microflora* 10:11-17, 1991

98 Meurman HJ et al, *Microbiol Ecology in Health & Disease* 7(6): 295-298, 1994

99 Agerbaek M et al, *Eur J Clin Nut* 49(5):346-352, 1995

100 Midolo PD et al, *J Applied Bacteriol* 79:475-479,1995

101 Harig JM et al, *New Eng J Med* 320:23-28, 1989

102 Roediger WEW, *Lancet* 2:712-717, 1980

103 Scheppach W et al, *Gastroenterology* 103:51-56, 1992

104 Vernia P et al, *Digest Dis Science* 40:305-307, 1995

105 Naurath HJ et al, *Lancet* 346:85-89, 1995

106 Shaw GM et al, *Epidemiology* 6(3):205-207, 1995

107 Jacob RA et al, *J Nutrition* 124(7):1072-1080, 1994

108 Lindenbaum J et al, *Am J Clin Nut* 60(1):2-14, 1994

109 Nichols HK, Basu TK, *J Am College Nut* 13(1):57-61, 1994

110 Stampfer MJ et al, *JAMA* 268:877-881, 1992

111 Pietrzik K et al, *Antioxidant Vitamins and Beta Carotene in Disease Prevention*, 2nd Intl Conference, Berlin 1994; Abs p93

112 Saavedra JM et al, *Lancet* 344:1046-1049, 1994

113 Mitsuoka T, *Intestinal Flora & Human Health*, 3rd Intl Symposium on Intestinal Flora, Yakult Bio-science Foundation, Amsterdam 1994; pp3-21

114 Mizutani T, Mitsuoka T, *Cancer Letters* 11:89-95, 1980

115 Mizutani T, Mitsuoka T, *J Natl Cancer Inst* 63:1365-1370, 1979

116 Cummings JH, *Food, People & Health: Past, Present & Future*, Royal Society of Medicine Conference, London 1995

117 Kheng HY et al, *J Infect Dis* 170:1209-1215, 1994

118 Kempf C et al, *J AIDS* 4:828-830, 1991

119 Raz R, Stamm WE, *New Eng J Med* 329:763-766, 1993

120 Reid G, Bruce AW, *Lancet* 346:1704, 1996

121 Gelissen IC, Eastwood MA, *Br J Nutrition* 74:221-228, 1995
122 Spiller RC, *Lancet* 347:415-416, 1996
123 Davidson MH et al, *JAMA* 265:1833-1839, 1991
124 Christl SU et al, *Gut* 33:1234-1238, 1992
125 Finegold SM, *Oral Pathogens as Contributors to Systemic Infections*, Eastman Dental Institute, London, 7-8th March 1996
126 Thompson L, Spiller RC, *Br J Nutrition* 74:733-71, 1995
127 Michetti P et al, *Gastroenterology* 108:SS, p166 1995
128 Deguchi Y et al, *Agricultural & Biological Chemistry*, 49:13-19, 1985
129 Bartram H-P et al, *Nutrition & Cancer* 25:71-78, 1996
130 Macknin ML et al, *Ann Intern Med* 125:81-88, 1996
131 Buddington RK et al, *Am J Clin Nut* 63:709-716, 1996
132 Perrin P et al, *C R Acad Sci (Life Sciences) Paris* 316:611-614,1993
133 Fabrice P et al, *Cancer Research* 57:225-228, 1997
134 Bezkorovainy A, *Biochem & Physiol of Bifido Bacteria*, CRC Press 1989; pp147-177
135 Lund EK et al, *Am J Clin Nut* 69: 250-255, 1999
136 Delzenne, N, Roberfroid, M, *Lebenson-Wiss. u Technol.* 27:1-6, 1994
137 Raa J, *Functional Foods* 2:25-27, 1999
138 Scheinin A, Makinen KK, *Acta Odent Scand* 33:S70, 1975
139 Lizho NN, *Die Nahrung* 31:5-6,, 443-447, 1987
140 Schultz F, Hartman H, *Gastrointestinale Mikroflora des Menschen*, JA Barth, Leipzig, 1980; pp221-224
141 Palmer RH, Hruban Z, *J Clin Invest* 45:1255-1267, 1966
142 Hill MJ et al, *Br J Cancer* 48:143, 1983
143 Vernitt S, *The Role of the Gut Flora in Toxicity and Cancer* (Ed.) Rowland IR, Academic Press, London, 1988; pp399-340
144 Miller HG et al, *Cereal Food World* 45:59-63, 2000

Chapter 8: Essential oils

1   Singh et al, *BMJ* 304:1015-9, 1992
2   Gissi-Prevenzione Investigators, *Lancet*, 354:447-445, 1999
3   Zhang J et al, *Prev Med* 28:520-529, 1999
4   Ziboh VA, *Lipids* 31:S249-S253, 1996
5   Rambjor GS, et al, *Lipids* 31:S45-S49, 1996
6   Feretti A, Flanagan VP, *Prostaglandins, Leukatrienes and Essential Fatty Acids* 54:451-455, 1996
7   Wander, RC, *Am J Clin Nut* 63:186-193, 1996
8   Eaton SB, *Food, People & Health: Past, Present & Future*, Royal Society of Medicine Conference, London, October 1995
9   Edwards IJ et al, *Clin Pharmacol Ther* 50:538-46,1991
10 Nordoy A et al, *Am J Clin Nut* 57:634-9, 1993
11 Pauletto P et al, *Lancet* 348:784-788, 1996
12 Takahashi K, Horrobin D, *Thrombosis Research* 47, 1987
13 Olsen EN et al, *Lancet* 339:1003-7, 1992
14 Troisi R et al, *Am J Clin Nut* 56:1010-24, 1992
15 Willett WC et al, *Lancet* 341:581-5, 1993
16 Min. of Agriculture, Fisheries & Food, *Food Information Surveillance Sheet 127*, HMSO, London
17 Horrobin D, personal communication
18 Bracco U, *Polyunsaturated Fatty Acids in Human Nutrition*, Eds. Bracco & Deckelbau, Nestlé Nutrition Workshop Series Vol 28, Nestec Ltd, Vevey/Raven Press Ltd, NY 199; pp147-158
19 Nestlé SA, European Patent Melange Anti-oxydant Synergique, 0326829_13.1.1989.
20 Nestle-Novo, Triglycerides composition WO 90/04013_10.10.1989
21 Innis S, *Dietary Omega 3 and Omega 6 Fatty Acids*, Eds. Galli C, Simopoulos AP, NATO ASI Series, 171:142, 1989
22 Spector AA, *Polyunsaturated Fatty Acids in Human Nutrition*, Eds. Bracco & Deckelbaum, Nestlé Nutrition Workshop Series Vol 28, Nestec Ltd, Vevey/Raven Press Ltd, NY 1992; pp1-12
23 James G, Olsen EN, *Biochemistry* 29:2623-2634, 1990
24 Lokesh BR et al, *J Lipid Res* 22:905-915, 1981
25 Spector AA, Yorek MA, *J Lipid Res* 26:1015-1035, 1985
26 Crawford MA et al, *Polyunsaturated Fatty Acids in Human Nutrition*, Eds. Bracco & Deckelbaum, Nestlé Nutrition Workshop Series Vol 28, Nestec Ltd, Vevey/Raven Press Ltd, NY 1992; pp93-110
27 Crawford MA, personal communication
28 Neuringer M, Connor WE, *Dietary Omega 3 & Omega 6 Fatty Acids: Biological Effects and Nutritional Essentiality*, Eds. Galli C, Simopoulos AP, Plenum Press, NY 1989; pp179-190
29 Feldman M et al, *Fetal and Neonatal Physiology*, Eds. Polin R, Fox W, Saunders WB, Toronto 1992; pp299-314
30 Clandidin MT et al, *Polyunsaturated Fatty Acids in Human Nutrition*, Eds. Bracco & Deckelbaum, Nestlé Nutrition Workshop Series Vol 28, Nestec Ltd, Vevey/Raven Press Ltd, NY 1992; pp111-119
31 Okuyama H, *Ibid*, pp169- 178
32 Gualde N, *Ibid*, pp195-209
33 Keys A, *Circulation* 41:11-211, 1979
34 Conference on Health Effects of Blood Lipids: Optimal distribution for populations *Prev Med* 8:612-678, 1979
35 Harris WS, *J Lipid Res* 30:785-807, 1989
36 Wong S, Nestel PJ, *Atherosclerosis* 64:139-146, 1987
37 Spady DK, Dietschy DM, *Proc Natl Acad Sci USA* 82:4526-4530, 1985
38 Nicolosi RJ et al, *Atherosclerosis* 10:119-128, 1990
39 Cheesman KH et al, *Toxicol & Pathol* 12(3):235-239, 1984
40 Stanley J, *Lipid Technology* May 99:61-64, 1999
41 Broughton KS et al, *Am J Clin Nut* 65:1011-1017, 1997
42 Visioli F, Galli C, *Biochem, Biophys Res Comm* 247:60-64, 1998
43 Dolicek TA, Grandita G, *World Review Nut Diet* 66, 205-216, 1991
44 Kromhout D et al, *New Eng J Med* 312, 1205-1207, 1985
45 Feskens EJM et al, *Diabetes Care* 16, 1029-1034, 1993
46 Shekelle RB et al, *New Eng J Med* 313:820, 1985
47 Addis PB et al, *Biochem Soc Sympsm* 61:259-271, 1995
48 Peng H et al, *Artery* 20:122-134, 1993
49 Osada T et al, *Lipids* 29:585-559, 1994
50 Aesbach R et al, *Antioxidants in Food*, Royal Soc Chemistry Meeting, London 2 Dec 1994
51 Yamamoto Y, *Ibid*
52 Genot C et al, *Ibid*
53 Nohl H et al, *Free Radicals in the Environment, Medicine & Toxicology*, Richelieu Press, London 1994; pp351-375
54 Hippeli S et al, *Ibid*, pp375-392
55 Bierenbaum ML et al, *Biochem International* 28:57-66, 1992
56 Hall DA, Burdett PE, *Biochem Soc Trans* 3:42-46, 1975
57 Wade E, Tsumita T, *Mech of Ageing & Dev* 27:287-294, 1984
58 Penzes L et al, *Mech of Ageing & Dev* 45:75-92, 1988
59 Deans SG, Svoboda, KP, *CAB AgBiotech News & Info* 2:211-216, 1990
60 Deans SG et al, *Experimental Gerontology, in Aspects of Ageing & Disease*, Eds. Knook & Hofeker, 9th Sympsm, Facultas Wien, 1994
61 Deans SG, Ritchie G, *Intl J Food Microbiol* 5:165-180, 1987
62 Deans SG et al, *Role of Free Radicals in Biological Systems*, Eds. Feher et al, Akademiai Kiado, Budapest 1993; pp159-165
63 Atkinson HAC, Maisey J, *Biochem Soc Trans* 23: 277S, 1995

REFERENCES

64 Yaqoob P et al, *Immunology* 82:603-610, 1994

65 Yaqoob P et al, *Immunology Letters* 41:241-247, 1994

66 Hubbard NE et al, *Leuk Biol* 49:592-598, 1989

67 Meydani SM et al, *Nut Clin Prac* 8:65-72, 1991

68 Hodgson J et al, *Am J Clin Nut* 58:228-234, 1993

69 Peterson J et al, *Lancet* 343:1528-1530, 1994

70 Rasmussen LB et al, *Am J Clin Nut* 59:572-577, 1994

71 Fernandes G, *Clin Immunol Immunopath* 72(2):193-197, 1994

72 Barth W, personal communication.

73 Mann GV, *Lancet* 343:1268-1271

74 Thomas LH, *Br J Prev Soc Med* 29:82-90, 1975

75 Senti FR Ed. *Health Aspects of Dietary Trans Fatty Acids*, August 1985, Bethesda Md & Fed Am Soc Experim Biol 1988 (contract no FDA 223-83-2020).

76 Enig MG et al, *J Am Oil Chem Soc* 60:1788-1794, 1983

77 Slover HT et al, *J Am Oil Chem Soc* 62:775-786, 1985

78 Holman RT et al, *Proc Natl Acad Science* 88:4830-4834, 1991

79 Mensink RPM, Katan MB, *New Eng J Med* 323:439-445, 1990

80 Zock PL, Katan MB, *J Lipid Res* 33:399-410, 1992

81 Thomas LH et al, *J Epidemiology Commun Health* 37:16-21, 1983

82 Willet WC et al, *Lancet* 341:581-585, 1993

83 Ascherio A et al, *Circulation* 89:94-101, 1994

84 Willett WC, Ascherio A, *Am J Pub Health* 84:722-724, 1994

85 COMA, *Nutritional Aspects of Cardiovascular Disease*, Dept. Health, UK 1994; p46

86 Koletzko B, *Acta Paediatric Care* 81:302-306, 1992

87 Claxson AWD et al, *FEBS Letters* 355:81-90, 1994

88 Anttolainen M et al, *Antioxidants & Disease Prevention: Biochem, Nut & Pharmacol Aspects*, ILSI Intl Symposium, Stockholm June/July 1993; p87

89 Addis PB, *Food & Nutrition News* 62:2-11, 1990

90 Sanders TAB, Hinds A, *Br J Nutrition* 68:163-173, 1992

91 Allard JP, *Antioxidants, Vitamins & Beta Carotene in Disease Prevention*, 2nd Intl Conf, Berlin 1994; Abs p47

92 Scherat T et al, *Ibid*; Abs p49

93 Vrana A et al, *Ibid*; Abs p66

94 Miner RW Ed. *Vitamin E, Ann NY Acad Science* 52:63-428, 1949

95 Willett WC et al, *New Eng J Med* 316(1):22-28, 1987

96 Willett WC et al, *New Eng J Med* 323(24):1664-1672, 1990

97 Kent S, *Geriatrics* 31:128-137, 1976

98 Burr M et al, *Lancet* 2:757-761, 1989

99 Powell J, Children's Hospital, Ladywood, Birmingham: personal communication

100 Nandy K, Bourne GH, *Nature* 210:313-314, 1966

101 Nandy K, *Mech of Ageing & Dev* 8:131-138, 1978

102 Hochschild R, *Experim Gerontology* 8:177-183, 1973

103 Mercer D, Hopkins SM, *Age & Ageing* 6:123-131, 1977

104 Jensen RG et al, *J Paediat Gastroent & Nutrition* 14:474-475; 1992

105 Kremer JN et al, *Arthritis & Rheumatism* 33:810; 1990

106 Uemara K, Pisa Z, *World Health Stats Quarterly* 41:155-177, 1988

107 Abbey M et al, *Am J Clin Nut* 59(5):995-999, 1994

108 Almendingen K et al, *J Lipid Research* 36:1370-1384, 1995

109 Loliger J, *Rancidity in Foods*, Eds. Allen JC & Hamilton RJ, Elsevier Applied Science, London 1989; p47

110 Schuler P, *Food Antioxidants*, Ed. Hudson BJF, Elsevier Applied Science, London 1990; p134

111 Gordon MH, Kourimská L, *J Science Food Agric* 68:347-353, 1995

112 Drevon CA et al, *Can J Cardiol* 11 Suppl G:47G-54G, 1995

113 Grey KF et al, *Am J Clin Nut* 53:3265-3345, 1991

114 Esterbauer H et al, *Chem per Toxicol* 3:77-92,1990

115 Steinberg et al, *New Eng J Med* 320:915-924, 1989

116 Sabate J et al, *New Eng J Med* 328(9):603-607, 1993

Omega 3

151 Bang HO, Dyerberg J, *Advances Nut Res* 3:1-40, 1980

152 Burr M et al, *Lancet* 2:757-761, 1989

153 Dolicek TA, Grandita G, *World Review Nut Diet* 66:155-216, 1991

154 Kromhout D et al, *New Eng J Med* 312:1155-1207, 1985

155 Feskens EJM et al, *Diabetes Care* 16:1029-1034; 1993

156 Shekelle RB et al, *New Eng J Med* 313:820, 1985

157 Hulley SB et al, *Circulation* 86:1026-1029, 1992

158 Stensvold I et al, *BMJ* 307:1322-1325, 1993

159 Steingart RM et al, *New Eng J Med* 325:226-230, 1991

160 Ayanian JZ, Epstein AM, *New Eng J Med* 325: 221-225, 1991

161 Takahashi R Horrobin D, *Thrombosis Research* 47: mm, 1987

162 Edwards IJ et al, *Atherosclerosis & Thrombosis* 11:1778-1785, 1991

163 Hirai A et al, *Thrombosis Research* 28:285-298, 1982

164 Van Houwelingen AC et al, *Atherosclerosis* 75:157-165, 1989

165 McVeigh J et al, *Diabetalogica* 36(1):33-38, 1993

166 Bonaa KH et al, *Am J Clin Nut* 55:1126-1134, 1992

167 Nordoy A et al, *Am J Clin Nut* 57:634-639, 1993

168 Chin J et al, *Hypertension* 21(1):22-28, 1993

169 Cobiac L et al, *Clin Experim Pharmacol Physiol* 18:265-268, 1991

170 McLellan PL et al, *Am Heart J* 116:709-712, 1988

171 Addis P, personal communication

172 Peng H et al, *Artery* 20:122-134, 1993

173 Osada T et al, *Lipids* 29:585-559, 1994;

174 Harris WS, *J Lipid Res* 30:785-807, 1989

175 Wong S, Nestel PJ, *Atherosclerosis* 64:139-146, 1987

176 Horrobin D, personal communication

177 Ashwell M, Ed. *Diet & Heart Disease – a round table of factors*, British Nutrition Foundation 1993; p50

178 British Nutrition Foundation, *Task Force Report Unsaturated Fatty Acids; Nut & Physiolog Significance*, Chapman & Hall, London, 1992

179 Kruger MC et al, *Prostaglandins,* 9th Intl Congress, Florence, June 4-9, 1994

180 Sakaguchi K et al, *Prostaglandins, Leukotrienes EFAs* 50:81-84, 1994

181 Schiff E et al, *Am J Obstet Gynecol* 168(1):122-124; 1993

182 Olsen EN at al, *Lancet* 339:1003-7, 1992

183 Prisco D et al, *Metabolism: Clin & Experim* 44(5):562-569, 1995

184 Garcia Osle M et al, *Ann Med Interna* (Spain) 11/10:473-478, 1994

185 Schwartz J, Weiss ST, *Eur Respir J* 7:1821-1824, 1994

186 Shahar E et al, *New Eng J Med* 331:228-233, 1994

187 Sharp DS et al, *Am J Respir & Crit Care Med* 150:983-987, 1994

188 Lau TF et al, *Br J Rheum* 32:82-89, 1993

189 Geusens P et al, *Arth & Rheum* 37:819-829, 1994

190 Morris MC et al, *Circulation* 88:523-533, 1993

191 Shimokawa H, Vanhoutte PM, *Circulation* 78:1421-1430, 1988

192 Leung W-H et al, *Lancet* 341:1496-1500, 1993

193 Chin JA et al, *J Clin Investig* 89:10-18, 1992

194 Salonen JT et al, *Lancet* 339:883-887, 1992

195 Ohara Y et al, *J Clin Investig* 91:2546-2551, 1993

196 Weber C et al, *Molec Aspects Med* 15:S97-S102, 1995

197 Chin JPF, Dart AM, *Clin Experim Pharmacol Physiol* 21(10):749-755, 1994

198 Chen LY et al, *Thrombosis Research* 76(4):317-322, 1994

199 Keli SO et al, *Stroke* 25(2):328-332, 1994

200 Sacks FM et al, *J Am College Cardiol* 25(7):1492-1498, 1995

201 Misso NLA, Thompson PJ, *Platelets (UK)* 6(5):275-282, 1995

202 Kremer JM et al, *Arthritis & Rheumatism* 38:1107-1114, 1995

203 Rhodes LE et al, *J Investig Dermatol* 105:532-535, 1995

204 Rees DC et al, *Lancet* 346:1133-1135, 1995

205 Siscovick DS et al, *JAMA* 274:1363-1367, 1995

206 Fortin PR et al, *J Clin Epidemiology* 48:1379-1390, 1995

207 Eritsland J et al, *Am J Cardiology* 77:31-36, 1996

208 Osterud B et al, *Lipids* 30:1111-1118, 1995

209 Parta E et al, *Mech of Ageing & Dev* 13:1-39, 1980

Chapter 9: Co-enzyme Q10

1 Kamei M et al, *Intl J Vit Nut Res* 56:57 1986

2 Hodges S et al, *Biofactors* 9:365-370, 1999

3 Mitchell P, *J Theoret Biol* 62:327-367, 1976

4 Littaru, GP, *Energy & Defence, Facts and Perspectives on Coenzyme Q10 in Biology and Medicine*, Casa Editrice Scientifica Internazionale, Rome, 1994

5 Buznakow E et al, *Biomed & Clin Aspects of Q*, Eds. Folkers K et al, Vol 3, Elsevier, Amersterdam 1988; pp311-323

6 Langsjoen H et al, *Am J Cardiology* 65:521-523, 1990

7 Langsjoen PH et al, *Proc Natl Acad Sci USA* 82:4240-4244, 1985

8 Morisco C et al, *Clin Investig* 71: S134-136 1993

9 Lockwood K et al, *Biomed and Biophys Res Comm*, 199(3):1504-1508, 1994

10 Nylander M et al, *Proc 8th Intl Sympsm Q10*, Stockholm 1993

11 Hanioka T et al, *Ibid*

12 Yamabe H et al, *Biomed & Clin Aspects of CoQ10*, Vol 6, Eds. Folkers K et al, Elsevier, Amsterdam 1991; pp535-540,

13 Zeppilli P et al, *Ibid*, pp 541-546

14 Fiorella P et al, *Ibid*, pp513-520

15 Hansen IL et al, *Res Commun Chem Path Pharm* 14:4:729-738, 1976

16 Nylander M, *Biomed* 4:6-11, 1991

17 Shizukuishi S et al, *Biomed & Clin Aspects of Q10*: 5:359-368, 1986

18 Wilkinson EG et al, *Biomed & Clin Aspects of Q10*: 1:251-266, 1977

19 Wilkinson EG et al, *Res Commun Chem Path Pharm* 14:4:715-719, 1976

20 Wilkinson EG et al, *Res Commun Chem Path Pharm* 12:1:111-123, 1975

21 Stocker R, *Antioxidants & Disease Prevention: Biochem, Nut & Pharmacol Aspects*, ILSI Intl Symposium, Stockholm June/July 1993; pp45-46

22 Ingold KU et al, *Proc Natl Acad Sci USA* 90:45-49, 1993

23 Stocker R et al, *Antioxidants, Vitamins & Beta Carotene in Disease Prevention*, 2nd Intl Conf, Berlin 1994; Abs p17

24 Ernster L et al, *BioFactors* 3:241-248, 1992

25 Forsmark P et al, *FEBS Letters* 285:39-43, 1991

26 Takayanagi R et al, *Biochemical J* 192:853-860, 1980

27 Takeshige K, Minakami S, *J Biochem* 77:1067-1073, 1975

28 Takeshige K et al, *Biomed & Clin Aspects Of CoQ10*, Vol 2, Eds. Folkers K, Yamamura , Elsevier, Amsterdam 1980; pp15-26

29 Mellors A, Tappel AL, *J Biol Chem* 241:4353-4356, 1966

30 Bäckström D et al, *Biochim Biophys Acta* 197:108-111, 1970

31 King TE, *CoQ: Biochem, Bioenergetics & Clin Actions of Ubiquinone*, Ed. Lenaz G, Wiley, NY 1985; p391

32 Kröger A, Klingenberg M, *Eur J Biochem* 34:358-368, 1973

33 Mellors A, Tappel AL, *Lipids* 1:282-284, 1966

34 Yuziriha T et al, *Biochim Biophys Acta* 759:286, 1983

35 Karlsson J et al, *Klinische Wochenschr* 71:S84-91, 1993

36 Mohr D et al, *Biochim Biophys Acta* 1126:247-254, 1992

37 Tomono Y et al, *Intl J Clin Pharmacol Tox* 24:536-541, 1986

38 Kishi H et al, *Biochem & Clin Aspects of CoQ10*, Vol 4, Eds. Folkers K et al, Elsevier, Amsterdam 1984; pp131-142

39 Lucker PF et al, *Ibid*, pp143-151

40 Greenberg SM et al, *Med Clin N Am* 72:243-258, 1988

41 Folkers K et al, *Proc Natl Acad Sci USA* 82:4513-4516, 1985

42 Beyer RE et al, *Mech of Ageing & Dev* 32:267-281, 1985

43 Apelqvist EL et al, *Biomed and Clinical Aspects of CoQ10*, Vol 6, Eds. Folkers K et al, Elsevier, Amsterdam 1991; pp141-150

44 Lenaz G et al, *Ibid*, pp11-18

45 Valls V et al, *Biomarkers of Ageing; Expression and Regulation*, Eds. Licastro F & Calderra CM, CLUEB, Bologna 1992; pp389-396

46 Kalen A et al, *Lipids* 24:579-584, 1989

47 Beyer RE, *Free Rad Biol Med* 5:297-303, 1988

48 Beyer RE et al, *Biomed & Clin Aspects of CoQ 10*, Vol 5, Eds. Folkers K , Yamamua Y, Elsevier, Amsterdam 1986; pp17-24

49 Lenaz G et al, *Klinische Wochenschr* 71:S71-75, 1993

50 Judy WV et al, *Biomed and Clinical Aspects of CoQ10*, Vol 5, Eds. Folkers K et al, Elsevier, Amsterdam, 1986; pp315-323

51 Hofman-Bang C et al, *J Am College Cardiol* 19:216A, 1992

52 Lampertico M, Comis S, *Klinische Wochenschr* 71:S129-133, 1993

53 Morisco B et al, *Clin Invest* 71 (8 Suppl):S134-S136, 1993

54 Permanetter B et al, *Eur Heart J* 13:1528-1533, 1992

55 Wilson MF et al, *Biomed and Clinical Aspects of CoQ10*, Vol 6, Eds. Folkers K et al, Elsevier Amsterdam, 1991; pp339-348

56 Baggio E et al, *Klinische Wochenschr* 71:S145-149, 1993

57 Oda T, *Ibid*, S150-154

58 Karlsson J et al, *Biomed and Clinical Aspects of CoQ10*, Vol 6, Eds. Folkers K et al, Elsevier Amsterdam, 1991

59 Karlsson J et al, *Eur Heart J* 13:758-762, 1992

60 Karlson J et al, *Highlights in Ubiquinone Research*, Eds. Lenaz G, Barnabei O, Rabbi A, Battino M, Taylor & Francis, London,1990

61 Karlsson J et al, *Ann Med* 23:339-344, 1991

62 Karlsson J, *Advances in Myochemistry*, Ed. Benzi G, Libbey, London, 1987

63 Kiessling K-H et al, *Coronary Artery Disease & Physical Fitness*, Eds. Larsen OA, Malmborg RO, Munksgaard, Copenhagen 1970

64 Kiessling K-H et al, *Clin Science* 44:547-554, 1973

65 Ernster L et al, *Eur J Biochem* 9:299-310, 1969

66 Folkers K et al, *Intl J Vit Res* 40:380-390, 1970

67 Littaru GP et al, *Proc Natl Acad Science* 68:2332-2335, 1971

68 Folkers K et al, *J Molec Med* 2:431-460, 1977

69 Iwamoto Y et al, *Biomed and Clinical Aspects of CoQ10*, Vol 3, Eds. Folkers K et al, Elsevier, Amsterdam 1981; pp109-119

70 Ernster L, Forsmark-Andrea P, *Clin Investig* 71:560-565, 1993

71 Awata N et al, *Biomed and Clinical Aspects of CoQ10*, Vol 2, Eds. Folkers K et al, Elsevier, Amsterdam 1980; pp247-253

72 Cacciapuoti F, Gentille S, *Ibid* Vol 6, 1991; pp481-488

73 Kawajiri K, Fujii-Kuriyama Y, *Jpn J Cancer Res* 82:1325-1335, 1991

74 Tawfiq N et al, *Eur J Cancer Prev* 3:285-292, 1994

75 Jollier P et al, *Intl J Clin Pharmacol Ther* 36:506-509, 1998

76 Ernster L, Stockholm Univ: personal communication

77 Weber C et al, *Molec Asp Med* 15:S97-S102, 1995

78 Folkers K et al, *Molec Asp Med* 15:S281-285, 1995

79 Bargossi AM et al, *Molec Asp Med* 15:S187-193, 1995

80 Shigenaga MK et al, *Proc Natl Acad Science* 91:23 (Nov 8 1994; pp10771-10778)

81 Chello M et al, *Ann Thoracic Surg* 58(5):1427-1432, 1994

REFERENCES

82 Vina J et al, *Antioxidants, Vitamins & Beta Carotene in Disease Prevention*, 2nd Intl Conf, Berlin 1994; Abs p95

83 Adembri C et al, *Histology & Histopathology* 9(4):683-690, 1994

84 Gugger ET, Erdman JW, *Antioxidants, Vitamins & Beta Carotene in Disease Prevention*, 2nd Intl Conf, Berlin 1994; Abs p53

85 Gonzales R et al, *Cancer Research* 44:4137-4139, 1984

86 Baum RM, *Chem Eng News* 20-26, Apr 9 1984

87 Ernster L, Dallner G, *Biochim Biophys Acta* 1271(1):195-204, 1995

88 Alleva R et al, *Proc Natl Acad Sci USA* 92:9388-9391, 1995

89 Lockwood K et al, *Biochem Biophys Res Comm* 212:172-177, 1995

90 Folkers K et al, *Biochem Biophys Res Comm* 192:241-245, 1993

91 Harman D, *Age* 18:51-62, 1995

92 Laaksonen R et al, *Eur J Applied Physiol & Occupational Physiol* 72:95-100, 1995

93 Stocker R, *Biomed & Clin Aspects of Coenzyme Q*, 9th Intl Symposium, Ancona, May 16-19, 1996; Abs pp16-17

94 Bowry WV et al, *J Biol Chem* 270:5756-5763, 1995

95 Alleva R et al, *Biomed & Clin Aspects of Coenzyme Q*, 9th Intl Symposium, Ancona, May 16-19, 1996; Abs pp18-19

96 Mortensen SA et al, *Ibid*, Abs p25

97 Langsjoen PH et al, *Ibid*, Abs p26

98 Oda T, *Ibid*, Abs p27

99 Soja AM, Mortensen SA, *Ibid*, Abs p29

100 Tarui S et al, *Ibid*, Abs p35

101 Ogasawara et al, *Neurology* 35:372, 1985

102 Ogasawara et al, *Neurology* 36:45, 1986

103 Suzuki Y et al, *Biomed & Clin Aspects of Coenzyme Q*, 9th Intl Symposium, Ancona, May 16-19, 1996; Abs p36

104 Wakabayashi T et al, *Ibid*, Abs p9

105 Sohal RS, *Ibid*, Abs p13

106 Lönnrot K et al, *Ibid*, Abs p53

107 Linane AW, *Ibid*, Abs pp45-46

108 Alho H et al, *Ibid*, Abs p20

109 Lewin A, *Ibid*, Abs p47

110 Kalen A et al, *Biochim Biophys Acta* 926:70-78, 1987

111 Lockwood K et al, *Biomed Biophys Res Comm*, 199(3):1504-1508, 1994

112 Lockwood K et al, *Biochem Biophys Res Comm* 212:172-177, 1995

113 Folkers K et al, *Biochem Biophys Res Comm* 192:241-245, 1993

114 Lockwood K et al, *Biomed & Clin Aspects of Coenzyme Q10*, 9th Intl Symposium, Ancona May 16-19, 1996; Abs p50

115 Beyer RE et al, *Ibid*, Abs p3-4

116 Crane FL, Navas P, *Ibid*, Abs p1

117 Lenaz G, *Ibid*, Abs p5

118 Nohl H, *Ibid*, Abs p6

119 Navas P, Villalba JM, *Ibid*, Abs p2

120 Kishi T et al, *Ibid*, Abs p12

121 Fritz IB, *Advances Lipid Research* 1:285-334, 1963

122 Greenhaff P, personal communication

123 Casey AD et al, *Am J Physiol* 271:E31-E37, 1996

124 Greenhaff PL et al, *Am J Physiol* 266:E725-E730, 1994

125 Greenhaff PL et al, *Clin Science* 84:565-571, 1993

126 Harris RC et al, *Clin Science* 83:367-374, 1992

127 Green AL et al, *Acta Physiol Scanda*, 158:2 195-202, 1996

128 Green Al et al, *Am J Physiol* 271:E821-E826, 1996

129 Hogan MC et al, *Med & Sci in Sports & Exercise* 27:371-377, 1995

130 McVeigh J, Lopaschuk GD, *Am J Physiol* 259:H1079-H1085, 1990

131 Jos OD et al, *Cardiovasc Research* 10:427-436, 1976

132 Higgins AJ et al, *Biochem Biophys Res Comm* 100:291-296, 1981

133 Dyck DJ et al, *Am J Physiol* 265:E852-E859, 1993

134 Putman CT et al, *Am J Physiol* 268:E1007-E1017, 1995

135 Timmons JA et al, *J Clin Investig* 97:879-883, 1996

136 Colombani P et al, *Eur J Applied Physiol & Occupational Physiol* 73:434-439, 1996

137 Lukaski HC et al, *Am J Clin Nut* 63:954-965, 1996

138 Malm C et al, *Acta Physiol Scandinavica* 157:511-512, 1996

139 Heinomen OJ, *Sports Med* 22:109-132, 1996

140 Hallmark MA et al, *Med & Science in Sports & Exercise* 28:139-144, 1996

141 Singh RB et al, *Cardiovasc Drugs & Therapy* 12:347-353, 1998

142 Scheinen A, Mäkinen KK, *Acta Odont Scand* 33:590, 1975

143 Khambanorida S et al, *J Bio Buccale* 11:255, 1983

144 Scheinen A et al, *Oral Health* 71:33, 1981

145 Mäkinen KK, *J Dent Res* 74:1904-1923, 1995

146 Mäkinen KK, personal communication

147 Bliznakov EG, *Proc Natl Acad Science*, 70:390-394 1973

148 Bliznakov EG, *Biomed Clin Aspects of Coenzyme Q10*, 1:73-84, 1984

149 Bliznakov EG, *Macrophages and Lymphocytes*, Pt A:361-369, 1980

150 Folkers K et al, *Biochem Biophys Res Comm* 192:214-245, 1997

151 Ihse I et al, *Biomed & Clin Aspects of Coenzyme Q10*, 8th Intl Symposium,1993; Abs p48

152 Lockwood K et al, *Biomed & Clin Aspects of Coenzyme Q10*, 8th Intl Symposium,1993; Abs p49

153 Lockwood K et al, *Biomed Biophys Res Comm* 212:172-177, 1995

154 Lockwood K et al, *Biomed & Clin Aspects of Coenzyme Q10*, 9th Intl Symposium,1996; Abs p50

155 Gugger ET, Erdman JW, *Antioxidants, Vitamins & Beta Carotene in Disease Prevention*, 2nd Intl Conf, Berlin 1994; Abs p53

Chapter 10: Amino sugars

1   King's Fund Report, *A Positive Approach to Nutrition as Treatment*, 1992

2   Prudden JF et al, *Surg Gynecol Obstet* 128:1321-1326, 1969

3   Prudden JF et al, *Am J Surg* 119:560-564, 1970

4   Campo RD, *Clin Orthop* 68:182-209, 1970

5   Lindahl U, Hook M, *Ann Review Biochem* 47:385-417, 1978

6   Kjellen L, Lindahl U, *Ann Review Biochem* 60:443-475, 1991

7   Born GVR, Palinksi W, *Br J Experim Path* 66:543-549, 1985

8   Zubay G, *Biochemistry*, 2nd edition, MacMillan, NY 1988; pp138-153

9   Setnikar I et al, *Pharmatherapeutica* 3(8):538-550, 1984

10 Setnikar I et al, *Arzneimittelforschung* 36(2): 729-736, 1991

11 Hodges S, personal communication

12 Viola RE et al, *Biochemistry* 19:3131-3157, 1980

13 Dycke PJ et al, *New Eng J Med* 319:542-548, 1988

14 Cohen-Forterre L et al, *Glomerular Basement Membrane*, Eds. Lubec & Hudson, J Libbey, London 1985; pp131-137

15 Croft DN et al, *Experim Med & Biol* 89:39-50, 1976

16 Burton AF, Anderson FH, *Am J Gastroenterol* 78:19-22, 1983

17 Murch et al, *Lancet* 341:711-714, 1993

18 Wesley AW et al, *Advances Experim Med & Biol* 144:145-146, 1981

19 Herring GM, *Clin Orthop* 60:261-299, 1968

20 Vaz A, *Current Med Res Opinion* 8:145-149, 1982

21 D'Ambrosio E et al, *Pharmatherapeutica* 2(8):504-508, 1981

22 Crolle G, D'Este E, *Current Med Res Opinion* 7:104-114, 1980

23 Klein NJ et al, *J Cell Science* 102:821-832, 1992

24 Naparstek Y et al, *Nature* 310:241-244, 1984

25 Fridman R et al, *J Cell Physiol* 130:85-92, 1987

26 McDermott RP et al, *J Clin Investig* 54:545-554, 1974

27 Goodman MJ et al, *Gut* 16:833-842, 1975

28 Malik AB et al, *J Investig Dermatol* 93:62S-67S, 1989

29 Sunergren KP et al, *J Applied Physiol* 63:1987-1992, 1987

30 Comper WD, Laurent TC, *Physiol Review* 58: 255-315, 1978

31 Mast BA et al, *Plast Reconstruct Surg* 89:503-509, 1992

32 Sawyer PN, Srinivasan S, *Bulltn NY Acad Med* 48:235-256, 1972

33 Gotloib L et al, *Resuscitation* 16:179-192, 1988

34 Vantrappen G, Geboes K, *Lancet* 341:730-731, 1993

35 Murch SH et al, *Lancet* 339:381-385, 1992

36 Lee JCL et al, *Gastroenterology* 54: 76-85, 1968

37 Burton AF, Anderson FH, *Am J Gastroenterol* 78:19-22, 1983

38 Tesoriere G et al, *Experientia* 28:770-771, 1972

39 Tsubura E et al, *Gann* 67(6): 849-856. 1976

40 Yamashita T et al, *Developments in Oncology* 4:127, 1980

41 Krueger GA, *Arzneimittel Praxis* 47:1796, 1967

42 Boyko EJ et al, *New Eng J Med* 316:707-710, 1987

43 Malik NS, Meek KM, *Biochem & Biophys Res Comm* 199:683-686, 1994

44 McKenzie LS et al, *Lancet* i:908-909, 1976

45 Vidal y Plana et al, *Pharmacol Res Comm* 10:557-569, 1978

46 Palmoski MJ, Brandt KD, *Arthritis Rheum* 23:1010-1020, 1980

47 Roden L, *Ark Kemi* 10:345-352, 1956

48 Karzel K, Domenjoz R, *Pharmacology* 5:337-345, 1971

49 Kim JJ, Conrad HE, *J Biol Chem* 249:3091-3097, 1974

50 Drovanti A et al, *Clin Ther* 3:260-272, 1980

51 Pujalte JM et al, *Current Med Res Opinion* 7:110-114, 1980

52 Block G, *Am J Clin Nut* 53:270S-282S, 1991

53 Harmand M-F et al, *Am J Med* 83(Suppl 5A):48-54, 1987

54 Barcelo HA et al, *Ibid*, pp55-59

55 Di Padova C, *Ibid*, pp60-65

56 Various authors, *Ibid*, pp1-110

57 Stramentinoli G, *Ibid*, pp35-42

58 Davie SJ et al, *Diabetes* 41:167-173, 1992

59 Mund-Hoym WD, *Z Allgemeinmed* 23:25-43, 1980

60 Eichler J, Noh E, *Orthop Praxis* 9:225, 1970

61 Tapadhinas MJ et al, *Pharmatherapeutica* 3:157-168, 1982

62 Setnikar I et al, *Arzneim-Forsch* 41:542-545, 1991

63 Kiecolt-Glaser J et al, *Lancet* 346:1194-1196, 1995

64 Murch SH et al, *Lancet* 347:1299-1301, 1996

65 Alpenfels WF, *Fed Proc* 43:680, 1984

66 Birchall JD, Espie AW, *Silicon Biochemistry*, Ciba Foundation Sympsm 121, 1986; pp140-159

67 Birchall JD, *Aluminium in Chem Biol & Med*, Ed. Nicolini M, Raven Press, NY 1991; p67

68 Leach RM, *Fed Proc* 30:991 1971

69 Freeland-Grames JH et al, *Nutritional Bio-availability of Manganese*, Ed. Kies C, Am Chem Soc, Washington 198; p90

70 Garrow J, *BMJ* 308:934, 1994

71 Avenall A, *BMJ* 308:1369, 1994

72 Royce C et al, *BMJ* 308:1370, 1994

73 Brooks PM et al, *J Rheumatol* 9:3-5, 1982

74 Newman NM, Ling RSM, *Lancet* 2:11-13, 1985

75 Soloman L, *J Bone Joint Surg* 55B:246-251, 1973

76 Senior K, *Lancet* 355:208, 2000

77 Awasthi S et al, *Am J Clin Nut* 64:761-766, 1997

Chapter 11: Betaine

1 Baker DH, *Handbook 1984, Nutrition Institute on Amino Acids*, NFIA, West Des Moines, Iowa, USA, 1984

2 Baker DH & Czarnecki GL, *J Nutrition* 115:1291, 1985

3 Barak AJ et al, *Alcohol* 11:501-503. 1993

4 Barak AJ et al, *Alcoholism: Clin & Experim Res* 17:552-555, 1994

5 Betafin Briefing Vol 1: FinnSugar BioProducts Inc, Schaumberg, 1996

6 Budavari S, *The Merck Index*, 11th edition, Ed. Rahway NJ, Merck & Co Inc, USA 1996; pp1201-1201

7 Chambers ST, *Clin Science* 88:25-27, 1995

8 Coelho-Sampio T, Ferreira ST, Castro EJ, Vieyra J, *Eur J Biochem* 221:1103-1110, 1994

9 Combs GF, *The Vitamins*, Academic Press Inc, NY 1992, pp393-456

10 Du Vigneaud V, Dyer HM, Kies MW, *J Biol Chem* 130:325, 1939

11 Du Vigneaud V, *Thesis*, Cornell University Press, 1952

12 Finkelstein JD, *J Nut Biochem* 1:228, 1990

13 Friedel HA, Goa KI, Benfield P, *Drugs* 38:389, 1989

14 Frontiera MS et al, *J Nut Biochem* 5:28, 1994

15 Hanson AD et al, *Proc Natl Acad Sci USA* 91:306-310, 1994

16 Konosu S, Hayashi T, *Bulltn Jap Soc Science Fish* 41:743-746, 1975

17 Konosu S, Yamaguchi K, *Chemistry & Biochemistry of Marine Food Products*, Eds. Flick GJ, Hebard CE, Ward DR, AVI Publishing Co, Westport CT, 1982; pp367-404

18 Lever M et al, *Clin Chim Acta* 230:69-79, 1994

19 LeRudulier DA, et al, *Science* 224:1064-1068, 1984

20 Lowry KR et al, *Poultry Science* 55:S135, 1987

21 Mann PJG et al, *Biochem J* 32:1024, 1938

22 Morrison H et al, *JAMA* 275:189-196, 1996

23 Motulsky AG, *Am J Human Genet* 58:17-20, 1996

24 Naurath HJ et al, *Lancet* 346:85-89, 1995

25 Newberne PJ, *J Nut Biochem* 4:618, 1993

26 Ortega RM et al, *J Am Col Nut* 13(1):68-72, 1994

27 Perry IJ et al, *Lancet* 346:1395-1398, 1995

28 Robinson K et al, *Cleveland Clin J Med* 61(6):438-450, 1994

29 Rogers AE, *Nut Biochem* 4:666, 1994

30 Saunderson CL, MacKinlay J, *Br J Nutrition* 63:339, 1990

31 Smolin LA & Benevenga, *Absorption & Utilisation of Amino Acids*, Ed. Friedman M. Vol 2, CRC Press Inc, Boca Raton, FL 1989

32 Storch KJ et al, *Am J Clin Nut* 54:386, 1991

33 Tiihonen J, *Cultor Technology Center Communications*, Helsinki, 1995

34 Tsiagbe VK et al, *Poultry Science* 66:1138, 1987a

35 Tsiagbe VK et al, *Poultry Science* 66:1147, 1987b

36 Yancey PH et al, *Science* 127:1214-1223, 1982

37 Yao Y et al, *Archives Family Med* 3(10):918-922, 1994

38 Malinow MR, *Clin Chem* 41:173-176, 1995

39 Ubbink JB et al, *J Nut* 124:1927-1933, 1994

40 Clayton R, Edinburgh Univ; personal communication

41 Kirke PN et al, *Lancet* 348:1037-1038, 1996

Chapter 12: Body weight, exercise

1 Coleman MP et al, *Atherosclerosis* 92:177-185, 1992

2 Royal College of General Practitioners (UK) Report, *Better Living, Better Life*, Primary Health Care Resource Pack, 1996

3 Royal College of Physicians of London, *Medical Aspects of Exercise, Benefits and Risks*, RCP, 1991

4 Allied Dunbar Fitness Survey, Sports Council & Health Education Authority (UK),1992

5 Blair SN et al, *Ann Review Public Health* 13:99-126, 1994

REFERENCES

6   Paffenberger PS et al, *New Eng J Med* 329:538-545, 1993

7   Lakka T et al, *New Eng J Med* 330:1549-1554, 1994

8   Shinton R et al, *BMJ* 307:231-234, 1993

9   Beatriz F et al, *Circulation* 89:2540-2544, 1994

10 Wood WG et al, *Metabolism* 32:31-39, 1983

11 Campaigne N et al, *Med & Science in Sports & Exercise* 25:1346-1351, 1993

12 Hardman A et al, *Med & Sci in Sports & Exercise* 25(5):S204, 1993

13 Kiens B et al, *J Clin Investig* 83:558-564, 1989

14 Blair SN et al, *Am J Clin Epidemiology* 129:1145-1156, 1989

15 Kannel WB et al, *Ann NY Acad Science* 382:3-20, 1982

16 Somers T et al, *Lancet* 337:1363-1368, 1991

17 Davies P et al, *Intl J Obesity* 19:6-10, 1995

18 Pedersen BK et al, *J Science & Med in Sport* 2(3):234-252, 1999

19 Peters EM et al, *Am J Clin Nut* 57:170-174, 1993

20 Fox KR, *Proc Children in Focus Conference*, NDC UK October 1993

21 Ji LL, *Free Rad Biol & Med* 18(6):1079-1086, 1995

22 Hartmann A et al, *Mutation Res Letters* 346(4):195-202, 1995

23 Karklin A et al, *Am J Clin Nut* 59(2):346-349, 1994

24 Rokitzki L et al, *Acta Physiol Scand* 151(2):149-158, 1994

25 Fentem PH, *Br J Med* 308:1291-1295, 1994

26 Clinton S, *Nut Review* 56:35-51,1998

27 Sumida S et al, *Intl J Biochem* 21:835-838, 1989

28 Rokitzki L et al, *Intl J Sport Nut* 4:253-264, 1994

29 Venitt S, Levy LS, *Nature* 250:493-495, 1974

30 Amit K, *Antioxidants, Vitamins & Beta Carotene in Disease Prevention*, 2nd Intl Conf, Berlin 1994; Abs p96

31 Lewis YS, Neelakantan S, *Phytochemistry* 4:619-625, 1965

32 Sreenivasan A, Venkataraman R, *Current Science* 4:151-152, 1959

33 Watson JA et al, *Archives Biochem & Biophys* 135:209-217, 1969

34 Watson JA, Lowenstein JM, *J Biol Chem* 245:5993-6002, 1970

35 Lowenstein JM, *Essays in Cell Metabolism*, Interscience, Wiley, NY 1970; pp153-166

36 Cheema-Dhadli S et al, *Eur J Biochem* 38:98-102, 1973

37 Sullivan AC et al, *J Biol Chem* 252:7583-7590, 1977

38 Lowenstein JM, *J Biol Chem* 246:629-632, 1971

39 Barth CJ et al, *FEBS Letters* 22:343-346, 1972

40 Berkhout T et al, *Biochem J* 272:181-186, 1990

41 Sullivan AC et al, *Lipids* 9:121-128, 1974

42 Brunengraber H, Lowenstein JM, *FEBS Letters* 36:130-132, 1973

43 Sullivan AC, Triscari J, *Am J Clin Nut* 30:767-776, 1977

44 Sullivan AC et al, *Am J Clin Nut* 30:777-784, 1977

45 Greenwood MRC et al, *Am J Physiol* 240:E72-E78, 1981

46 Sullivan AC, Triscari J, *Hunger: Basic Mechanisms & Clinical Implications,* Eds. Novin D, Wyriwicka W, Bray G, Raven Press, NY 197; pp115-125

47 Sullivan AC et al, *Intl J Obesity* 8:S241-S248, 1984

48 Conte A, *The Bariatrician* Summer:17-19, 1993

49 Colquhoun E, *Possible new pharmacological approaches to the management of obesity*, 2nd Scientific Meeting of the Australian Society for the Study of Obesity, Melbourne, July 1993.

50 Lee NA, Reasner CA, *Diabetes Care* 17(12):1449-1452, 1994

51 Underwood EJ, *Trace Elements in Human & Animal Nutrition*, 4th edition, 1977

52 Mertz W, Schwartz K, *Am J Physiol* 209:489-494, 1959

53 Saner G, *Am J Clin Nut* 34:853-855, 1981

54 Mahalko JR, Bennion M, *Am J Clin Nut* 29:1069-1072, 1976

55 Anderson RA, *Science Total Environ* 17:13-29, 1981

56 Hopkins LL et al, *Am J Clin Nut* 21:203-211, 1986

57 Liu VJ, Morris JS, *Am J Clin Nut* 31:972-976, 1978

58 Offenbacher EG, Pi-Sunyer FX, *Diabetes* 29:919-925, 1968

59 Sherman L et al, *Metabolism* 17:439-422, 1968

60 Anderson RA, *Chromium in Human Health & Disease*, Proc 1st Meeting Intl Trace Element Res, Palm Springs USA, Dec 1986

61 Clausen J, *Biol Trace Element Res* 17:229-236, 1988

62 Mahdi G, Naismith DJ, *Ann Nut Metab* 35:65-70, 1991

63 Anderson RA, Kozlovsky, *Am J Clin Nut* 41:1177-1183, 1985

64 Naismith DJ et al, *Ann Nut Metab* 35:61-64, 1991

65 Bibow K et al, *Näringsforskning* 3:84-88, 1984

66 Kozlovsky AS et al, *Metabolism* 35:515-518, 1986

67 Campbell WW, Anderson RA, *Sports Med* 4:9-18, 1987

68 Anderson RA et al, *Metabolism* 36:351-355, 1987

69 Clouatre D, Rosenbaum ME, *Diet & Health Benefits of HCA*, Keats Publishing Inc, New Canaan, CT 1994

70 Tucek S et al, *J Neurochem* 36:1331-1337, 1981

71 Sullivan AC, Gruen RK, *Fed Proc* 44:139-144, 1985

72 Brunengraber H et al, *Eur J Biochem* 82:373-384, 1978

73 Sullivan AC, Triscari J, *Recent Advances in Obesity Research 2*, Eds. Bray G, Technomic Publishing Co, Westport, CT 1977; pp442-452

74 Anderson RA et al, *Metabolism* 32, 894-899; 1983

75 Anderson RA et al, *J Applied Physiol* 64, 249-252; 1988

76 Mertz W, *Physiol Review* 49:163, 1969

77 Levis AG, *Br J Cancer* 37:386, 1978

78 Dekkers JC et al, *Sports Med* 21:213-238, 1996

79 Hemila H, *Int J Sports Med* 17:379-383, 1996

80 Roberts L, Haycox A, *About the Size of It*, DHSS, London,

81 Seidell JC, *Intl J Obesity* 19:S13-S15, 1995

82 Colditz GA, *Am J Clin Nut* 55:S503-S507, 1992

83 Jeffrey RW et al, *Am J Clin Nut* 55:641-644, 1992

84 Lissner L et al, *New Eng J Med* 324:1839-1844, 1991

85 Weeks D, personal communication

86 Castell L, *Proc Amino Acids & Athletic Performance*, St Catherine's College, May, 1998

Smoking

95 *The Smoking Epidemic; Counting the Cost in England*, London, HEA 1991

96 General Household Survey: Cigarette Smoking 1972-1990 OPCS Monitor SS91/3; 26.11.1991

97 Jick H et al, *Lancet* 1:1354-1355, 1977

98 *Smoking and the Young*, A Report of a Working Party of the Royal College of Physicians, London, RCP 1992

99 Barry M, *New Eng J Med* 28 March 1991

100 *World Tobacco*, May 1987

101 *Save the Rainforests*, WHO Bulltn, IUCN 11(5), 1980

102 Whidden P, *Green Magazine*, Jan 1991

103 Mathews JD et al, *Lancet* 2:254-258, 1973

104 Brewerton D, *All About Arthritis*, Harvard Press, 1992

105 Riemersma R, Duthie SJ, personal communication

106 *Health Benefits of Smoking Cessation – a Report of the Surgeon General*, US Dept Health & Human Services, 1990

107 Doll R et al, *BMJ* 309:901-911, 1994

108 Peto R, *BMJ* 309:937-939, 1994

109 Ryberg D et al, *Cancer Research* 54(22):5801-5803, 1994

110 Cross CE et al, *Antioxidants, Vitamins & Beta Carotene in Disease Prevention*, 2nd Intl Conf, Berlin 1994; Abs p37

111 Brown KM et al, *Ibid,* Abs p47

112 Grinberg-Funes RA et al, *Ibid, Abs p48*
113 Doll R, *Ibid, Abs p9*
114 Rahman I et al, work in progress in Dept Medicine, University of Edinburgh (Reported at Royal Biochem Soc Annual Conference, Brighton Dec 1994)
115 Church T, Pryor WA, *Env Health Perspec 64:111-126, 1985*
116 Duthie SJ et al, work in progress at Rowett Research Institute, Aberdeen (Reported at Royal Biochem Soc Annual Conference, Brighton Dec 1994)
117 Dawson EB et al, *Fertility & Sterility 58(5):1034-1039, 1992*
118 Fraga CG et al, *Proc Natl Acad Science 88:11003-11006, 1991*
119 Tribble DL et al, *Am J Clin Nut 58:886-890, 1993*
120 Allard JP et al, *Am J Clin Nut 59(4):884-890, 1994*
121 McPhillips JB et al, *Am J Diet Assoc 94:287-292, 1994*
122 Schwartz J, Weiss ST, *Eur Respir J 7:1821-1824, 1994*
123 Shahar E et al, *New Eng J Med 331:228-233, 1994*
124 Sharp DS et al, *Am J Respir & Crit Care Med 150:983-987, 1994*
125 Quitman data (unpublished)
126 Thurnham DI, *Proc Nutrition Society 53:77-87, 1994*
127 Chow CK et al, *J Am College Nut 5:305-312, 1986*
128 Ortega RM et al, *J Am College Nut 13(1):68-72, 1994*
129 Hopper JL, Seeman E, *New Eng J Med 330(6):387-392, 1994*
130 Pamuk ER, et al, *Lancet 347:1450-1451, 1996*
131 Mezzeti A et al, *Atheroscelerosis 112:91-99, 1995*
132 Van Antwerpen VL et al, *Free Rad Biol Med 18:935-941, 1995*
133 Sohn SO et al, *Archives Toxicol 67:667-673, 1993*
134 Schwartz J, Weiss ST, *Am J Clin Nut 59:110-114, 1994*
135 Fuller CR et al, *Atherosclerosis 119:139-150, 1996*
136 Lapenna D et al, *Free Rad Biol & Med 19:849-852, 1995*
137 Duthie SJ et al, *Cancer Research 56:1291-1295, 1996*
138 Steinberg FM, Chait A, *Am J Clin Nut 68:319-327, 1998*
139 Hoshino E et al, *J Paren Ent Nut 14:399-305, 1990*
140 Chow CK et al, *Environ Research 34:8-17.1984*
141 Marangon K et al, *Am J Clin Nut 67:231-239, 1998*
142 Klesges LM et al, *Am J Epidemiology 147:127-135, 1998*
143 Hendelman GJ et al, *Am J Clin Nut 63:559-565, 1996*
144 Brown AJ, *J Nut Biochem 7:29-39, 1996*
145 McPhillips JB et al, *J Am Diet Assoc 94: 287-292, 1994*
146 Zondervan KT et al, *Intl J Epidemiol 25:70-79, 1996*
147 ATBC Prevention Study Group, *New Eng J Med 330: 1029-1035, 1994*
148 Omenn GS et al, *New Eng J Med 334:1150-1155, 1996*

DIETS WHICH FIGHT DISEASE
Chapter 13: Cancer

1   Editorial, *Lancet 345:874-875, 1995*
2   Block G, *Epidemiology 3(3):189-191, 1992*
3   Anon, *Diet, Nutrition & Cancer*, Natl Academic Press, Wash DC 1982; p358
4   Steinmetz KA, Potter JD, *Cancer Causes Control 2:325-357, 1991*
5   Weisburger JH, Williams GM, *Cancer Medicine*, 2nd edition, chaps 1-4, Lea & Febiger, Philadelphia 1982
6   Weisburger JH, *Macronutrients; Investigating their Role in Cancer*, Marcel Dekker Inc, NY, 1992
7   Paganelli GM et al, *JNCI 84:47-51, 1992*
8   Cahill RJ et al, *Gut 34:963-967, 1993*
9   Muto Y et al, *Antioxidants, Vitamins & Beta Carotene in Disease Prevention*, 2nd Intl Conf, Berlin 1994; Abs p73
10 Meyskens FL et al, *Ibid, Abs p27*
11 Lamm DL et al, *J Urol 151(1):21-26, 1994*
12 Steinmetz KA, Potter JD, *Cancer Causes Control 2:325-357, 1991*
13 Block G et al, *Nut & Cancer 18(1):1-26, 1992*
14 Tomatis L (Ed), *Cancer: Causes, Occurrence and Control*, IARC Scientific Pub No 100, Lyon 1990
15 Blott WJ et al, *J Natl Cancer Inst 85,15th Sep 1993*
16 Gridley G et al, *Am J Epidemiology 135:1083-1092, 1992*
17 Horrobin D, personal communication
18 Spector AA, Yorek MA, *J Lipid Research 26:1015-1035, 1985*
19 Gualde N, *Polyunsaturated Fatty Acids in Human Nutrition*, Eds. Bracco & Deckelbaum, Nestlé Nutrition Workshop Series Vol 28, Nestec Ltd, Vevey/Raven Press Ltd, NY 1992; pp195-209
20 Cheesman KH et al, *Toxicol & Pathol 12(3):235-239, 1984*
21 Wolfson N et al, *Experimental Cell Research 10:566-568, 1956*
22 Cheesman KH et al, *FEBS Letters 209:191-196, 1986*
23 Gerber M et al, *Cancer Investigations 9(4): 421-428, 1991*
24 Lash ED, *Archives Biochem Biophys 115:332-336, 1966*
25 Duchesne J, *J Theoret Biol 66:137-145, 1967*
26 Das UN et al, *Free Rads in Biol & Med 3:9-14, 1987*
27 Dunbar LM, Bailey JM, *J Biol Chem 250:1152-1154, 1975*
28 Bailey JM, *Lipid Metabolism in Mammals*, Ed. Snyder F, Plenum Press, NY 1977; pp352-364
29 Eggens I et al, *Br J Pathology 69:671-683, 1988*
30 De Antueno RJ et al, *Biochimica International 16:413-420, 1988*
31 Bartoli GM et al, *Biochim Biophys Acta 620:205-211 ,1980*
32 Roos DS, Choppin PW, *J Cell Biol 101:1578-1590, 1985*
33 Roos DS, Choppin PW, *J Cell Biol 101:1591-1598, 1985*
34 Schroder F, Gardiner JM, *Cancer Research 44:3262-3269, 1984*
35 Dahiya R et al, *Biochimica International 27(4):567-577, 1992*
36 Pritchard GA et al, *Br J Surgery 76:1069-1073, 1989*
37 Pritchard GA, Mansel RE, *Omega 6 Fatty Acids; Pathophysiol & Roles in Clin Med*, Ed. Horrobin D, Alan Liss, NY 1990; pp379-390
38 Falconer JS et al, *New Approaches to Cancer Treatment*, Ed. Horrobin D, Churchill Communications Europe 1994; pp68-78
39 Reynolds PD et al,*Ibid, pp79-83*
40 Fearon KCH et al, *Ibid, pp84-87*
41 Diplock AT et al, *Biochim Biophys Acta 962:42-50, 1988*
42 Schauenstein E, *J Lipid Research 8:417-428, 1967*
43 Horrobin DF, *Omega 6 Fatty Acids; Pathophysiol & Roles in Clin Med*, Ed. Horrobin D, Alan Liss, NY 1990; pp351-378
44 Begin ME et al, *J Natl Cancer Inst 80:188-194, 1988*
45 Begin ME, *Chemistry & Physics of Lipids 45:269-313, 1987*
46 Takeda S et al, *Med Science Research 20:203-205, 1992*
47 Takeda S et al, *Anticancer Research 12:329-334, 1992*
48 Takeda S et al, *Intl J Oncology 1:759-63, 1992*
49 Hopewell JW et al, *New Approaches to Cancer Treatment*, Ed. Horrobin D, Churchill Communications Europe 1994; pp88-108
50 Ohnishi T, *Gann 49:233-248, 1952*
51 Utsumi K et al, *Biochim Biophys Acta 105:368-371, 1965*
52 Slater TF et al, *Free Radicals in Molecular Biology, Ageing and Disease*, Ed. Slater TF, Raven Press NY 1994
53 Porta E et al, *Mech of Ageing & Dev 13:1-39, 1980*
54 Rose DP et al, *J Natl Cancer Inst 85(21):1743-1747, 1993*
55 Dolcek TA, *Proc Soc Experim Biol Med 200(2):177-182, 1992*
56 Roebuck BD, *Lipids 27(10):804-806, 1992*
57 Galeotti T et al, *Xenobiotica 21:1041-1051, 1991*
58 Hockenberry DM et al, *Cell 75:241-251, 1993*
59 Work in progress, Cancer Research Campaign at Aston University, UK

REFERENCES

60 Roos DS, Choppin PW, *Proc Natl Acad Sci USA* 81:7622-7626, 1984

61 Herblin WF et al, *Experim Opinion Ther Patents* 4(6):641-654, 1994

62 Oikawa T et al, *Cancer Letters* 51:181-186, 1990

63 Lovegrove JA et al, *Gut* 34:203-207, 1993

64 Gardner ML, *Ann Review Nut* 8:329-350, 1988

65 Sanderson JR, Walker WA, *Gastroenterology* 104:622-639, 1993

66 Luer CA, *Tumour Biology* 45(4):(4624) p949, 1986

67 Messina MJ et al, *Nutrition & Cancer* 21(2):113-131, 1994

68 Pagliacci MC et al, *Eur J Cancer* 30A:1675-1682, 1994

69 Lund E K et al, *Am J Clin Nut* 69:250-5, 1999

70 Billings PC et al, *Cancer Letters* 62:191-197, 1992

71 Jonadet M et al, *J Pharmacol* (Paris) 17:21-27, 1986

72 Kuppusamy UR, Das NP, *Experientia* 47(11-12):1196-1200, 1991

73 Herbage D, *Phlebologie* 44:873-880, 1991

74 Kuppusamy UR et al, *Biochem Pharmacol* 40(2):397-401, 1990

75 Tixier JM et al, *Biochem Pharmacol* 33(24):3933-3940, 1984

76 Troll W, Yavelow J, *Diet, Nutrition & Cancer: From Basic Research to Policy Implication*, Ed. Roe DA, Alan R Liss, NY 1983; pp167-176

77 Tawfiq N et al, *Eur J Cancer Prevn* 3:285-292, 1994

78 Mukhtar H et al, *Cancer Research* 44:2924-2928, 1984

79 Dunnick JK et al, *Fund Applied Toxicol* 2:114-120, 1982

80 Graham S et al, *J Natl Cancer Inst* 3:709-714, 1978

81 Poulsen HE et al, *Antioxidants, Vitamins & Beta Carotene in Disease Prevention*, 2nd Intl Conf, Berlin 1994; Abs p75

82 Nijhoff WA, Peters WHM, *Food & Cancer Prevention: Chem & Biol Aspects*, Eds. Waldron, Johnson, Fenwick, Royal Soc Chem, 1993; pp138-139

83 Krinsky NI, *Antioxidants & Disease Prevention: Biochem, Nut & Pharmacol Aspects*, ILSI Intl Symposium, Stockholm June/July 1993; pp27-29

84 Zhang YH et al, *Carcinogenesis* 12:2109-2114, 1991

85 Krinsky NI, *Am J Clin Nut* 52:238S-246S, 1991

86 Bendich A, *Proc Nutrition Society* 50:263-274, 1991

87 Connett JE et al, *Cancer* 64:126-134, 1989

88 Garewal H, Shamdas GJ, *Micronutrients in Health & Disease*, Ed. Bendich & Butterworth, Dekker, NY, 1991; pp127-140

89 Wolf G, *Nut Review* 50:270-274, 1993

90 Menkes MS et al, *New Eng J Med* 315:1250-1254, 1986

91 Bertram J, *Antioxidants, Vitamins & Beta Carotene in Disease Prevention*, 2nd Intl Conf, Berlin 1994; Abs p13

92 Garewal H, *Ibid*, Abs p26

93 Meyskens FL et al, *Ibid*, Abs p27

94 Yamanushi T et al, *Ibid*, Abs p53

95 Nir Z, *Ibid*, Abs p74

96 Sharoni Y, Levy J, *Ibid*, Abs p80

97 Stahl W et al, *Antioxidants & Disease Prevention: Biochem, Nut & Pharmacol Aspects*, ILSI Intl Symposium Stockholm June/July 1993; pp23-24

98 Gollnick H et al, *Proc Intl Life Sci Inst*, Europe, 1993; pp88-89

99 Sugimura T, *Environ Health Perpsect* 67:5, 1986

100 Reddy BS et al, *Cancer Research* 51:487, 1991

101 Carroll KK, Braden LN, *Nut Cancer* 6:254, 1984

102 Pell JD et al, *Food & Cancer Prevention: Chem & Biol Aspects*, Eds. Waldron, Johnson, Fenwick, Royal Soc Chem, 1993; pp295-299

103 Skog KI, Jagerstad, *Ibid*, pp87-91

104 Huang M-T et al, *Ibid*, pp209-213

105 Bianchi-Santamaria A et al, *Ibid*, pp75-81

106 Wattenberg LW, *Ibid*, 1993, pp12-23

107 Zhang Y et al, *Ibid*, pp416-420

108 Lee BH et al, *Ibid*, pp53-61

109 Rumney CJ, Rowland IR, *Ibid*, pp0-74

110 Willett WC et al, *New Eng J Med* 316(1):22-28, 1987

111 Willett WC et al, *New Eng J Med* 323(24):1664-1672, 1990

112 Van Bladeren PJ, *Food & Cancer Prevention: Chem & Biolog Aspects*, Eds. Waldron, Johnson, Fenwick, Royal Soc Chem, 1993; pp64-174

113 Yang CS et al, *FASEB J* 6:737, 1992

114 Belman S, *Carcinogenesis* 4:1063, 1983

115 Horwitz N, *Med Tribune* Aug 12 1981

116 Bradlow HL et al, *Food & Cancer Prevention: Chem & Biolog Aspects*, Eds. Waldron, Johnson, Fenwick, Royal Soc Chem, 1993; pp270-274

117 Leighton T et al, *Ibid*, pp23-232

118 Hayatsu H et al, *Mutation Research* 202:429, 1988

119 Holman PCH, Venema DP, *Food & Cancer Prevention: Chem & Biolog Aspects*, Eds. Waldron, Johnson, Fenwick, Royal Soc Chem, 1993; pp203-208

120 Smart RC et al, *Carcinogenesis* 7:1663, 1986

121 Waldron KW, Selvendran RR, *Food & Cancer Prevention: Chem & Biolog Aspects*, Eds. Waldron, Johnson, Fenwick, Royal Soc Chem, 1993; pp307-326

122 Kawamura Y, Muramoto M, *Ibid*, pp331-335

123 Pontz BF et al, *Biochem Pharmacol* 31:3581-3589, 1982

124 Schlebusch H, Kern D, *Angiologia* 9:248-256, 1972

125 De Luca G et al, *Ital J Biochem* 29:305-306, 1980

126 Cameron E et al, *Cancer Research* 39:663-681, 1979

127 Matsushima T et al, *Artery* 14(6):316-337, 1987

128 Luer CA, *Fed Proc* 45(4):949, 1986

129 Wei H et al, *Proc Soc Experim Biol Med* 208(1):124-130, 1995

130 Hirano T et al, *Life Science* 55(13):1061-1069, 1994

131 Lamartiniere CA et al, *Proc Soc Experim Biol Med* 208(1):120-123, 1995

132 Monti E, Sinha BK, *Anticancer Research* 14(3A):1221-1226, 1994

133 Yanagihara K et al, *Cancer Research* 53(23):5815-5821, 1993

134 Constantinou A, Huberman E, *Proc Soc Experim Biol Med* 208(1):109-115, 1995

135 Spinozzi F et al, *Leukaemia Research* 18(6):431-439, 1994

136 Gorczyca W et al, *Cancer Research* 53(13):3186-3192, 1993

137 Bergan R et al, *Clin Exp Metastasis* 14(4):389-398, 1996

138 Peterson G, Barnes S, *Prostate* 22(4):335-345, 1993

139 Scholar EM, Toews ML, *Cancer Letters* 87(2):159-162, 1994

140 Garewal HS, Schantz S, *Archives Otolaryngol Head Neck Surg* 121(2):141-144, 1995

141 Work in progress, Cancer Research Campaign at Aston University, UK

142 Palozza P et al, *Acta Medica Romana* 32(4):623-632, 1994

143 Rogers MAM et al, *Cancer Epidemiol Biomarkers Prevn* 4(1):29-36, 1995

144 Goldin BR et al, *New Eng J Med* 307:1542-1547, 1982

145 Gorbach SL, Goldin BR, *Prevn Med* 16:525-529, 1987

146 Van't Veer P et al, *Intl J Cancer* 47:649-653, 1991

147 Rose DP et al, *Am J Clin Nut* 54:520, 1991

148 Schultz TD, Howie BJ, *Nut Cancer* 8:141, 1986

149 Delzenne N et al, 1st Orafti Research Conference, Université Catholique de Louvain, Jan 17th 1995; pp275-278

150 Tzischinsky O et al, *Sleep* 17(7):638-645, 1994

151 Cos S et al, *USA J Pineal Res* 17(1):25-32, 1994

152 Nersessian AK, *Food & Cancer Prevention: Chem & Biolog Aspects*, Eds. Waldron, Johnson, Fenwick, Royal Soc Chem, 1993; pp62-63

153 Howarth JM et al, *Am Review Respir Dis* 123:496-499, 1981

154 Scheider JF et al, *Proc 3rd Intl Conf on Stable Isotopes*, Eds. Klein & Klein, Acad Press, NY 1974; pp507-516

155 Reich R et al, *Biochem Biophys Res Comm* 160(2):559-564, 1989

156 ATBC Cancer Prevention Study Group, *New Eng J Med* 330(15):1029-1035, 1994

157 Feng W et al, *New Zealand Med J* 106:319-322, 1993

158 Schreinemachers DM, Everson RB, *Epidemiology* 5(2):138-146, 1994

159 Folkman J, *J Natl Cancer Inst* 82:4-6, 1990

160 Folkman J, *Nature Med* 1:27-31, 1995

161 Ellis LM, Fidler IJ, *Lancet* 346:388-389, 1995

162 Stevens RG, *Iron Nutrition in Health & Disease*, Swedish Nutrition Foundation 20th Intl Symposium, Stockholm August 1995; p44

163 Halliday JW, *Ibid*, p41

164 Ascherio A, Willett WC, *Ibid*, p47

165 McGlynn KA et al, *Ibid*, p66

166 Boushey CJ et al, *Ibid*, p68

167 Knekt P et al, *Ibid*, p67

168 Rossander-Hulthén L, *Ibid*, p25

169 Lapin V, Ebels I, *J Neurol Trans* 50:275-282, 1981

170 Neri B et al, *Oncol Rep* 1:1-13, 1994

171 Cagoni ML et al, *Lancet* 346:1229-1230, 1995

172 Blount BC, Ames BN, *Baillières Clinical Haematology (UK)*, 8/(3):461-478, 1995

173 Johnson EJ et al, *Am J Clin Nut* 62:598-603, 1995

174 Buring JE, Hennekens CH, *J Cell Biochem* 58S:226-230, 1995

175 Lipkin M, Newmark H, *J Cell Biochem* 58S:65-73, 1995

176 Bostick RM et al, *J Natl Cancer Inst* 87:1307-1315, 1995

177 Baron JA et al, *J Natl Cancer Inst* 87:1303-1307, 1995

178 Jacobsen EJ et al, *Biochemie* 77:394-398, 1995

179 Pukkala E et al, *BMJ* 311:649-652, 1995

180 Palan PR et al, *Gynecol Oncol* 55:72-77, 1994

181 Block G, Langseth L, *Food Technol* 48:80-84, 1994

182 Lockwood K et al, *Biomed Biophys Res Comm* 199(3):1504-1508, 1994

183 Lockwood K et al, *Biochem Biophys Res Comm* 212:172-177, 1995

184 Folkers K et al, *Biochem Biophys Res Comm* 192:241-245, 1993

185 Nagabhushan M, *The Toxicologist* 10:166, 1990

186 Grønbæk M et al, *BMJ* 310:1165-1169, 1995

187 Renaud S, De Lorgeril M, *Lancet* 339:1523-1526, 1992

188 Klatsky AL, Armstrong MA, *Am J Cardiology* 71:467-469, 1993

189 St Leger AS et al, *Lancet* 2:1017-1020, 1979

190 Gerdes L, *Ugeskr Lager* 154:3580-3586, 1992

191 Sælan H et al, *Alcohol & Drug Abuse 1992*: 21st edition, Copenhagen, Natl Board of Health, 1993

192 Giovanucci E et al, *J Natl Cancer Inst* 87:1767-1773, 1995

193 Morris DL et al, *JAMA*, 272:1439-1441, 1994

194 Le Marchand L et al, *Cancer Epidem* 2:185-187, 1993

195 Seddon JM et al, *JAMA* 272:1413-1420, 1994

196 Trannier H, *Current Aspects of Light Protection and Skin Physiology*, Univ of Witten/Herdecke, Germany, 1995

197 Wang X-D et al, *JNCI* 91:60-66, 1999

198 Reddi K et al, *Cytokine* 7:287-290, 1995

199 Murakoshi M et al, *J Nat Cancer Inst* 81:1649-1652, 1989

200 Murakoski M et al, *Cancer Research* 52:6583-6587, 1992

201 Di Mascio P et al, *Arch Biochem Biophys* 272:532-538, 1989

202 Dorant E et al, *Gastroenterology* 110:12-20, 1996

203 Bertram JS, Bortkiewicz H, *Am J Clin Nut* 62:S1327-S1336, 1995

204 Duthie SJ et al, *Cancer Research* 56: 1291-1295, 1996

205 Freudenheim JL et al, *J Natl Cancer Inst* 88:340-348, 1996

206 Paraskeva C et al, *Cancer Research*, May 1996

207 Franchesci S et al, *Lancet* 347:1351-1356, 1996

208 Van Antwerpen VL et al, *Intl J Vit Nut Res* 65:231-235, 1995

209 Le Marchand L et al, *Intl J Cancer* 63:18-23, 1995

210 Zheng W et al, *Am J Epidemiology* 142:955-960, 1995

211 Negri E et al, *Intl J Cancer* 65:140-144, 1996

212 Hodges S et al, *Biofactors* 9:365-370, 1999

213 Peterson K, *Science* 271:4411, 1996

214 Cao G et al, *J Agri & Food Chem* 44:3426-3431, 1996

215 Wang H et al, *J Agri & Food Chem* 44:701-705, 1996

216 Prior RL, Cao G, *J Am Nutraceutical Assoc* 2:46-56, 1999

217 Mayne ST et al, *J Natl Cancer Inst* 86:33-38, 1994

218 Hennekens CH et al, *New Eng J Med* 334:1145-1149, 1996

219 Greenberg ER et al, *JAMA* 275:699-703, 1996

220 Mares-Perelman JA et al, *Archives Opthalmol* 113:1518-1523, 1995

221 Ziegler RG et al, *J Natl Cancer Inst* 88:612-615, 1996

222 Pool-Zobel BL et al, *Carcinogenesis* 18:1847-1850, 1997

223 Huang CY et al, *Am J Diet Assoc* 85:17-18, 1995

224 Heinonen O et al, *JNCI* 90:440-446, 1998

225 Smedman AGM et al, *Anticancer Research Abs* 82:1656, 1995

226 Levy J et al, *Anticancer Research Abs* 80:1655, 1995

227 Thun M et al, *New Eng J Med* 325:1593-1596, 1991

228 Elder DJE et al, *Cancer Research* 56:2273-2276, 1996

229 Shiff SJ et al, *J Clin Inv* 96:491-503, 1995

230 Mizutani T, Mitsuoka J, *Cancer Letters* 11:89-95, 1980

231 Umegaki K et al, *Carcinogenesis* 18:1943-1947, 1997

232 Chen BP et al, *Anticancer Research* 16:3689-3694, 1997

233 Zheng W et al, *Cancer Epidemiol Biomark Prec* 8:35-40, 1999

234 Clark L et al, *JAMA* 276:1957-1963, 1996

235 Rayman MP, *BMJ* 314:387, 1997

236 Van Damme EJ et al, *Eur J Biochem* 245:648-655, 1997

237 Rooprai HK et al *Inhibition of Matrix Metalloproteases; Therapeutic Applications*, Eds. Greenwald RA, Zucker S, Golub LM, *Ann NY Acad Sci* Vol 878:654-658, 1999

238 Dexter D and Rooprai H, personal communication

239 Dexter D, personal communication

240 Emonard H et al, *Inhibition of Matrix Metalloproteases; Therapeutic Applications*, Eds. Greenwald RA, Zucker S, Golub LM. *Ann NY Acad Sci* 878:647-653, 1999

241 Jang M et al, *Science* 275:218-220, 1997

242 Clifford AJ et al, *Am J Clin Nut* 64:748-756, 1996

243 Ames, BN et al, *Science* 236:271-280, 1987

244 Fontham EG, *Intl J Epidemiol* 19 suppl 1:S32-S42, 1990

245 Lichtenstein P et al, *New Eng J Med*, 13 July, 2000

246 Dimberg LH et al, *Cereal Chem* 70:637, 1993

247 Collins FW et al, *J Agric Food Chem* 68:184-187, 1991

248 Collins FW et al, *J Agric Food Chem* 37:60-64, 1989

249 Chan JM et al, *Cancer Causes Control* 9:559-566, 1998

250 Rooprai HK, personal communication

Shark cartilage

251 Lane B, Comac L, *Sharks Don't Get Cancer*, Avery Publishing Group, NY

252 Langer R et al, *Science* 193:70, 1976

253 Langer R et al, *Proc Soc Natl Acad Science USA*, 77:4331, 1980

254 Langer R, Murray J, *J Applied Biochem & Biotech* 8:9, 1983

REFERENCES

255 Langer R and Lee A, *Science* 221:1185-1187, 1983

256 Luer CA et al, *Fed Proc* 45:949, 1986

257 Durie BGM et al, *J Biol Response Modifiers* 4:590-595, 1985

258 Prudden JF, *J Biol Response Modifiers* 4:551-584, 1985

269 Prudden JF, Balassa LL, *Seminars in Arthritis and Rheumatism* 3:287-321, 1974

260 Rosen J et al, *J Biol Response Modifiers* 6:355-366, 1987

261 Rosen J et al, *J Biol Response Modifiers* 7:498-512, 1988

262 Brohult A et al, *Acta Chem Scand* 24:730, 1970

263 Brohult A et al, *Experientia* 28: 954, 1972

264 Brohult A, *Nature* 193:4822, 1962

265 Brohult A, *Acta Radiol* 1963, Suppl 223.

266 Brohult A et al, *Acta Obstet Gynecol Scand* 56: 441-448, 1977

267 Brohult A et al, *Acta Obstet Gynecol Scand* 65:779-785, 1986

Lycopene

271 Albanes D et al, *Am J Clin Nut* 62:1427S-1430S, 1995

272 ATBC Cancer Prevention Study Group, *New Eng J Med* 330(15):1092-1035, 1994

273 Aviram M, Personal Communication (Lipid Research Laborary, Technion Faculty of Medicine, Haifa, Israel)

274 Batieha AM et al, *Cancer Epidemiol Biomarkers & Prevention* 2:335-339, 1993

275 Bendich A, *Proc Nutrition Society* 50:263-264, 1991

276 Bertram JS et al, *Am J Clin Nut* 62(S) 1995

277 Bertram JS, *Antioxidants, Vitamins & Beta Carotene in Disease Prevention*, 2nd Intl Conf, Berlin 1994; Abs p13

278 Buring JE, Hennekins CH, *J Cell Biochem* 58S:226-230, 1995

279 Clinton SK, et al, *FASEB J* 10:A242, 1996

280 Clinton SK et al, *J Cancer Epidemiology, Biomarkers & Prevention* 5:823-833, 1996

281 Connett JE et al, *Cancer* 64: 126-134, 1989

282 Franchesci S et al, *Intl J Cancer* 59:181-184, 1994

283 Garewal HS, Shandas, GJI, *Micronutrients in Health & Disease*, Eds. Bendich & Butterworth, Dekker, NY 1991; pp127-140

284 Di Mascio P et al, *Archives Biochem Biophys* 274:532-538, 1989

285 Fuhrman B et al, *Biochem Biophys Res Comm* 233:658-662, 1997

286 Garewal HS, *Antioxidants, Vitamins & Beta Carotene in Disease Prevention*, 2nd Intl Conf, Berlin 1994; Abs p26

287 Garewal HS, Schantaz S, *Archives Otolaryngol Head Neck Surg* 121(2):141-144, 1995

288 Gerster H, *Intl J Vit Nut Res* 63:93-121, 1993

289 Gerster H, *J Am College Nut* 16:109-126, 1997

290 Giovanucci E et al, *J Natl Cancer Inst* 87:1767-1773, 1995

291 Greenberg ER et al, *New Eng J Med* 331:141-147, 1994

292 Greenberg ER et al, *JAMA* 275:699-703, 1996

293 Hennekens CH et al, *New Eng J Med* 334:141-147, 1994

294 Johnson EJ et al, *Am J Clin Nut* 62:598-603, 1995

295 Kohlmeier L et al, *Am J Epidemiology* 146:618-626, 1997

296 Krinsky NI, *Antiox & Disease Prevention: Biochem, Nut & Pharmacol Aspects*, ILSI Intl Sympsm, Stockholm June/July 1993; pp27-29

297 Krinsky NI, *Am J Clin Nut* 52:238S-246S, 1991

298 Kucuk O, 12th Intl Carotenoid Sympsm, Cairns, July 1999

299 Levy J et al, *Nut & Cancer* 24:257-267, 1995

300 Levy J et al, *Anticancer Research Abs* 80:15:1655, 1995

301 Kobayashi et al, *Anti-cancer Drugs* 7:195-198, 1996

302 McLennan R, *J Natl Cancer Inst* 87:1760-1766, 1995

303 Menkes MS et al, *New Eng J Med* 315: 1250-1254, 1986

304 Meyskens FL et al, *Antioxidants, Vitamins & Beta Carotene in*

Disease Prevention, 2nd Intl Conf, Berlin 1994; Abs p27

305 Slater T et al, *Biochem J* 265:51-59, 1990

306 O'Driscoll D, Salford Hope Hospital UK, paper presented at Br Thoracic Soc Meeting, Winter 1994/5.

307 Knekt P et al, *Iron Nutrition in Health & Disease*, Swedish Nutrition Foundation, 20th Intl Symposium, Stockholm August 1995; p67

308 Nagasawa H et al, *Anticancer Research* 15:1173-1178, 1995

309 Narisawa T et al, *Cancer Letters* 107:137-142, 1996

310 Nir Z, *Antioxidants, Vitamins & Beta Carotene in Disease Prevention*, 2nd Intl Conf, Berlin 1994; Abs p74

311 Palan PR et al, *Clin Cancer Research* 2:181-185, 1996

312 Peterson K, *Science* 271:4411, 1996

313 Seddon JM et al, *JAMA* 272:1413-1420, 1994

314 Sharoni Y et al, *Proc 16th Intl Cancer Congress*, Eds. Rao RS et al, 1:641-645, 1994

315 Smedman AEM, et al, *Anticancer Research Abs* 82:15:1656, 1995

316 Stahl W, Sies H, *J Nutrition* 122:2161-2166, 1992

317 Stahl W et al, *Archives Biochem Biophys* 294:173-177, 1992

318 Tonucci LH et al, *J Agric Food Chem* 43:579-586, 1995

319 Van Eenwyck J et al, *Intl J Cancer* 48:34-38, 1991

320 Wolf G, *Nut Review* 50:270-274, 1993

321 Zhang LX et al, *Carcinogenesis* 122:109-2114, 1991

322 Zhang LX et al, *Cancer Research* 52:5707-5712, 1992

323 Zhang S et al, *Am J Clin Nut* 66: 626, 1997

324 Newton R et al, *Lancet* 347:1450-1451, 1996

325 Hughes DA et al, *Biochem Soc Trans* 25:S206, 1997

326 Chan JM et al, *Science* 279:563-566, 1998

327 Hankinson SE et al, *Lancet* 351:1396-1397, 1998

328 Zhang SM et al, *Am J Clin Nut* 66:626-632, 1997

329 Levy J et al, *Lycopene & Cancer, Functional Foods: Overview & Disease Prevention*, Eds. Shibamato T et al, Am Chem Soc., Wash DC

330 Sharoni Y et al, *Cancer Detect Prevn* 21:118-123, 1997

331 Roos DS, Choppin PW, *Proc Natl Acad Sci USA* 81:7622-7626, 1984

332 Chiappe LE et al, *Lipids* 9:489-490, 1974

333 Bostick RM et al, *Cancer Research* 53(18):4230-4237, 1993

Chapter 14: Heart disease

1 Miettinen TA et al, *Lancet* 2:1261, 1988

2 Sing CF et al, *World Review Nut Diet* 63:220-235, 1990

3 Barker DJP et al, *BMJ* 306:422-426, 1993

4 Gordon T et al, The Framingham Study, *Am J Med* 62(5):707-714, 1977

5 British Heart Foundation Report 1994

6 Coleman MP et al, *Atherosclerosis* 92:177-185, 1992

7 Wing R et al, *Am J Clin Nut* 55:1086-1092, 1992

8 Royal College of General Practitioners 1992

9 Report of the Surgeon General, *Health Benefits of Smoking Cessation*, US Dept Health & Human Services

10 Stampfer M et al, *New Eng J Med* 328:1444-1450, 1993

11 Rimm EB et al, *New Eng J Med* 283:1450-1457, 1993

12 Chopra M, Thurnham DI, *Proc Nutrition Society* 58(3):663-671 1999

13 Landi L et al, *Biochim Biophys Acta* 902:200-206, 1987

14 Littarru GP et al, *Highlights of Ubiquinone Research*, Eds. Taylor & Francis, 1990; pp254-257

15 Suadicani P et al, *Atherosclerosis* 96:33-42, 1992

16 Frankel EN et al, *Lancet* 341:454-457, 1993

17 Burr M et al, *Lancet* 2:757-761, 1989

18 Mensink RM et al, *New Eng J Med* 323:439-445, 1990

19   Ascherio MD et al, *Circulation* 89:94-101, 1994

20   Willett WC et al, *Lancet* 34:581-585, 1994

21   Troisi R et al, *Am J Clin Nut* 56:1019-1204, 1992

22   Hulley SB et al, *Circulation* 86:1026-1029, 1992

23   Stensvold I et al, *BMJ* 307:1322-1325, 1993

24   Ramsay LE et al, *BMJ* 308:953-957, 1991

25   Stampfer MJ et al, *New Eng J Med* 325:756-762, 1991

26   Dimsdale JE, *New Eng J Med* 318:1110-1132, 1988

27   Kannel WB et al, *Am Heart J* 112:825-83, 1986

28   Thom DH et al, *JAMA* 268:68-72, 1992

29   Saikku P et al, *Annals Intern Med* 116:273-278, 1992

30   Lissner L et al, *New Eng J Med* 324(26):1839-1844, 1991

31   Frankel EN et al, *Lancet* 341:454-457, 1993

32   Renaud S et al, *Lancet* 339:1523-1526, 1992

33   Hulley SB et al, *Circulation* 86:1026-1029, 1992

34   Addis P, personal communication

35   Willett J et al, *Lancet* 341:581-555, 1993

36   Harris J et al, *Br J Nutrition* 61:519-529, 1989

37   Peng H et al, *Artery* 20:122-134, 1993

38   Osada T et al, *Lipids* 29:585-559, 1994;

39   Aesbach R et al, *Antioxidants in Food*, Royal Soc Chemistry Meeting, London, 2 December 1994

40   Yamamoto Y, *Ibid*

41   Genot C et al, *Ibid*

42   Mitchinson MJ, *Br J Clin Prac* 48:147-151, 1994

43   Rice-Evans C, Bruckdorfer KR, *Molec Aspects of Medicine* 13:1-111, 1992

44   Nohl H et al, *Free Radicals in the Environment: Medicine & Toxicology*, Richelieu Press, London 1994; pp351-375

45   Hippeli S et al, *Ibid*, pp375-392

46   Bierenbaum ML et al, *Biochem Intl* 28:57-66, 1992

47   Hallfrisch J et al, *Am J Clin Nut* 60(1):100-105, 1994

48   Baltimore Longtitudinal Ageing Study, *Am J Clin Nut* 60:100-105, 1994

49   Chopra M et al, *Antioxidants, Vitamins & Beta Carotene in Disease Prevention*, 2nd Intl Conf, Berlin 1994; Abs p56

50   Nakano M et al, *Biochem Biophys Res Comm* 142:919-924, 1987

51   Ingold KU et al, *Proc Natl Acad Sci USA* 90:45-49, 1993

52   Rifici VA et al, *J Am College Nut* 12:631-637, 1993

53   Rimm EB et al, *New Eng J Med* 328:1450-1457, 1993

54   Enstrom JE et al, *Epidemiology* 3:194-202, 1992

55   Takahashi R et al, *Thrombosis Research* 47(2):135-146, 1987

56   Edwards IJ et al, *Atherosclerosis & Thrombosis* 11:1778-1785, 1991

57   Hirai A et al, *Thrombosis Research* 28:285-298, 1982

58   Van Houwelingen AC et al, *Atherosclerosis* 75:157-165, 1989

59   McVeigh J et al, *Diabetalogica* 36(1):33-38, 1993

60   Bonaa KH et al, *Am J Clin Nut* 55:1126-1134, 1992

61   Nordoy A et al, *Am J Clin Nut* 57:634-639, 1993

62   Chin J et al, *Hypertension* 21(1):22-28, 1993

63   Chopra M et al, *Proc Intl Life Sci Inst*, Europe, p92, 1993

64   Esterbauer H et al, *Am J Clin Nut* 53:314S-321S, 1991

65   Stocker R, personal communication

66   Stocker R, *Antioxidants & Disease Prevention: Biochem, Nut & Pharmacol Aspects*, ILSI Intl Symposium, Stockholm June/July 1993; pp45-46

67   Ingold KU et al, *Proc Natl Acad Sci USA* 90:45-49, 1993

68   Stocker R et al, *Antioxidants, Vitamins & Beta Carotene in Disease Prevention*, 2nd Intl Conf, Berlin 1994; Abs p17

69   Steiner M, *Ibid*, Abs p22

70   Hodis HN et al, *Ibid*, Abs p59

71   Biacs P et al, *J Agric Food Chem* 40:363, 1992

72   Camejo G, *Antioxidants & Disease Prevention: Biochem, Nut & Pharmacol Aspects*, ILSI Intl Symposium, Stockholm June/July 1993; pp66-67

73   Frankel EN et al, *Lancet* 341:454-457, 1993

74   Renaud S et al, *Lancet* 339:1523-1526, 1992

75   Moroney M-A et al, *J Pharmacol* 40:787-792, 1988

76   Maxwell S, *Lancet* 344:193-194, 1994

77   Muller CJ et al, *Lancet* 343:1428-1429, 1994

78   Afanaslev IB et al, *Biochem Pharmacol* 38:1763, 1989

79   Thompson M et al, *Anal Chim Acta* 85:375, 1976

80   Takahama U, *Phytochemistry* 24:1443-1446, 1985

81   Harper KA et al, *J Food Technol* 4:255, 1969

82   Laughton MJ et al, *Biochem Pharmacol* 42:1673-1681, 1991

83   Hagerman AE, Butler LG, *J Biol Chem* 256:4494, 1981

84   Tixier JM et al, *Biochem Pharmacol* 33:3933-3939, 1984

85   Kuttan R et al, *Experientia* 37:221-223, 1981

86   Masquelier J et al, *Acta Therapeutica* 7:101-105, 1981

87   Kakegawa H et al, *Chem Pharmacol Bulltn* 33:5079 1985

88   Thompson EB et al, *J Pharmaceutical Sciences* 63:1936-1937, 1974

89   Rewerski W et al, *Arzneimittelforschung* 21:886-888, 1971

90   Rodale JI, *The Hawthorn Berry for the Heart*, Rodale Books, Emmaus PA, 1971

91   Werbach, MR & Murray MT, *Botanical Influences in Illness: A Sourcebook of Clinical Research*, Third Line Press, Tarzana, CA 1994

92   Calzada C et al, *Free Radical Res* 23(5):489-503, 1995

93   Gaziano JM et al, *Atherosclerosis* 112(2):187-195, 1995

94   Selhub J et al, *New Eng J Med* 332(5):286-291, 1995

95   Malinow MR, *Clin Chem* 41(1):173-176, 1995

96   Ubbink JB at al, *J Nutrition* 124(10):1927-1933, 1994

97   Schroeder HA, *JAMA* 172:1902-1908, 1960

98   Gawaz M et al, *Thromb Haemost* 72(6):912-918, 1994

99   Klevay LM, *Am J Clin Nut* 28:764-774, 1975

100   Vitale JJ, *Lancet* 340:1223-1224, 1992

101   Eisenberg MJ, *Am Health J* 124:544-548, 1992

102   Stampfer MJ at al, *JAMA* 268:877-881, 1992

103   Pietrzik K et al, *Antioxidant Vitamins & Beta Carotene in Disease Prevention,* 2nd Intl Conference, Berlin 1994; Abs p93

104   Martin A et al, *Ibid*, Abs p61

105   Sack MN et al, *Lancet* 349:269-270, 1994

106   Sempos CT et al, *New Eng J Med* 330:1119-1124, 1994

107   Sabate J et al, *New Eng J Med* 329:603-607, 1993

108   Robinson K et al, *Cleveland Clin J Med* 61(6):438-450, 1994

109   Morrison HI et al, *Epidemiology* 5(2):243-246, 1994

110   Yao Y et al, *Archives Family Med* 3(10):918-922, 1994

111   Ortega RM et al, *J Am Col Nut* 13(1):68-72, 1994

112   Carrasquedo F et al, *Free Rad Biol Med* 26:1587-1590, 1999

113   Ascherio A et al, *Circulation* 89(3):969-974, 1994

114   Morrison HI et al, *Epidemiology* 5(2):243-246, 1994

115   Naurath HJ et al, *Lancet* 346:85-89, 1995

116   Shaw GM et al, *Epidemiology* 6(3):205-207, 1995

117   Jacob RA et al, *J Nutrition* 124(7):1072-1080, 1994

118   Lindenbaum J et al, *Am J Clin Nut* 60(1):2-14, 1994

119   Nichols HK, Basu TK, *J Am College Nut* 13(1):57-61, 1994

120   Gould KL et al, *Lancet* 346:750-753, 1995

121   Salonen JT, *Iron Nutrition in Health & Disease*, Swedish Nutrition Foundation 20th Intl Symposium, Stockholm August 1995; p46

REFERENCES

122 Rossander-Hulthén L, *Ibid*, p25

123 Hershko C, *Ibid*, p39

124 Gey KF, *Food, People & Health: Past, Present & Future*, Royal Society of Medicine Conference, London, October 1995

125 Stevens RG, *Iron Nutrition in Health & Disease*, Swedish Nutrition Foundation 20th Intl Symposium, Stockholm August 1995; p44

126 Arnesen E et al, *Intl Epidemiology* 24:704-709, 1995

127 Gaziano JM et al, *Annals Epidemiology* 5:255-260, 1995

128 Boushey CJ et al, *JAMA* 274:1049-1057, 1995

129 Misso NLA, Thompson PJ, *Platelets (UK)* 6:275-282, 1995

130 Blount BC, Ames BN, *Baillières Clinical Haematology (UK)*, 8/(3):461-478. 1995

131 Keaney JF, Vita JA, *Progress in Cardiovasc Dis* 38:129-154, 1995

132 Metz J, *Med J Aust* 163:231-232, 1995

133 Ubbink JB, *Nutrition Review* 53:173-175, 1995

134 Lijnen P, Petrov V, *J Hypertension* 13:875-882, 1995

135 Gillman MW et al, *J Pediatrics* 127:186-192, 1995

136 Jacobsen EJ et al, *Biochemie* 77:394-398, 1995

137 Loliger J, *Rancidity in Foods*, Eds. Allen JC & Hamilton RJ, Elsevier Applied Science, London 1989; p47

138 Schuler P, *Food Antioxidants*, Ed. Hudson BJF, Elsevier Applied Science, London 1990; p134

139 Gordon MH, Kourimská L, *J Sci Food Agric* 68:347-353, 1995

140 Satyavati GC, *Indian J Med Res* 87:327-335, 1988

141 Nityanand S et al, *J Assoc Phys India* 37:323-328, 1989

142 Mester L et al, *Planta Med* 37:357-369, 1979

143 Perry IJ et al, *Lancet* 346:1395-1398, 1995

144 Landgren F et al, *J Intern Med* 237:381-388, 1995

145 Mackness MI, Durrington PN, *Atherosclerosis* 115:243-253, 1995

146 Mackness MI, Durrington PN, *Lancet* 346:856, 1995

147 Ruiz J et al, *Lancet* 346:869-872, 1995

148 Hattersley J, *Intl J Alt & Comp Med* 13:22-24, 1995

149 Harpel PC et al, *Proc Natl Acad Sci USA* 89:10193-10197, 1993

150 Parthasarathy S, *Biochim Biophys Res Acta* 917:337-340, 1977

151 Nygard O et al, *JAMA* 274:1526-1533, 1995

152 Kritchevsky SB et al, *Circulation* 92:2142-2150, 1995

153 Jialal I, Fuller CJ, *Can J Cardiol* 11-Suppl G:97G-103G, 1995

154 Winklhofer-Roob BM et al, *Free Rad Biol & Med* 19:725-733, 1995

155 Morrison H et al, *JAMA* 275:189-196, 1996

156 Trovata A et al, *Phytomedicine* 2:221-227, 1996

157 Maggi E et al, *Kidney International* 45:876-883, 1994

158 Jackson P et al, *Clin Chem* 41:1135-1138, 1995

159 Austin MA et al, *J Am Med Assoc* 260:1971-1921, 1988

160 Dejager S et al, *J Lipid Res* 34:295-308, 1993

161 De Graaf J et al, *Arteriosclerosis Thromb* 11:298-306, 1990

162 Alleva R et al, *Biomed & Clin Aspects of Coenzyme Q*, 9th Intl Symposium, Ancona May 16-19, 1996; Abs pp18-19

163 Serebruany VL et al,*Ibid*, Abs p37

164 Gissi-Prevenzione authors, *Lancet* 354:447-455, 1999

165 Butcher HC et al, *JAMA* 275:1016-1022, 1996

166 Butcher HC et al, *JAMA* 275:1113-1117, 1996

167 Waterhouse AL et al, *Lancet* 348:834, 1996

168 Lieff O, van Bergman K, *Gut* 26:32-37, 1985

169 Lieff O, van Bergman K, *Fette, Zeifen und Anstrichmiddel 85*, Issue 2, pp599-603, 1983

170 Lieff O, van Bergman K, *Verh Dtsch GEF/INN/Med* 89:668-672, 1983

171 Hordinsky BZ, Hordinsky DW, *Arzneitherapie* 3/1:45-51, 1979

172 Hordinsky BZ, *Z Therapie* 13:262-267, 1975

173 Bell GD et al, *Atherosclerosis* 36:47-54, 1980

174 Chatterjee SS et al, *Arzneimittelforschung* 47(7):821-825, 1997

175 Scussler M et al, *Arzneimittelforschung* 45(8):842-845, 1995

176 Loew D, *Proc 2nd Intl Congress Phytomedicine*, Munich 1996

177 Kontush A et al, *FEBS Letters* 341:69-73, 1994

178 Leha HA et al, *Proc Natl Acad Science* 91:7688-7692, 1994

179 Kirke PN et al, *Lancet* 348:1037-1038, 1996

180 Negre-Salvayre A, Salvayre R, *Free Rad Biol Med* 12:101-106, 1992

181 Gey KF et al, *Am J Clin Nut* 45:1368-1377, 1987

182 Sayhoun NR et al, *Am J Epidemiology* 144:501-511, 1996

183 Vitoux D et al, *Annales de Biologie Clinique* 54:181-187, 1996

184 Motulsky AG, *Am J Human Genetics* 58:17-20, 1996

185 Kohlmeir L et al, *Am J Epidemiology* 146:618-628, 1997

186 Davey PJ et al, *Am J Cardiology* 82:414-417, 1998

187 Chan AC, *J Nutrition* 128:1593-1596, 1998

188 Mietus-Sayder M, Malloy MJ, *J Paediat* 133:35-40, 1998

189 Leha HA et al, *Prov Natl Acad Science* 91:7688-7692, 1994

190 Carpenter KLH et al, *Gerontology*, 41:S53-S57, 1995

191 Poston R, Johnson-Tidey R, *Am J Path* 149:207-211, 1996

192 Wei ZH et al, *Redox Report* 3:219-224, 1997

193 He J et al, *JAMA*, 282:2027-2034, 1999

194 Ibrahim W et al, *J Nutrition* 127:1401-1406, 1997

195 Bell GD et al, *Proc Br Pharm Society*, 17-10 Dec 1979; pp309-310

196 Benson RT et al, *Proc Am Acad Neurol*, 51st Annual Meeting, Toronto, Apr 20, 1999

197 Devaraj S, Jialal L, *Arteriosclerosis, Thrombosis & Vascular Biol* 19:1125-1133, 1999

198 Facino MR et al, *Arzneimittelforschung* 44: 592, 1994

199 Fitzpatrick DF et al, *J Cardiovasc Pharmacol* 32:509-515, 1998

200 Karppinen, Mervaala E, *J Human Hypertens* 10 Suppl 1:S57-S61, 1996

201 Stephens NG et al, *Lancet* 347:781-786, 1996

202 Bao DQ et al, *Hypertension* 32:710-717, 1998

203 Fitzpatrick DF et al, *J Cardiovascular Pharmaco* 32:509-515, 1998

204 Williams JK, Clarkson TB, *Coronary Artery Disease* 9:759-764, 1998

205 Jie KG et al, *Calcif Tissue Intl* 59:352-356, 1996

206 Jie KG et al, *Atherosclerosis* 116:177-123, 1995

207 Agarwal S, Rao AV, *Lipids* 33:981-984, 1998

208 Upstone JM et al, *FASEB J* 13:977-994, 1999

209 Karppinen H et al, *J Cardiovascular Pharmacol* 6:S236-S243, 1984

210 Geleijnse JM et al, *BMJ* 309:436-440, 1994

211 Mervaala E et al, *Hypertension* 19:535-540, 1992

212 Peggy CW et al, *New Eng J Med* 342:1-8, 2000

Chapter 15: Bones

1 Hodges SJ et al, *J Bone Mineral Res* 8:1241-1245, 1993

2 Hodges SJ et al, *Clin Science* 78:63-66, 1990

3 Hodges SJ et al, *Bone* 12:387-389, 1991

4 Knapen MJH et al, *Ann Intern Med* 111:1001-1005, 1989

5 Plantelech L et al, *J & Bone Mineral Res* 6: 1211-1216, 1991

6 Hodges SJ, personal communication, 1997

7 Hodges SJ et al, *J Bone & Mineral Res* 8:1005-1008, 1993

8 Ralston SH et al, *J Bone & Mineral Res* 5:983-988, 1990

9 Hermann E et al, *Clin Experim Rheumatol* 7: 411-414, 1989

10 Rawlinson A et al, *J Clin Periodontol* 25:662-665, 1998

11 Hirano T et al, *Immunology Today* 11:443-449, 1990

12 Coetzer H et al, *Prostaglandins Leukotrienes EFAs* 50:257-266, 1994

REFERENCES

13   Buck AC et al, *J Urol* 146:188-194, 1991

14   Buck AC et al, *J Urol* 149:253A, 1993

15   Sakaguchi K et al, *Prostaglandins Leukotrienes EFAs* 50:81-84, 1994

16   Kruger MC et al, *Proc 9th Intl Congress Prostaglandins*, Florence June 4-9, 1994

17   Melhus H et al, *J Bone Min Res* 14:129-135, 1999

18   Miller SC, Marks SC, *Bone* 14:143-151, 1993

19   Buck AC et al, *J Urol* 149:499A, 1993

20   Silberberg M et al, *Gerolologia* 11:179-187, 1965

21   Lippiello L, Fienhold M, *Arthritis Rheum* 36: S165, 1993

22   Neil Ward, Univ Surrey, personal communication.

23   Blumenthal NC, Posner AS, *Calcified Tissue Intl* 36:439-441, 1984

24   Nyholm NEI, *Env Research* 26:363-371, 1981

25   Skinner HB et al, *J Bone Joint Surg* 65A: 843-847, 1983

26   Edwardson J et al, *Lancet* July 24th 1993

27   Casserly UM et al, *Biochem Soc Trans* 23: 385S, 1995

28   Sebastian A et al, *New Eng J Med* 330:1776-1781, 1994

29   Olsen JH et al, *BMJ* 308:895-896, 1994

30   Nielson FH, *FASEB J* 1:394-397, 1987

31   Yamazaki I et al, *Life Science* 38:951-958, 1986

32   Yamazaki I et al, *J Bone Min Metab* 3:205-210, 1986

33   Shino A et al, *J Bone Min Metab* 3:27-37, 1986

34   Rondelli I et al, *Intl J Clin Pharmacol Res* X1:183-192, 1991

35   Melis GB et al, *Bone Mineral* 19:S49-56, 1992

36   Melis GB et al, *J Endocrinol Investig* 15:755-761, 1992

37   Brandi ML, *Am J Med* 95:(S5A), 69-74, 1993

38   Agnusdei D et al, *Bone Mineral* 19(S):43-48, 1992

39   Passeri M et al, *Bone Mineral* 19(S):57-62, 1992

40   Agnusdei D et al, *Drugs Expt Clin Res* XV:97-104, 1989

41   Agnusdei D et al, *Curr Ther Res* 51:82-91, 1992

42   Agnusdei D et al, *Bone Mineral* 19(S):35-42, 1992

43   Scali G et al, *Curr Ther Res* 49:1004-1010, 1991

44   Brandi ML, *Bone Mineral* 19(S):3-14, 1992

45   Bonucci E et al, *Bone Mineral* 19(S):15-25, 1992

46   Notoya K et al, *Calcified Tissue Intl* 51(S):3-6, 1992

47   Azria M et al, *Calcified Tissue Intl* 52:16-20, 1993

48   Ozawa H et al, *Calcified Tissue Intl* 51(S):21-26, 1992

49   Notoya K et al, *Calcified Tissue Intl* 51(S):16-20, 1992

50   Moberg A, Karolinska Institute, personal communication

51   Baber R, *Patient Management* pp63-69, 1992

52   Robins SP et al, *Eur J Clin Investig* 21:310-315, 1991

53   Robins SP et al, *J Bone & Mineral Res* 9(Suppl 1):S278, 1994

54   Robins SP et al, *J Bone & Mineral Res* 9:1643-1649, 1994

55   Uebelhart D et al, *Bone Mineral* 8:87-96, 1990

56   Cummings SR et al, *Epidemiology Review* 7:178-208, 1985

57   Riggs BL, *West J Med* 154:63-77, 1991

58   Felson DT et al, *New Eng J Med* 329:16-19, 1993

59   *Scientific American Medicine* (Updated): chapter 15, Scientific American Inc, NY; p9

60   Stepan JJ et al, *J Clin Endocrin Metab* 69:523-527, 1989

61   Finkelstein JS et al, *J Clin Endocrin Metab* 69:49-52, 1989

62   Prior JC, Vigna YM, *New Eng J Med* 323:12221-12227, 1990

63   Prior JC, *Endocrine Reviews* 11:386-398, 1990

64   Manolagas SC et al, *Science* (3) 257:88-91, 1992

65   Lee JR, *Intl Clin Nut Review* 10:384-911, 1990

66   Lee JR, *Lancet* 336:1327, 1990

67   Lee JR, *Medical Hypotheses* 35:316-318, 1991

68   Lee JR, *Intl Clin Nut Rev*, Sydney Aus, June 1990

69   Peat RF, *Progesterone in Orthomolecular Medicine*, Foundation for Hormonal & Nutrition Research, Portland, OR

70   Cowan LD et al, *Am J Epidemiology* 114:2-19, 1981

71   Setchell K, personal communication

72   Tenover JS, *J Clin Endocrin Metab* 75:1092-1098, 1992

73   Gordon T et al, *Am Med J* 62:707, 1977

74   Ross RK et al, *Lancet* 1:858, 1981

75   Ottoson UB et al, *J Obstet Gynecol* 151:746-750, 1985

76   Hargrove JT et al, *J Obstet & Gynecol* 73:606-612, 1989

77   Michan H, Zander J, *J Steroid Biochem* 2:1467-1470, 1979

78   Dalton K, *Br J Psychiat* 129:438-442, 1976

79   Dalton K, *Neuropharmacology* 29:1267-1269, 1981

80   Mencioni T, Polvani F, *Calcitonin*, Ed, Pecile A, Elsevier NY 1985; pp297-305

81   Snow GR, Anderson C, *Calcified Tissue Intl* 39:198-205, 1986

82   Prior JC et al, *Can J Obstet & Gynocol* 3:178-184, 1991

83   Munk-Jensen N et al, *BMJ* 296:1150-1152, 1988

84   Rosen CJ et al, *J Clin Endocrinol Metab* 79:854-857, 1994

85   *Proc Workshop on Osteoporosis & Oral Bone Loss*, Leesburg, VA, Aug 26-28, 1992, *J Bone Min Res* 8(Suppl 2):S443-606, 1993

86   Jeffcoate MK, Chesnut CK, *J Am Dental Assoc* 124:49-56, 1993

87   Houki K et al, *J Bone & Mineral Res* 9(Suppl 1): S211, 1994

88   Iskenderov GB, *Farmatsiya* 39(6):37-41, 1990

89   Mowrey D, *The Scientific Validation of Herbal Medicine*, Keats Publishing, 1990

90   Namba T et al, *Planta Med* 55(6):501-505, 1989

91   Jones CJP et al, *SA Mediese Tydskrif* 66:907-910, 1984

92   Cetta G et al, *Connect Tissue Res* 5:51-58, 1977

93   Stoss H et al, *Dtsch Med Wochenschr* 104:1774-1778, 1979

94   Maugeri D et al, *Archives Gerontol Geriatr* 19(3):253-263, 1994

95   Sojka JE, Weaver CM, *Nut Reviews* 53(3):71-74, 1995

96   Dawson-Hughes B et al, *Am J Clin Nut* 61(5):1140-1145, 1995

97   Chan GM et al, *J Pediatrics* 126(4):551-556, 1995

98   Niedelson FH, *Environ Health Perspectives* (USA) 102(Suppl 7): 59-63, 1994

99   Kassem M et al, *Growth Regulation* 4(3):131-135, 1994

100   Newnham RE, *Environ Health Perspectives* (USA) 102(Suppl 7): 83-85, 1994

101   Conly J, Stein K, *Clin Investig Med* 17(6):531-539, 1995

102   Kannus P et al, *Lancet* 346:50-51, 1995

103   Feldman DL et al, *Endocrinology* 96:29-36, 1975

104   Snow GR, Anderson C, *Calcified Tissue Intl* 37:282-286, 1985

105   Karambolova KK et al, *Calcified Tissue Intl* 38:239-243, 1986

106   Weinstein RS, Bell NH, *New Eng J Med* 319:1698-1702, 1988

107   Prior JC, *Intl Proc J* 1:70-73, 1989

108   Johnston CC et al, *Osteoporosis 2*, Ed. Barzel E, Grune & Stratton, NY 1980; pp91-100

109   Grecu E et al, *Calcified Tissue Intl* 48:239-243, 1991

110   Roof BS et al, *Clin Res* 31:546A, 1983

111   Selby PL, Peacock M, *New Eng J Med* 314:1481-1485, 1986

112   Horowitz M et al, *Archives Intl Med* 147:681-685, 1987

113   Visser JJ, Hoekman K, *Med Hypotheses* 43(5):339-342, 1994

114   Maugeri D et al, *Archives Gerontol Geriatr* 19(3):253-263, 1994

115   Valente M et al, *Calcified Tissue Intl* 54(5):377-380, 1994

116   Orimo H et al, *Calcified Tissue Intl* 54(5):370-376, 1994

117   Van der Wielen RJP et al, *Lancet* 346:207-210, 1995

118   Hurson M et al, *J Parenteral & Enteral Nutrition* 19(3):227-230, 1995

119   Price P et al, *Proc Natl Acad Science* (USA) 73:1447-1451, 1976

REFERENCES

120 Price P et al, *Biochim Biophys Res Acta* 117:765-771, 1983
121 Maillard C et al, *Endocrinol* 130:1599-1604, 1992
122 Brown JP et al, *Lancet* 1:1091-1093, 1984
123 Eastell R et al, *J Clin Endocrinol Metab* 67:741-748, 1988
124 Szulc P et al, *J Clin Investig* 91:1769-1774, 1993
125 Szulc P et al, *J Bone Mineral Res* 9:1591-1596, 1994
126 Kanis et al, *Eur J Clin Metab* 48:833-841, 1995
127 Dawson-Hughes et al, *New Eng J Med* 323:878-883, 1990
128 Riis et al, *New Eng J Med* 316:173-177, 1987
129 Chapuy et al, *BMJ* 308:1081-1082, 1994
130 Pak CYC et al, *Ann Intern Med* 123:401-408, 1995
131 Devogelaer JP, de Deuxchaisnes CT *Clin Rheumatol* 14(S3):26-31, 1995
132 Seeman E et al, *Bone* 17S:23-29, 1995
133 Citron JT et al, *Osteoporosis International* 5:228-233, 1995
134 Vermeer C et al, *Ann Review Nut* 15:1-22, 1995
135 Keane EM et al, *Br J Clin Prac* 49:301-303, 1995
136 Gloth FM et al, *J Am Ger Soc* 43:1269-1271, 1995
137 Brazier M et al, *J Bone Min Res* 10:1753-1761, 1995
138 Fardellone P et al. *Rev de Rheuma* 62:576-581, 1995
139 Barrow GW, Saha S, *Am J Sports Med* 16:209-216, 1988
140 Leach RM, *Fed Proc* 30:99, 1971
141 Chapuy M-C et al, *J Clin Endocrin & Metab* 81:1129-1133, 1996
142 Chapuy M-C et al, *Revue de Rheumatisme* 63:135-140, 1996
143 Rizzoli R, Bonjour JP, *Lancet* 347:1274-1276, 1996
144 Fujita T et al, *Calcified Tissue Intl* 58:226-230, 1996
145 Anderson FH et al, *Bone* 18:171-177, 1996
146 Lips P et al, *Ann Intern Med* 124:400-406, 1996
147 Clayton P, Hodges S, unpublished trial results.
148 Smith R, *Update* 51:357-361, 1995
149 Agnusdei D et al, *Calcified Tissue Intl* 61:523-527, 1997
150 McCarron DA et al, *Am J Nephrol* 1:84-90, 1981
151 Devine A et al, *Am J Clin Nut* 62:740-745, 1995
152 McParland BE et al, *BMJ* 299:834-835, 1989
153 Matkovic V et al, *Am J Clin Nut* 62:417-425, 1995
154 Silver J et al, *Lancet* ii:484-486, 1983
155 Pak CYC et al, *J Urol* 131:850-852, 1984
156 Macgregor GA et al, *J Hypertens* 11:781-785, 1993
157 Izawa Y et al, *Calcified Tiss Intl* 37:605-607, 1985
158 LaCroix AZ et al, *New Eng J Med* 322:286-290, 1990
159 Antonios TFT, MacGregor GA, *Lancet* 348:250-251, 1996
160 Klesges RC et al, *JAMA* 276:226-230, 1996
161 Orimo H et al, *Clin Eval* 20:45-100, 1992
162 Brown JP et al, *Lancet* 1:1091-1093, 1984
163 Delmi M et al, *Lancet* 335:1013-1016, 1990
164 Eastell R et al, *J Clin Endocrin Metab* 67:741-748, 1988
165 Hara K et al, *Bone* 16: 179-184, 1993
166 Hara K et al, *J Bone & Mineral Res* 8:535-541, 1995
167 Hart JP et al, *J Clin Endocrin Metab* 60:1268-1269, 1985
168 Moscarini M et al, *Gynecol & Endocrinol* 8:203-207, 1994
169 Barrett-Connor E et al, *New Eng J Med* 315:1519-1524, 1986
170 Coleman DI et al, *Diabetes* 31:830-833, 1982
171 Daynes RA, Araneo BA, *J Immuno Ther* 12:174-179, 1992
172 Daynes RA et al, *J Immunology* 150:5219-5230, 1993
173 Foldes J et al, *Eur J Endocrinol* 136:277-281, 1997
174 Gordon GB et al, *Advances Enzym Reg* 26:355-382, 1987
175 Indrayeno G et al, *An Prof Drug Subs & Excipient* 23:99-124, 1994
176 Jilka RL et al, *Science* 257:88-91, 1992

177 Kalimi M, Regelson W, *Biochem Biophys Res Comm* 156 :22-29, 1988
178 Kalimi M et al, *The Biologic Role of DHEA*, Walter de Gruyter, NY; pp397-404
179 Kalimi M et al, *Molec Cell Biochem* 131:99-104, 1994
180 Labrie F et al, *J Clin Endrocinol & Metal* 82:3498-3505, 1997
181 Li S et al, *Breast Cancer Research Treat* 29:203-217, 1993
182 McEwan EG, Kurzman D, *J Nutrition* 121:S51-S65, 1991
183 Nestler JE et al, *J Clin Endocrinol Metab* 66:57-61, 1988
184 Regelson W, Kalimi M, *Ann NY Acad Science* 719:564-575, 1994
185 Schelock ED et al, *J Clin Endocrinol Metab* 66:1329-1331, 1988
186 Shafagoj Y et al, *Am J Physiol* 263:210-213, 1992
187 Spector TD et al, *Clin Endocrinol* 34:37-42, 1991
188 Schwartz AG et al, *Toxicol Pathol* 14:357-362, 1986
189 Michelson D et al, *New Eng J Med* 335:1176-1181, 1996
190 Van Papendorp DH et al, *Nutrition Research* 15/3:325-334, 1995
191 Nawata H et al, *J Steroid Biochem Mol Biol* 53(1-6):165-174, 1995
192 Melton et al, *Calcified Tissue Intl* 14:57-64, 1987
193 Passeri M et al, *Ital J Min Electrolyte Metab* 9:137-144, 1995
194 Carlisle EM, *Fed Proc* 33: 1758-1766, 1974
195 Natl Res Council, *Recommended Dietary Allowances*, 9th edition, 1980
196 Schwarz K et al, *Nature* 239:333-334, 1972
197 Carlisle EM, *Fed Proc* 33:1758-1766, 1974
198 Carlisle EM, *Science* 167:179-180, 1970
199 Schwarz K, *Biochemistry of Silicon & Related Problems*, Eds. Bendz G, Lindqvist I, Plenum Press, NY 1978
200 Anderson A et al, *Lancet* 355:1967-1968, 2000
201 Wyshak G et al, *Arch Ped Adolescent Med* 15:610-617, 2000
202 Magklara A et al, *Clin Chem* 45:1774-1780, 1999
203 Chan JM et al, *Cancer Causes Control* 9:559-566, 1998
204 Giovanicci E, *Advances Exp Med Biol*, 472:29-42, 1999

Chapter 16: Diabetes

1   Karjalainen J et al, *New Eng J Med* 327:302-307, 1992
2   Savilahti E et al, *Diabetes Research* 7:137-140, 1988
3   Elliott RB, Martin JM, *Diabetologica* 26:297-299, 1984
4   Daneman D et al, *Diabetes Research* 5:93-97, 1987
5   Virtanen SM et al, *Diabetes Care* 14:415-417, 1991
6   Glerum M et al, *Diabetes Research* 10:103-107, 1989
7   Monte WC et al, *J Am Diet Assoc* 94:313-315, 1994
8   Mayer EJ et al, *Diabetes* 37:1625-1632, 1988
9   Garcia Osle M et al, *An Med Interna (Spain)* 11/10:473-478, 1994
10   Weber C et al, *Molec Aspects Med* 15:S97-S102, 1995
11   Eibl NL et al, *Diabetes Care* 18(2):188-192, 1995
12   Reaven PD, *Antioxidants, Vitamins & Beta Carotene in Disease Prevention*, 2nd Intl Conf, Berlin 1994; Abs p36
13   Roeback JR Jr, et al, *Annals of Intern Med* 115(12):917-924, 1991
14   Thomas VI, Gropper SS, *Biol Trace Elemts Res* 55(3):297-305, 1996
15   Mertz W, *J Nutrition* 123:626-633, 1993
16   Anderson RA et al, *Am J Clin Nut* 51:864-868, 1990
17   Vrana A et al, *Antioxidants, Vitamins & Beta Carotene in Disease Prevention*, 2nd Intl Conf, Berlin 1994; Abs p66
18   Deckert T et al, *Diabetologica* 14:363-370, 1978
19   Diabetic Control & Complications Trial Res Group, *New Eng J Med* 329:977-986, 1993
20   Strain JJ, *Proc Nutrition Society* 50:591-604, 1991
21   Wolff SP, *BMJ* 49:642-652, 1993
22   Pai LH, Prasad AS, *Nutrition Res* 8:889-897, 1988

REFERENCES

23 Williams NR et al, *The Analyst* 120(3):887-890, 1995

24 Murty et al, *Diabetes Res Clin Pract* 18:11-16, 1992

25 Irene Green, Biochemistry & Molecular Genetics, University of Sussex, personal communication

26 Amiel SA, *BMJ* 307:881-882, 1993

27 Wang PH et al, *Lancet* 341:1306-1309, 1993

28 Jain SK et al, *Antioxidants, Vitamins & Beta Carotene in Disease Prevention*, 2nd Intl Conf, Berlin 1994; Abs p85

29 Report from Unit of Metabolic Medicine, UMDS, Guy's Campus, London 1994

30 Nourooz-Zadeh J et al, *Antioxidants, Atherosclerosis & Diabetes*, William Harvey Research Conference, London October 1994

31 Addis P, personal communication

32 Peng H et al, *Artery* 20:122-134, 1993

33 Stevens E, Dept Pharmacology, Queen Mary & Westfield College, London, personal communication

34 Paolisso G et al, *Am J Clin Nut* 57(5):650-656, 1993

35 Paolisso G et al, *Diabetes Care* 16(11):1433-1437, 1993

36 Lavy A et al, *Ann Nut Metab* 38/5:287-294, 1994

37 Vitamin and Mineral Nutrition Lab, *National Dietary Survey*, Human Nut Res Centre, US Dept Agric, Beltsville MD, 1993

38 Shah H, Dept Nutrition, King's College, London, personal comm.

39 Gawaz M et al, *Thromb Haemost* 72(6):912-918, 1994

40 Williams C, School Biological Science, University of Surrey; personal communication

41 Bonaa KH et al, *Am J Clin Nut* 55, 1126-1134, 1992

42 Nordoy A et al, *Am J Clin Nut* 57, 634-639, 1993

43 Wadworth AN, *Drugs* 44(6):1013-1032, 1992

44 Passwater R, *The New Super-Antioxidant*, Keats Publishing, New Canaan, CT 1992

45 Lee NA, Reasner CA, *Diabetes Care* 17(12):1449-1452, 1994

46 Underwood, EJ, *Trace Elements in Human & Animal Nutrition*, 4th edition, 1977

47 Mertz W, Schwartz K, *Am J Physiol* 209:489-494, 1959

48 Saner G, *Am J Clin Nut* 34:853-855, 1981

49 Mahalko JR, Bennion M, *Am J Clin Nut* 29:1069-1072, 1976

50 Anderson RA, *Science Total Environ* 17:13-29, 1981

51 Hopkins LL et al, *Am J Clin Nut* 21:203-211, 1986

52 Liu VJ, Morris JS, *Am J Clin Nut* 31:972-976, 1978

53 Offenbacher EG, Pi-Sunyer FX, *Diabetes* 29:919-925, 1968

54 Anderson RA, *Chromium in Human Health & Disease*, Proc 1st Meeting Intl Trace Element Res, Palm Springs, FL, Dec 1986.

55 Clausen J, *Biol Trace Element Res* 17:229-236, 1988

56 Mahdi G, Naismith DJ, *Ann Nut Metab* 35:65-70, 1991

57 Anderson RA, Kozlovsky AS, *Am J Clin Nut* 41:1177-1183, 1985

58 Naismith DJ et al, *Ann Nut Metab* 35:61-64, 1991

59 Bibow K et al, *Näringsforskning* 3:84-88, 1984

60 Kozlovsky AS et al, *Metabolism* 35:515-518, 1986

61 Campbell WW, Anderson RA, *Sports Med* 4:9-18, 1987

62 Anderson RA et al, *Metabolism* 36:351-355, 1987

63 Martin BC et al, *Lancet* 340:925-929, 1992

64 Clausen JO et al, *Lancet* 346:397-402, 1995

65 Murphy MC et al, *Br J Nutrition* 70:727-736, 1993

66 Zampelas P et al, *Eur J Clin Nutrition* 48:88-96, 1994

67 Zampelas P et al, *Br J Nutrition* 71:401-410, 1994

68 Knekt P et al, *J Intl Med* 245:99-102, 1999

69 Ford ES et al, *Am J Epidemiol* 149:168-176, 1999

70 Badmaer V et al, *J Alt Comp Med* 5:273-291, 1999

71 Ceriello A et al, *Diabetes Care* 20: 1589-1593, 1997

72 Simen CH, Eriksson UJ, *Diabetes* 46:1054-1061, 1997

73 Fitzpatrick DF et al, *J Cardiovasc Pharmacol* 32:509-515, 1998

74 Konrad T, et al *Diabetes Care* 22:280-287, 1999

75 Clin G et al, *Am J Clin Nut* 55:1161-1167, 1992

76 Ingermann RL et al, *Am J Physiol* 250:c637-c641, 1986

77 Pecovaro RG, Chen MS, *Ann NY Acad Science* 498:248-258, 1987

78 Murphy MC et al, *Eur J Clin Nut* 49(8):578-588, 1995

79 Das UN, *Prostaglandins, Leukotrienes and Essential Fatty Acids* 52(6):387-391, 1995

80 Bonnema SJ et al, *Diabetes, Nutrition & Metabolism – Clin & Experim* 8(2):81-87, 1995

81 Reaven PD et al, *Diabetes Care* 18(6):807-816, 1995

82 Wilson BE, Gondy A, *Diabetes Res & Clin Prac* 28:179-184, 1995

83 Kajanachumpol S et al, *J Med Assoc Thailand* 78:344-349, 1995

84 Kumpulainen J et al, *Bioinorg Chem* 8:419-429, 1978

85 Davies DM et al, *Biochem Med* 33:297-303, 1985

86 Shepherd PR et al, *Biol Trace Elem Res* 32:109-113, 1992

87 Uusitupa M et al, *Am J Clin Nut* 38:404-410, 1983

88 Gondy A, Wilson BE, *FASEB J* 8:A194 (abstract no 1121), 1994

89 Simonoff M et al, *Biol Trace Elem Res* 32:25-38, 1992

90 Mertz W, *J Nutrition* 123:626-633, 1993

91 Paolisso G et al, *Am J Nutrition* 55:1161-1167, 1992

92 Paolisso G et al, *J Clin Endocrin Metab* 78:1510-1514, 1994

93 Corica F et al, *Magnesium Research* 7:43-47, 1994

94 Ghannam N, *Hormone Res* 24:288-294, 1986

95 Srivastava Y et al, *Phytotherapy Res* 7:285-289, 1993

96 Sharma RD, *Nutrition Research* 6:1353-1364, 1986

97 Cunningham JJ et al, *J Am College Nut* 13:344-350, 1994

98 Salonen JT et al, *BMJ* 311:1124-1127, 1995

99 Dandona P et al, *Lancet* 347: 444-445, 1996

100 Armstrong D et al, *Free Rad Biol Med* 11:433-436, 1991

101 Vertommen J et al, *Phytotherapy Research* 8:430-432, 1994

102 Gertstein HC, Yusuf S, *Lancet* 347:949-950, 1996

103 Ripa S, Ripa A, *Minerva Medica* 86:415-412, 1995

104 Ravina A et al, *J Trace Elements in Experim Med* 8:183-190 1995

105 Jovanovic-Peterson L, Peterson CM, *J Am College Nut* 15:14-2, 1996

106 Reading SA, Wecker L, *J Florida Med Assoc* 83:29-31, 1996

107 Kantterud GL et al, *JAMA* 217:777-784, 1971

108 Jain SK et al, *Lipids* 31:S87-S90, 1996

109 Perry IJ et al, *BMJ* 310:560-564, 1995

110 Rimm EB et al, *BMJ* 310:555-559, 1995

111 Eriksson J, Kohvakka A, *Ann Nut Metab* 39:217-223, 1995

112 Fuller CJ et al, *Am J Clin Nut* 63:753-759, 1996

113 Davie SJ et al, *Diabetes* 41:167-173, 1992

114 Ceriello A et al, *Diabetes Care* 14:68-72, 1991

115 Scott FW et al, *Diabetes Care* 19:379-383, 1996

116 Paolisso G et al, *Am J Clin Nut* 59:1291-1296, 1994

117 Cavallo MG et al, *Lancet* 348:926-928, 1996

118 Maezaki Y et al, *Biosci Biotech Biochem* 57:1439-1444, 1993

119 Sugano M et al, *Nut Reports Intl* 18:531-537, 1978

120 Jennings CD et al, *Proc Experim Biol Med* 189:13-20, 1988

121 Kobayashi T et al, *Nut Rep Intl* 19:327-334, 1979

122 Sugano M et al, *Am J Clin Nut* 33:787-793, 1980

123 Kapeghian JC, Verlangien AJ, *Life Science* 34:577-584, 1984

124 McGrath LT et al, *Atherosclerosis* 121:275-283, 1996

125 Maxwell SRJ et al, *Eur J Clin Investig* 27:484-490, 1997

REFERENCES

126 Low PA et al, *Diabetes* 46:538-542, 1997
127 Kohler W et al, *The Role of Anti-oxidants in Diabetes Mellitus*, Eds. Gries FA, Wessel K, Verl Gruppe 1993; pp33-53
128 Tutuncu NB et al, *Diabetes Care* 21:1915-1918, 1998
129 Ziegler D, Gries FA, *Diabetes* 46:562-566, 1997
130 Awasthi S et al, *Am J Clin Nut* 64:761-766, 1997
131 Mann GV, *Perspectives Biol Med* 17:210-217, 1974
132 Mann GV, Newton P, *Ann NY Acad Science* 258:243-252, 1975
133 Verlangien AJ, Sestito J, *Life Science* 29: 5-9, 1981
134 Tremble J, Donaldon D, *J Royal Soc Promotion Health* 119:235-239, 1999

Chapter 17: A healthy brain

1   Grundke-Iqbal I et al, *J Biol Chem* 261:6084-6089, 1986
2   Grundke-Iqbal I et al, *Proc Natl Acad Sci USA* 83: 4913-1917, 1986
3   Iqbal K et al, *Lancet* 2:421-426, 1986
4   Iqbal K et al, *Proc Natl Acad Sci USA* 86:5646-5650, 1989
5   Alonso A del C et al, *Proc Natl Acad Sci USA* 91:5562-5566, 1994
6   Braak E et al, *Acta Neuropathol (Berl)* 87:554-567, 1994
7   Gong C-X et al, *J Neurochem* 61:921-927, 1993
8   Gong C-X et al, *J Neurochem* 62: 803-806, 1994
9   Gong C-X et al, *Neuroscience* 1:765-774, 1994
10 Gong C-X et al, *FEBS Letters* 341:94-98, 1994
11 Iqbal K, personal communication.
12 Nash RJ et al, *Phytochemistry* 345:1281-1283, 1993
13 Menzies JS et al, *Southwestern Vet* 32:45, 1979
14 Molyneux RJ, James LF, *Science* 216:190, 1982
15 Wallace RW et al, *Flavonoids in Med & Biol 3: Current Issues in Flavonoid Res*, Ed. Das NP, Natl Univ Singapore 1990; pp369-380
16 Rewerski W et al, *Arzneimittelforschung* 21:886-888, 1971
17 Scherat T et al, *Antioxidants, Vitamins & Beta Carotene in Disease Prevention*, 2nd Intl Conf, Berlin 1994; Abs p49
18 Dorling PR et al, *Neuropath Applied Neurobiol* 4:285, 1978
19 Renwick JH, *Br J Prevn Soc Med* 26:76, 1972
20 Morales AJ et al, *J Clin Endocrinol Metab* 78:1360-1367, 1994
21 Lee VMY et al,*Science* 251:675-678, 1991
22 Lai RYK et al, *Neurobiol Ageing* 16(3):443-445, 1995
23 Wischik CM et al, *Neurobiol Ageing* 16(3):409-417, 1995
24 Mann DMA, *Neurobiol Ageing* 10:397-399, 1989
25 Yankner BA et al, *Science* 25:279-282, 1990
26 Behl C et al, *Biochem Biophys Res Comm* 186:944-952, 1992
27 Behl C et al, *Brain Research* 645:253-264, 1994
28 Behl C et al, *Cell* 77:817-827, 1994
29 Deans SG, Svoboda, KP, *CAB Ag Biotech News & Info* 2:211-216, 1990
30 Deans SG et al, *Experimental Gerontology, in Aspects of Ageing & Disease*, Eds. Knook & Hofeker, 9th Symposium, Facultas Wien, 1994
31 Deans SG, Ritchie G, *Intl J Food Microbiol* 5:165-180, 1987
32 Deans SG et al, *Role of Free Radicals in Biological Systems*, Eds. Feher, Blazovics, Matkovics and Mezes, Akademiai Kiado, Budapest 1993, pp159-165
33 Harrington CR et al, *Dementia* 5:215-228, 1994
34 Harrington CR et al, *Am J Path* 14:1472-1484, 1994
35 Harrington CR et al, *Lancet* 343:993-997, 1994
36 Lannfelt L et al, presented at *Alzheimer's Disease: Molecular Aspects*, Cavendish Conference Centre, London, 6-7 March 1995
37 Loo DT et al, *Proc Natl Acad Sci USA* 90:7951-7955, 1993
38 Copeland RL et al, *Arch Intl Pharmacodynamics* 252:113-123, 1981
39 Emmenegger H et al, *Pharmacology* 1:65-78, 1968
40 Yoshikawa M et al, *J Am Geriatric Soc* 31:1-7, 1983
41 Hughes JR et al, *J Am Geriatric Soc* 24:490-497, 1976
42 Thompson TL et al, *New Eng J Med* 323:445-448, 1990
43 Davis JB, presented at *Alzheimer's Disease: Molecular Aspects*, Cavendish Conference Centre, London, 6-7 March 1995
44 Linane A, personal communication
45 Edlund C et al, *Neurochem Intl* 25:35-38, 1994
46 Evans PH et al, *Dementia* 3:1-6, 1992
47 Amaducci L, Lippi A, *Intl J Geriat Psychiat* 7:383-388, 1992
48 Jorm AF et al, *Intl J Epidemiology* 20 (Suppl 2):43-47, 1991
49 Broe GA et al, *Neurology* 40:1699-1707, 1990
50 French SL et al, *Am J Comm Psychol* 20:243-252, 1992
51 Sapolsky RM et al, *Endocrin Review* 7:285-301, 1986
52 Sapolsky RM, Plotsky PM, *Biol Psychiatry* 27:937-952, 1990
53 Dodt C et al, *J Clin Endocrin Metab* 72:272-276, 1991
54 Plumb GW et al, *Biochem Soc Trans* 23:254S, 1995
55 Olanow CW, *Trans Neurosci* 16:429-444, 1993
56 Fox RM et al, *Biochem Soc Trans* 258S, 1995
57 Imagawa M et al, *Alzheimer's Disease & Dementia of Alzheimer Type: Basic mechanisms, diagnosis & strategies*, Eds. Iqbal K et al, New York, Wiley 1991; pp649-651
58 Orentreich N et al, *J Clin Endocrin Metab* 75:1002-1004, 1992
59 Blauer KL et al, *Endocrinology* 129:3174-3179, 1991
60 Casson PR et al, *Am J Obstet Gyne* 169:1536-1539, 1993
61 Daynes RA et al, *Eur J Immunol* 20:793-802, 1990
62 Krieger D et al, *Lancet* 346:270-274, 1995
63 Kosenko E et al, *J Neurochem* 63:2172-2178, 1994
64 Nelson K et al, *Br J Ind Med* 50:510-513, 1993
65 Ritchie K, Kildea D, *Lancet* 346:931-934, 1995
66 Henderson AS et al, *Lancet* 346:1387-1390, 1995
67 Skoog I et al, *Lancet* 347:1141-1145, 1996
68 Thomas T et al, *Nature* 380:168-171, 1996
69 Bradbury J, *Lancet* 347:750, 1996
70 Kalaria RN, Hedera P, *Lancet* 347:1492-1493, 1996
71 Gurwitz D, *Lancet* 347:1492, 1996
72 Wagner SL et al, *Proc Natl Acad Sci* 86:8284-8288, 1989
73 Ayotte P, Plaa GL, *Biochem Pharmacol* 34:3857-3865, 1985
74 Plaa GL et al, *Biochem Pharmacol* 31:3698-3701, 1982
75 Henderson V et al, *Archives Neurol* 51:896-900, 1994
76 Tang MX et al, *Lancet* 348:429-433, 1996
77 Gould E et al, *J Neuroscience* 10:1286-1291, 1990
78 Jama JW et al, *Am J Epidemiology* 1444:275-280, 1996
79 Perrig WJ et al, *J Am Geriat Soc* 45:718-724, 1997
80 Paleologeos et al, *Am J Epidemiology* 148:45-50, 1998
81 Sano M et al, *New Eng J Med* 336:1216-1222, 1997
82 Drachman and Leber, *New Eng J Med* (editorial) 336:1245-1247, 1997
83 Socci DJ, et al, *Brain Research* 693:88-94, 1995
84 Meydeni SM et al, *Nutrition Research* 5:1227-1236, 1985
85 Ingold KU et al, *Lipids* 22:163-172, 1987
86 Burton GW et al, *Acc Chem Res* 19:194-201, 1986
87 Britton HJ et al, *Lancet* 344:357-361, 1994
88 Toffano G, *Lecithin, Technological, Biological and Therapeutic Aspects*, Ed. Hanin I, Ansell GB, NY Plenum Press, 1987; pp1376-146
89 Aporti F et al, *Neurobiol of Ageing* 7(2):115-120, 1986
90 Cairella M, et al, *Lecithin Consumption in the W European Diet: Lecithin & Health Care*, Eds. Paltauf F, Lekim D, Semmelweis Verlag, Austria
91 Carpenter D, *Sem Neurol* 5, 283-287, 1985
92 Cohen SA, Mueller WE, *Brain Research* 584:174-180, 1992

93   Crook TH et al, *Psychopharmacol Bulltn* 28:61-66, 1992

94   Crook TH, et al, *Neuorology* 412:644-649, 1991

95   Delwaide PJ, Gysetnynck-Mambourg et al, *Acta Neurol Scand* 73:136-140, 1986

96   Goss-Sampson et al, *J Neurol Science* 87:25-35, 1988

97   Nandy K et al, *Lipofucsin: State of the Art*, Ed. Nagy I, Elsevier Scientific, Amsterdam, 1988; pp289-304

98   Nunzi MG et al, *Neurobiol of Ageing* 8:501-510, 1987

99   Nunzi MG et al, *Phospholipids: Biochemical, Pharmaceutical and Analytical Considerations*, Eds. Hanin I Pepeu G, Plenum Press, NY 1990

100 Palmieri G et al, *Clinical Trials J* 24:73-83, 1987

101 Shukla A et al, *Free Rad Res* 22:303-308, 1995

102 Sokol RJ, *Ann Review Nut* 8:351-373, 1988

103 Van der Worp HB et al, *Stroke* 29:1002-1006, 1998.

104 Morris MC et al, *Alzheimer's Disease and Related Disorders* 12:121-126, 1998

105 Schmidt R et al, *J Am Geriat Soc* 46:1407-1410, 1998

106 Dexter D et al, *Lancet* ii:639-640, 1986

107 Dexter D et al, *Lancet* ii:1219-1220, 1987

108 Gorman AM et al, *J Neurol Science* 139:S45-52, 1996

109 Halliwell B, Gutteridge JMC, *Trends Neuroscience* 8:22-29, 1985

110 Olanow CW, *Ann Neurol* 32:S2-9, 1992

111 Olanow CW, *Trends Neuroscience* 16:439-444, 1993

112 Slivka A et al, *Brain Research* 409:275-284, 1987

113 Gale CR et al, *BMJ* 316:608-611, 1996

114 Foy CJ et al, *Am J Med* 92: 39-45, 1999

115 Uchida S et al, *Plant Flavonoids in Biol & Med II; Biochem, Cellular & Med Properties*, Eds. Cody V et al, Alan Liss Inc., NY 1987; pp135-138

116 Driscoll C, *Environ Health Perspec* 66:93-104, 1985

117 Witters HD, *Aqua Tox* 8:197-210, 1986

118 Birchall JD et al, *Nature* 338:146-148, 1989

119 Birchall JD, *Aluminium in Chemistry, Biology and Medicine*, Eds. Nicolini M et al., Raven Press, NY, 1991; pp53-69

120 Edwardson JA, et al, *Ibid*; pp85-96

121 Rifat SL, et al, *Lancet* 336:1162-1165, 1990

122 Moon W, Univ of Virginia, personal communication

123 Flaten TP, *Environ Geochem Health* 12:152-167, 1990

124 Birchall JD, Chappell JF, *Lancet* 313:953, 1989

125 Martyn CN , *CIBA Foundation Symposium* 169:69-86, Wiley, 1992

126 Perl DP, Brodie AR, *Science* 208:297-299, 1980

127 Candy JM et al, *Lancet* 293:354-357, 1986

128 Clayton RM et al, *Life Science* 51:1922-1928, 1992

129 Laviola G et al, *Psychopharmacology* 113:388-394, 1994

130 Slanina P et al, *Food Chem Tox* 22:391-397, 1984

131 Taylor GA et al, *Age and Ageing* 21:81-90, 1992

132 Day JP et al, *Lancet* 337:1345, 1991

133 Edwardson JA et al, *Lancet* 342:211-212, 1993

134 Editorial *J Roy Soc Med* 85:69-70, 1992

135 Ward N, Univ of Surrey, personal communication

136 Bowen HJM, Peggs A, *J Sci Food Agric* 35:1225-1229, 1984

137 Carlisle, EM, Curran MJ, *Alzheimer's Disease and Assoc Disorders* 1:82-89, 1987

138 Schafagoj Y et al, *Am J Physiol* 263:210-213, 1992

139 Regelson W, Kalimi M, *Ann NY Acad Sci*, 719:569-575, 1994

140 Kalimi M et al, *Mol Cell Biochem* 131:99-104, 1999

141 Labrie F et al, *J Clin Endocrinol* 82:3498-3505, 1997

142 Kerr DNS, Ward, MK, *Metal Ions in Biological Systems 24: Aluminium & its role in Biology*, Eds. Sigel H, Sigel A, Marcell Dekker Inc 1988; pp217-258,

Intelligence

143 Lanting CI et al, *Lancet* 344:1319-1322, 1994

144 Leaf A et al, *J Paediat Gastro Nut* 14:300-308, 1992

145 Lucas A, *Lancet* 339: 1992

146 Bjerve KS et al, *Nutrition* 8:130-132, 1992

147 Innis S, *Dietary Omega 3 and Omega 6 Fatty Acids*, Eds. Galli C, Simopoulos AP, NATO ASI Series, 171:142, 1989

148 Crawford M, Doyle W, Human Nutrition, Homerton Hospital London, personal communication

149 Crawford M, Doyle W, *Eur J Clin Nut* 46:S51-S62, 1992

150 Clandidin MT et al, *Polyunsaturated Fatty Acids in Human Nutrition*, Eds. Bracco & Deckelbaum, Nestlé Nutrition Workshop Series Vol 28, Nestec Ltd, Vevey/Raven Press Ltd, NY 1992; pp111-119

151 Okuyama H, *Ibid*, pp 169-178

152 Crawford MA et al, *Ibid*, pp 93-110

153 Crawford MA, personal communication

154 Neuringer M, Connor WE, *Dietary Omega 3 & Omega 6 Fatty Acids: Biological Effects and Nutritional Essentiality*, Eds Galli C, Simopoulos AP, Plenum Press, NY 1989; pp179-190

155 Olsen EN at al, *Lancet* 339:1003-7, 1992

156 Schiff E et al, *Am J Obstet Gynecol* 168(1): 122-124, 1993

157 Benton D, Roberts G: *Lancet* 1:140-143, 1988

158 Schoenthaler S et al, *Controlled trial of vitamin-mineral supplementation on non-verbal intelligence of incarcerated males aged 18-25*: unpub'd

159 Schoenthaler S, Eysenk H et al, *Ibid*, unpublished

160 Nelson M et al, *Br J Nutrition* 64:13-22, 1990

161 Carroll HCM, *Personal Indiv Diff* 16(5):6469-6475, 1995

162 Schoenthaler S et al, *Personal Indiv Diff* 12:343-362, 1991

163 Crombie S et al, *Lancet* 335:744-747, 1990

164 Benton D, Butts J, *Lancet* 335:1158-1160, 1990

165 Benton D, Cook R, *Personal Indiv Diff* 12:1151-1158, 1991

166 Schoenthaler S et al, *Altn Complement Medicine* 6(1):19-29, 2000

167 Benton D et al, *Psychopharmacol* 117(3):298-305, 1995

168 Harman D, *Age* 7:111-131, 1984

169 Kent S, *Geriatrics* 31:128-137, 1976

170 Clausen J et al, *Biol Trace Element Res* 20:135-151, 1989

171 Nagy I, Floyd R, *Archives Gerontol & Geriatrics* 3:297-310, 1984,

172 Hochschild R, *Experimental Gerontology* 8:177-183, 1973

173 Nandy K, Bourne GH, *Nature* 210:313-314, 1966

174 Nandy K, *Mech of Ageing & Dev* 8:131-138, 1978

175 Personal observation

176 Carlson S, Dept Paediatrics, Obstetrics and Gynecology, Univ Tennessee, ongoing work

177 Shaw GM et al, *Epidemiology* 6(3):219-26, 1995

178 Kirke PN et al, *Quarterly J Med* 86:703-708, 1993

179 Makrides M et al, *Lancet* 345:1463-1468, 1995

180 Halama P, *Nervenheilkunde* 10:250-253, 1991

181 Woelk H, *Der Allgemeinarzt* 11:662-668, 1993

182 Schmidt U, *Fortschritte der Medizin* 19:339-342, 1993

183 Murphree HB et al, *Clin Pharmacol & Therapeutics* 1:303-310, 1960

184 Oettinger L, *J Pediatrics* 3:671-675, 1958

185 Osvaldo R, *Curr Ther Res* 16:1238-1242, 1974

186 Pfeiffer CC, *Science* 126:610-611, 1959

187 Shaw GM et al, *Epidemiology* 6(3):205-207, 1995

188 De-Kun Li et al, *Epidemiology* 6(3):212-218, 1995

189 Shaw GM et al, *Lancet* 346:393-396, 1995

190 Hallfrisch J et al, *Am J Clin Nut* 60(2):176-182, 1994

191 Makrides M et al, *Lancet* 345:1463-1468, 1995

REFERENCES

192 Tolarova M, Harris J, *Teratology* 51(2):71-78, 1995
193 Jacob H, Beckmann H, *J Neurol Trans* 65:303-326, 1986
194 Arnold SE et al, *Archives Gen Psychiatry* 48:25-632, 1991
195 Benes FM et al, *Archives Gen Psychiatry* 48:990-1001, 1991
196 Akbarian S et al, *Archives Gen Psychiatry* 50:169-177, 1993
197 Weinberger D, *Lancet* 346:552-557, 1995
198 Mednick SA et al, *Archives Gen Psychiatry* 45:189-192, 1988
199 Hoek HW et al, *Am J Psychiatry* 153(12):1637-1639, 1996
200 Gottesman II, *Schizophrenia Genesis*, WH Freeman, NY 1991
201 McGuffin P et al, *Lancet* 346:678-682, 1995
202 Walter T, *Iron Nutrition in Health & Disease*, Swedish Nutrition Foundation 20th Intl Symposium, Stockholm August 1995; p38
203 Hershko C, *Ibid*, p39
204 Saarinen UM, Kajosaari M, *Lancet* 346:1065-1070, 1995
205 Ubbink JB, *Nutrition Review* 53:173-175, 1995
206 Benton D et al, *Neuropsychobiology* 32:98-105, 1995
207 Rothman KJ et al, *New Eng J Med* 333:1369-1373, 1995
208 Van Houwelingen AC et al, *Br J Nutrition* 74:723-731, 1995
209 Williams J et al, *Lancet* 347:1294-1296, 1996
210 Scholl TO et al, *Am J Clin Nut* 63:520-525, 1996
211 Uauy R et al, *Lipids* 31:S167-S176, 1996
212 Wartanowicz M et al, *Ann Nut Metab* 28:186-191,1984
213 Tolonen M et al, *Biol Trace Element Res* 17:221-228, 1988
214 Tolonen M et al, *Biol Trace Element Res* 7:161-168, 1985
215 Riggs, KM et al, *Am J Clin Nut* 63:306-314, 1996
216 Monji A et al, *Brain Research* 634:62-68, 1994
217 Deans SG et al, *Age* 16:71-74, 1993
218 Deans SG et al, *Acta Horticulturae* 324:237-241, 1993
219 Recsan Z et al, *Proc Nutritional Soc* 54:149, 1995
220 Deans SG et al, *Proc Nutritional Soc* 54:150, 1995
221 Penzes LG et al, *Archives Parmacol* 345:20-21, 1996
222 Keli SI et al, *Archives Intern Med* 156:637-642, 1996
223 Wald NJ et al, *Br J Obstet & Gynecol* 103:319-324, 1996
224 Broadhurst CL et al, *Br J Nutrition* 79:3-21, 1998
225 Mikhail MS et al, *Am J Obstet Gynecol* 171:150-158, 1994
226 Jain SKJ, *Molec Cell Biochem* 151:33-38, 1995
227 Shaaraway M, *Intl J Gynecol & Obstet* 60:123-128, 1998
228 Gratacos E et al, *Am J Obstet Gynecol* 178:1072-1076, 1998
229 Willatts P et al, *Lancet* 352:688-691, 1998
230 Gale CR, Merton CN, *Lancet* 347:1072-1075, 1996
231 Bell KM et al, *Acta Neurol Scand* Suppl 154:15-18, 1994
232 Berlanga C et al, *Psychiatric Research* 44:257-262, 1992
233 Bottiglieri T et al, *J Neurol Neurosurg Psychiat* 53:1096-1098, 1990
234 Rosenbaum JF et al, *Acta Neurol Scand* 81:432-436, 1990
235 Kagan BL et al, *Am J Psychiat* 147:591-595, 1990
236 Bressa GM et al, *Acta Neurol Scand* Suppl 154:7-14, 1994
237 Sparling RJ et al, *J Clin Invest* 91:651-660, 1993
238 Stoll AL et al, *Arch Gen Psychiat* 56:415-416, 1999
239 Calabrese JR et al, *Arch Gen Psychiat* 56:413-414, 1999
240 Feldman M et al, *Fetal and Neonatal Physiology*, Eds. Polin R, Fox W, WB Saunders, Toronto 1992; pp299-314

Chapter 18: Skin

1 Kune JF et al, *Nut & Cancer* 18/(3):237-44, 1992
2 Fenical W, *J Natural Products* 50:1001-1008, 1987
3 Gers-Barlag H et al, *Antioxidants, Vitamins & Beta Carotene in Disease Prevention*, 2nd Intl Conf, Berlin 1994; Abs p69

4 Jonadet M et al, *J Pharmacol* (Paris) 17:21-27, 1986
5 Kuppusamy UR, Das NP, *Experientia* 47(11-12):1196-1200, 1991
6 Kuppusamy UR et al, *Biochem Pharmacol* 40(2):397-401, 1990
7 Herbage D, *Phlebologie* 44:873-880, 1991
8 Tixier JM et al, *Biochem Pharmacol* 33(24):3933-3940, 1984
9 Pontz BF et al, *Biochem Pharmacol* 31:3581-3589, 1982
10 Schlebusch H, Kern D, *Angiologia* 9:248-256, 1972
11 De Luca G et al, *Ital J Biochem* 29:305-306, 1980
12 Garmyn M et al, *Experim Dermatol* 4(2):104-111, 1995
13 Bohm F et al, *J Am Chem Soc* 119:621-622, 1997
14 Keller KL, Fenske NA, *J Am Ac Dermatol* 39:611-625, 1998
15 Lopez-Torres M et al, *Br J Derm* 138:207-215, 1998
16 Eberlein-Koenig B et al, *J Am Ac Dermatol* 38:45-48, 1998
17 Stahl W, Heinrich U, *J Nutrition* 128:903-907, 1998
18 *The Maillard Reaction in Foods & Medicine*, Eds. O'Brian J, Nursten HE, Crabbe MJC, Ames JM, Royal Soc Chemistry, Special Publication No 223, June 1998
19 Vertommen J et al, *Phytotherapy Res* 8:430-432, 1994
20 Ceriello A et al, *Diabetes Care* 14:68-72, 1991
21 Awarthi S et al, *Am J Clin Nut* 64:761-766, 1997
22 Verlangieri AJ, Selvidge LA, *Proc Fed Am Socs Experim Biol* 46: 572, 1987
23 Alpenfels WF, *Fed Proc* 43:680, 1984
24 Viola RE et al, *Biochemistry* 19:3131-3157, 1980
25 Birchal JD, *Silicon Biochemistry*, Ciba Foundation Sympsm 121
26 Birchall JD, *Aluminium in Chem Biol & Med*, Ed. Nicolini M, Raven Press, NY 1991; p67
27 Ibbotson et al, *J Investig Dermatol*, 113:933-938, 1999
28 Watson R et al, *J Investig Dermatol*, 112:782-787, 1999
29 Pilkington G, personal communication

DIETS WHICH PROMOTE HEALTH
Chapter 19: Functional foods

1 Ichikawa T, *Functional Foods*, Ed. Goldberg I, Chapman & Hall, NY & London 1994; pp453-468
2 Milner JA, *Foods & Cancer: Functional Foods*, Ed. Goldberg I, Chapman & Hall 1994, pp39-70
3 Mackness MI, Durrington PN, *Lancet* 346:856, 1995
4 Pfeifer A, *Antioxidants & Disease Prevention: Biochem, Nut & Pharmacol Aspects,* ILSI Intl Sympsm, Stockholm June/July 1993; pp63-65
5 Aruoma OI et al, *Xenobiotica* 22:2:257-268, 1992
6 Guillot F et al, *Polyunsaturated Fatty Acids, Eicosanoids and Antioxidants in Biology & Human Diseases*, IFSC Meeting, May 1993, p2428
7 Soc Prod Nestlé, Eur Pt 0.307.626; 13.08.1988
8 Soc Prod Nestlé, Eur Pt 0480077; 6.10.1990
9 Soc Prod Nestlé, Eur Pt 0.201.000, 1986
10 Soc Prod Nestlé, Green tea rich in catechins, Patent pending.
11 Tietyen J, *J Am Diet Assoc* 95:1-55, 1995

Chapter 20: Ageing

1 Karppinen M et al, *J Human Hypertension*, 10:231-238, 1996
2 Farquhar JW et al, Abs from 18th Conf on Cardiovascular Disease, *Epidemiology*, 1998
3 Trujillo EB, *J Vasc Nursing* 11(1):12-18, 1993

INDEX

INDEX

INDEX

bronchitis, chronic 136, 182
Brussels sprouts 194
bulimia, and osteoporosis 246
butyric acid 108, 109, 110, 112

C

C43 (connexin 43) protein 204–5, 217
cabbage 189, 194
CAD *see* heart disease/coronary artery disease (CAD)
caffeic acid 81, 92
calcitonin 253
calcium 237
    absorption 110, 256
    and cancer 218
    doses 257, 258
    excretion 256–7
    foods containing 258
    and osteoporosis 246, 248, 249, 257–8
    in sweat 246
    weight in the body 242
calories
    daily intake 5
    percentage by source 11
cancer 19
    anti-cancer agents 188–91, 195, 331–2
        anti-oxidants as 187, 188–9, 211
        bifidobacteria 108
        carnosic acid 216
        carotenoids 203–6, 206, 207, 218, 331
        DHEA 256
        flavonoids 81, 90–4, 189, 195, 201, 202, 206, 207, 213
        folic acid 215
        garlic 92
        genistein 92, 94, 97, 98, 191, 196, 199, 202–3, 205, 213
        lycopene 6, 94, 204, 206
        melatonin 69
        pre-biotics 108, 109, 215, 218, 219
        Q10 148, 190, 212, 219
        selenium 95, 217, 218
        soy products 13, 94, 95–7, 98, 201, 202–3, 213, 218, 219
        turmeric/curcumin 92, 214, 216
        Vitamin E 6, 218
        Vitamin K 250
        see also angiostats
    anti-cancer diet 214–17
        cancer avoidance 187, 188–90, 192–5, 213, 215, 221

cancer containment 190–1, 195–206, 213, 215, 221
cancer killing 187, 206–12, 213, 221
bladder 36, 96, 101, 211
bowel *see* colon/bowel
brain 199
breast 219
    anti-cancer agents 13, 95, 96, 97, 109, 148, 199, 203, 206, 219
    and calcium/magnesium 257
    and dietary deficiency 6
    and frequent air travel 219
    and fruit/vegetables 188
    and MMPs 201
    and oestrogen 98, 219
    remission/regression 148, 190
causes 186–7
cervical 36, 199, 205, 206, 211
colon/bowel
    anti-cancer agents 13, 96, 108, 110, 203, 209, 215, 218
    and fats 108, 216
    and fibre 13, 110, 215, 218
    and fruits/vegetables 188, 194
    and iron 217
colorectal 51, 194, 216, 331
counterbalancing the risks 220
defence plan against 213
development 31
and exercise 78
and folate deficiency 236
gastrointestinal 205, 206
genetic risk factors 97
growth 196–200
and the immune system 32, 94, 192
incidence 36
    increased incidence 31, 36
and iron 51, 216, 217
kidney 36
liver 108, 188, 216
lung
    anti-cancer agents 96, 199, 204, 205, 209, 217
    and beta carotene 204
    and gender 36, 179
    and iron 216
    and smoking 223
mouth *see* oral cancer cavity/mouth
oesophagus 96, 188, 205
oral cavity/mouth 96, 188, 205
ovary 188

INDEX

INDEX

INDEX

INDEX

INDEX

INDEX

INDEX